CLINICAL
APPLICATIONS
OF MEDICAL IMAGING

CLINICAL APPLICATIONS OF MEDICAL IMAGING

Jeffrey Bisker, M.D.
Humana Hospital–University
University of Louisville
Louisville, Kentucky

PLENUM MEDICAL BOOK COMPANY
NEW YORK AND LONDON

Library of Congress Cataloging in Publication Data

Bisker, Jeffrey.
  Clinical applications of medical imaging.

  Includes bibliographies and index.
  1. Diagnostic imaging. I. Title. [DNLM: 1. Nuclear Magnetic Resonance—diagnostic use. 2.
Radionuclide Imaging. 3. Tomography, X-Ray Computed. 4. Ultrasonic Diagnosis. WN 445
B622c]
RC78.7.D53B58   1986   616.07′57   86-15093
ISBN-13: 978-1-4684-5085-9

ISBN-13: 978-1-4684-5085-9   e-ISBN-13: 978-1-4684-5083-5
DOI: 10.1007/978-1-4684-5083-5
© 1986 Plenum Press, New York
 Softcover reprint of the hardcover 1st edition 1986
A Division of Plenum Publishing Corporation
233 Spring Street, New York, N.Y. 10013

This book is lovingly dedicated to

JILL, ESTHER, and SOLOMON,

without whose support this book
could never have been written.

Preface

The primary purpose of this book is to bridge the gap between the practice of clinical medicine and diagnostic radiology. It is intended primarily for utilization by medical students in training and by nonradiologist physicians.

In this world of rapidly expanding knowledge in the many specialties of medicine, it is becoming increasingly difficult for many physicians to stay abreast of the newer and constantly changing modalities of diagnosis as well as the therapeutic regimens of the common as well as the less common disease processes within their realm of practice.

This book will enable the busy clinician to utilize the consultative services offered by his or her colleagues in diagnostic radiology with maximum effectiveness. The most common clinical applications of the more recent imaging modalities (i.e., nuclear medicine, ultrasound, computerized tomography, and magnetic resonance imaging) have been categorized and condensed into a format that will be both comprehensible and useful on a daily basis for those physicians routinely requesting these diagnostic examinations for their patients. For simplicity, the book is divided, whenever feasible, into organ systems and subdivided into the multiple classifications of pathologic states (i.e., congenital, trauma or iatrogenic, inflammatory, and neoplasm). In addition, there are brief comments related to the specific advantages and disadvantages as well as the cost effectiveness of each modality.

Although the actual diagnostic criteria employed for interpretation of each study are well beyond the scope of this book, the volume may also prove useful as an introduction to medical imaging for junior radiology residents prior to beginning their subspecialty rotations.

I wish to thank my former and present colleagues at the New York Medical College and the University of Louisville, who have, through their thoughtfulness and wisdom, both encouraged and indirectly assisted me in the preparation of this book. I would also like to include a special note of thanks to Dr. Michael Goldman for supplying copies of interesting cardiac cases and to Mrs. Shirley Brown for her competence and patience in the typing of the manuscript.

Jeffrey Bisker

Louisville, Kentucky

Contents

CLINICAL APPLICATIONS OF MEDICAL IMAGING

1 Gastrointestinal System

The barium swallow has long been the radiographic method of choice for evaluation of lesions of the esophagus or in the evaluation of patients presenting with dysphagia. This examination still remains the primary screening procedure although recently other diagnostic imaging modalities have been utilized to supplement the findings on fluoroscopic examinations.

Radionuclide studies have shown increasing utility in evaluation of clinical problems related to esophageal motility and in the detection or quantitation of gastroesophageal reflux. The patient is asked to swallow 10 ml of water that contains [99m Tc] sulfur colloid. The peristaltic activity can be monitored utilizing a gamma camera, and following construction of region-of-interest curves by computer, gross esophageal motility and rate of clearance of the radioactive tracer can be assessed. Esophageal transit time studies have demonstrated a higher sensitivity in the detection of esophageal motor disturbances than either manometric or radiographic methods.[5]

Scanning patients following ingestion of acidified orange juice with radioactive tracer material can also successfully detect and quantitate the presence of gastroesophageal reflux (Fig. 1-1). This study can be performed with or without artificially increasing abdominal pressure gradients simulating physiologic changes such as those produced by exercise or wearing tight garments. This procedure

GASTROINTESTINAL DISEASES
Esophagus

Nuclear Medicine

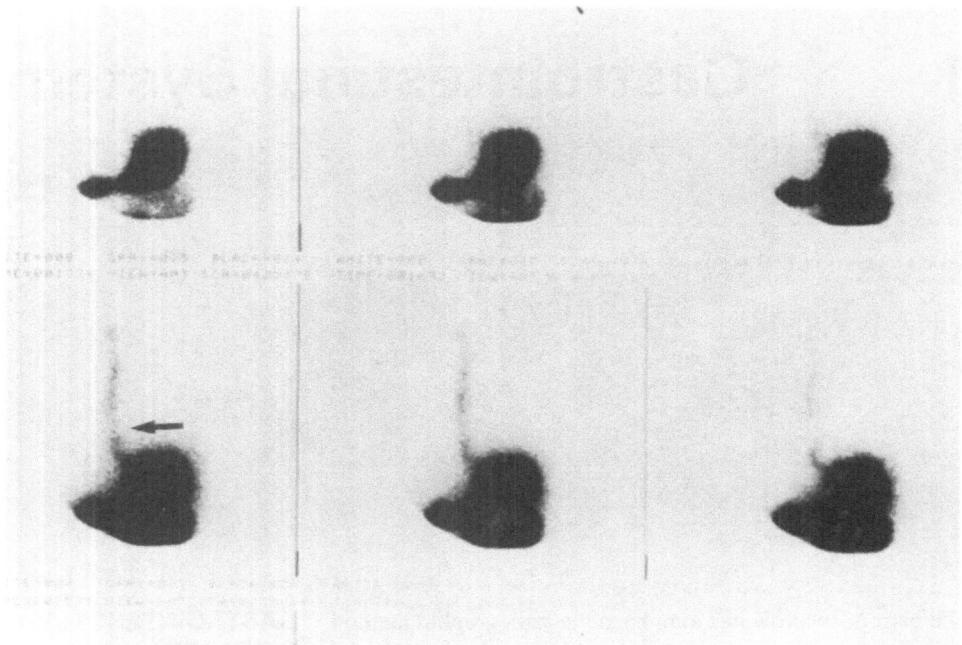

Figure 1-1. Scintigram of upper abdomen reveals free reflux of tagged gastric contents into esophagus (arrow).

has been found to be more sensitive in detecting smaller quantities of reflux than that utilizing fluoroscopic examination of the esophagus.[7] In addition, occasionally tiny esophageal diverticula or fistulae can be detected as incidental findings.

Computerized Tomography

Computerized tomography (CT) of the esophagus is a very valuable means of staging esophageal tumors, evaluating local invasion as well as detecting the presence of hilar or mediastinal lymphadenopathy[8] (Figs. 1-2 to 1-4). Pulmonary parenchymal metastases can also be detected. In addition to the initial staging of tumors, serial scans can be obtained following therapy to evaluate the possible recurrence or regression of the tumor. CT is also a useful means by which radiation portals can be constructed. Occasionally, unsuspected lesions of the esophagus, such as achalasia, large diverticula, or congenital anomalies, can be detected incidentally on thoracic scans performed for other indications. Mucosal disease of the esophagus, however, is still best evaluated utilizing the barium swallow.

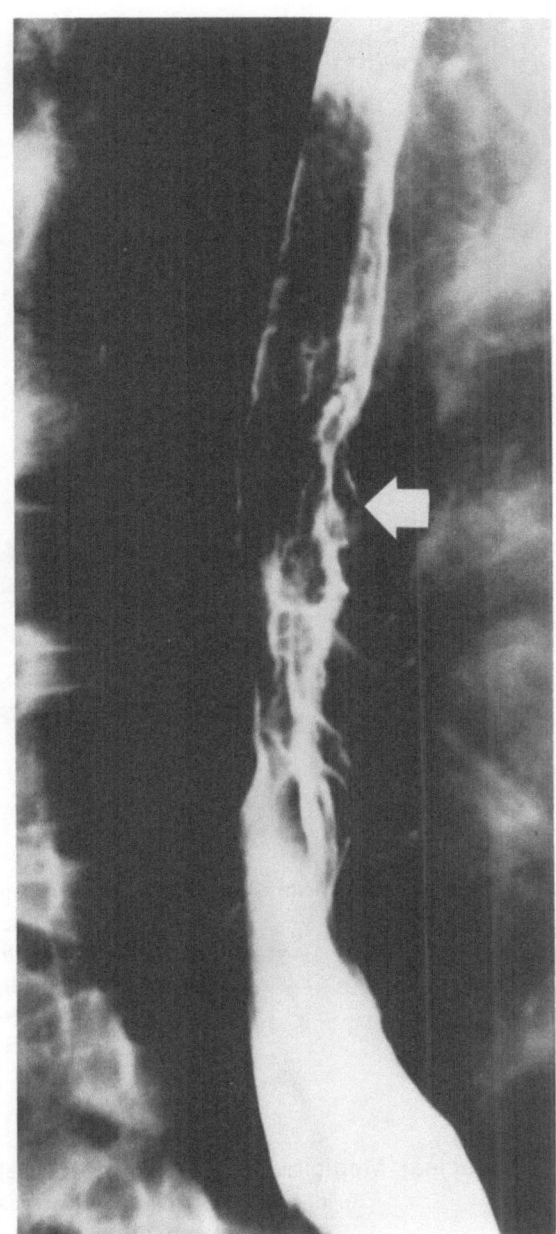

Figure 1-2. Barium esophagram demonstrates large segment of mucosal destruction by tumor (arrow).

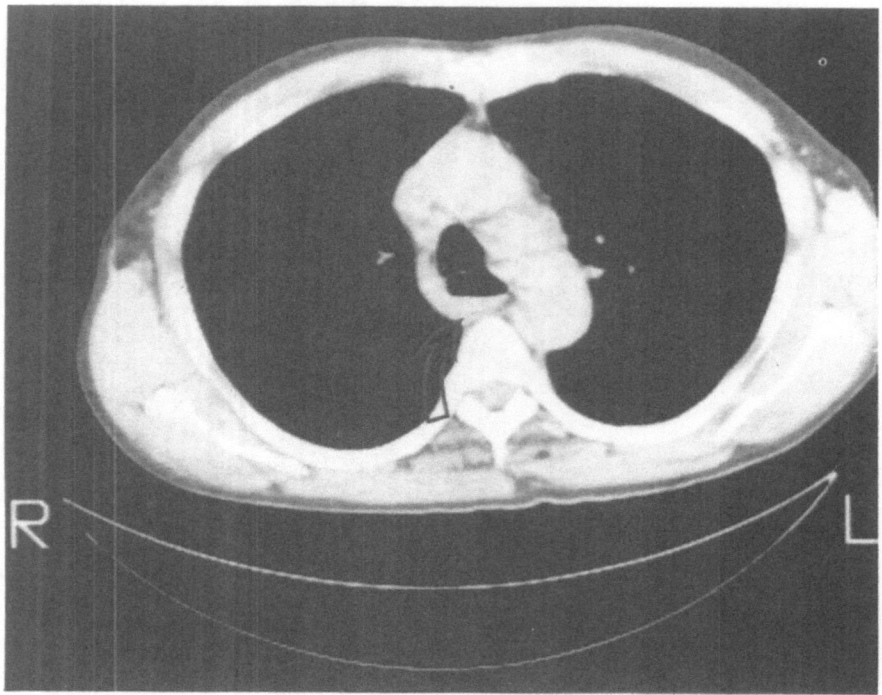

Figure 1-3. Dilated upper thoracic esophagus with fluid (arrow) secondary to obstructing tumor in lower segment.

Stomach   The initial means of radiographic evaluation of the stomach has been the fluoroscopic gastrointestinal series, which still remains the screening procedure of choice in patients with upper-digestive-tract disturbances. Within recent years, other modalities have been utilized to supplement the routine barium study in helping to evaluate the extramucosal extent of lesions detected on fluoroscopic procedures.

Nuclear Medicine   Abnormally accelerated or delayed emptying of gastric contents may be assessed in patients with ulcer disease or other motility disorders such as that in patients with diabetes or postoperative patients. Since solid food and liquids empty at different rates, one can evaluate both solid and liquid gastric half-emptying times utlizing different isotopes that are tagged to solid or liquid contents of meals.

Because the mucosa of the stomach concentrates free

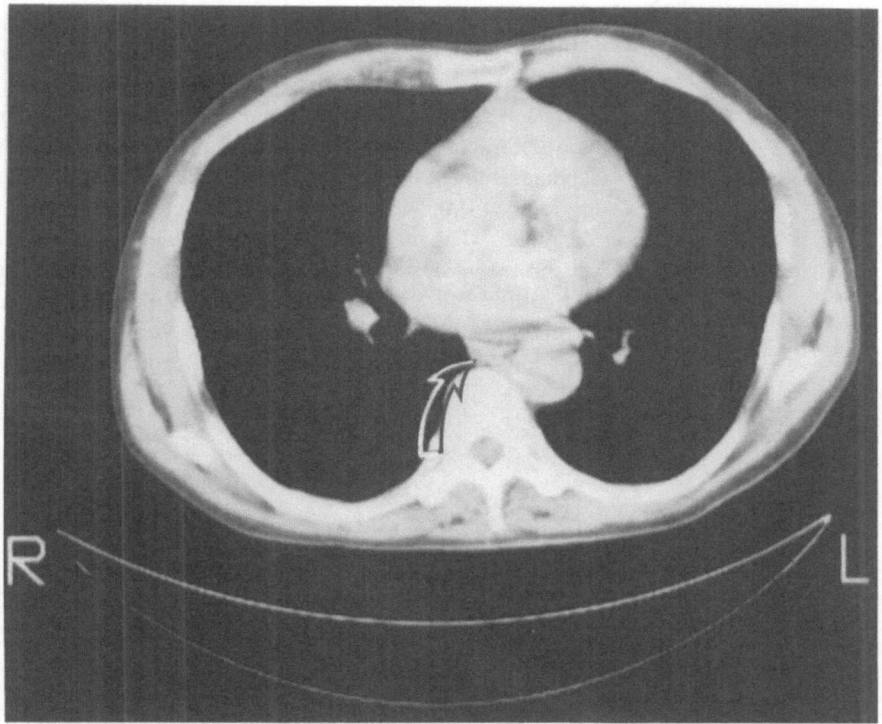

Figure 1-4. Posterior mediastinal mass (arrow) representing extramucosal extent of esophageal mass (arrow) on CT.

pertechnetate, patients can be injected with technetium pertechnetate resulting in localization of retained gastric antrum following a Billroth procedure for ulcer disease or in localization of ectopic gastric mucosa in either a Barrett's esophagus or Meckel's diverticulum scan.[4]

Gastrointestinal Bleeding

Acute gastrointestinal hemorrhage is often a medical or surgical emergency. Prompt recognition and localization of the bleeding site is necessary for early therapy resulting in increased chances for survival. Endoscopy and angiography have traditionally been the procedures of choice in these patients. However, selective angiography is invasive and expensive and in many instances may be difficult to perform. Two methods of imaging have now become standardized, one utilizing intravenous technetium sulfur colloid and the other using tagged red blood cells. *In vivo* or *in vitro* methods of tagging have been formulated that result in a high efficiency of tagging. The sulfur colloid examination is most useful in fairly active bleeding and specifically in lower-gastrointestinal hemorrhage, since the rapid accumulation of tracer within the liver and spleen can obscure more cephalad sites of bleeding. It has also been found that bleeding rates at 0.05–0.1 ml/min can be detected utilizing this technique.[1] The other method involves tagging of red blood cells to technetium pertechnetate. This study is more useful than sulfur colloid in detecting the site of upper gastrointestinal bleeding (Figs. 1-5 and 1-6). It is also more useful in patients with chronic intermittent bleeding since the im-

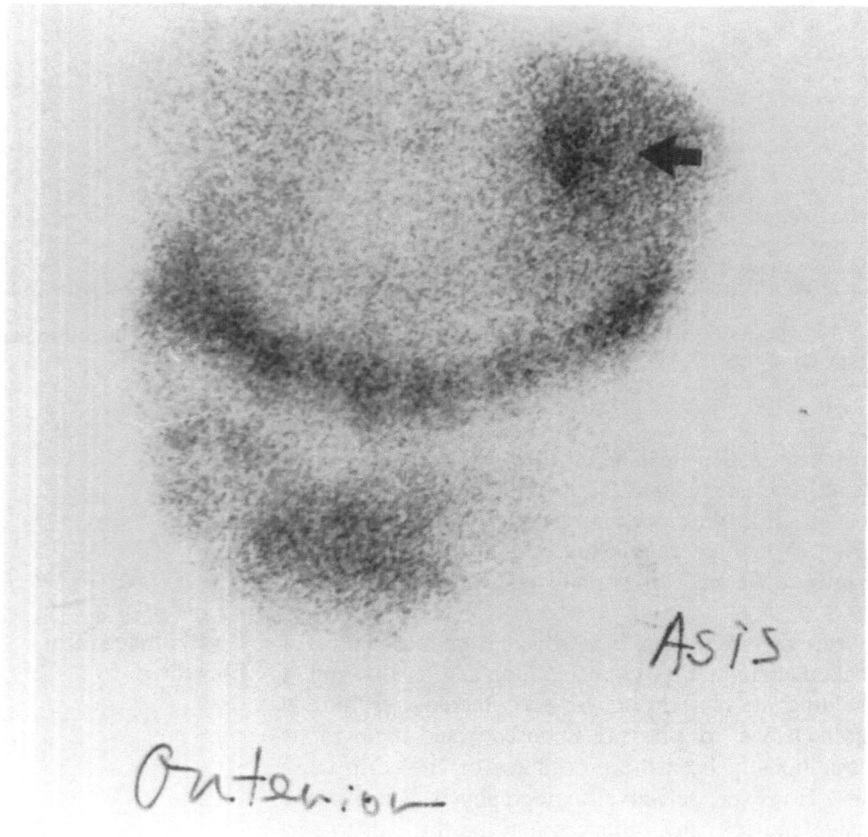

Figure 1-5. Tagged red blood cell study demonstrates increased activity in stomach and colon at 24 hr representing gastric (arrow) hemorrhage.

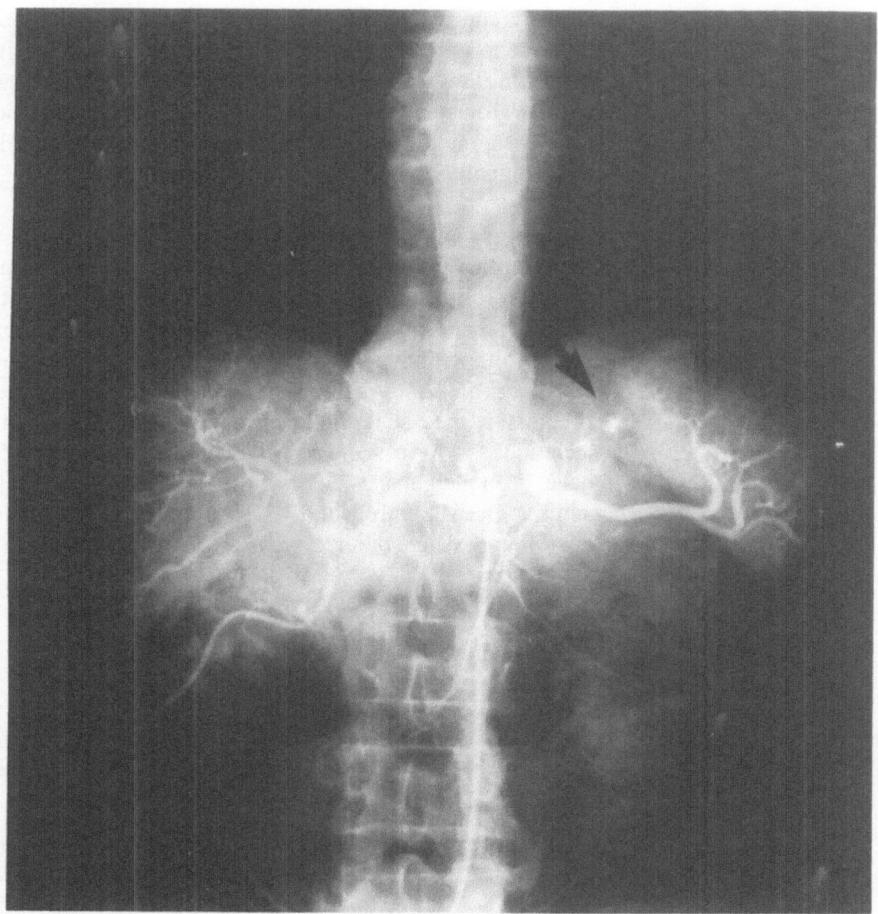

Figure 1-6. Angiography confirms bleeding site in stomach (arrow) from left gastric artery.

ages can be obtained over longer periods of time lasting up to 24 hr whereas the sulfur colloid examination is only useful for 15–20 min following the tracer administration.

Meckel's diverticulum is a congenital abnormality resulting from failure of closure of the omphalomesentric duct, which usually occurs as an outpouching in the distal ileum and in many cases may contain ectopic gastric mucosa. The most common symptom is rectal bleeding secondary to ulceration by the hydrochloric acid produced by the gastric mucosa. Since the technetium pertechnetate is

Meckel's Scan

actively concentrated and secreted by the gastric mucosa, diverticula will localize as an area of increased activity in the right lower quadrant in a fairly high percentage of cases.[3] However, false positives such as hyperemic bowel lesions or intussusception have been reported in the literature reducing the specificity of the procedure.

Small and Large Bowel

Ultrasound

Ultrasound of the small and large bowel has a very limited role being mainly utilized in patients with palpable masses or in children to whom one wishes to limit the radiation exposure. Numerous instances of abscesses or bowel tumors have been detected utilizing ultrasound.[2] However, the sonographic appearance of neoplastic and inflammatory disease is similar, limiting the usefulness of this technique. Pyloric stenosis (Fig. 1-7) and intussusception have been diagnosed successfully in children as well as adults.[9] Occasionally, solid visceral tumors will be incidentally found when other organs are being evaluated (Fig.

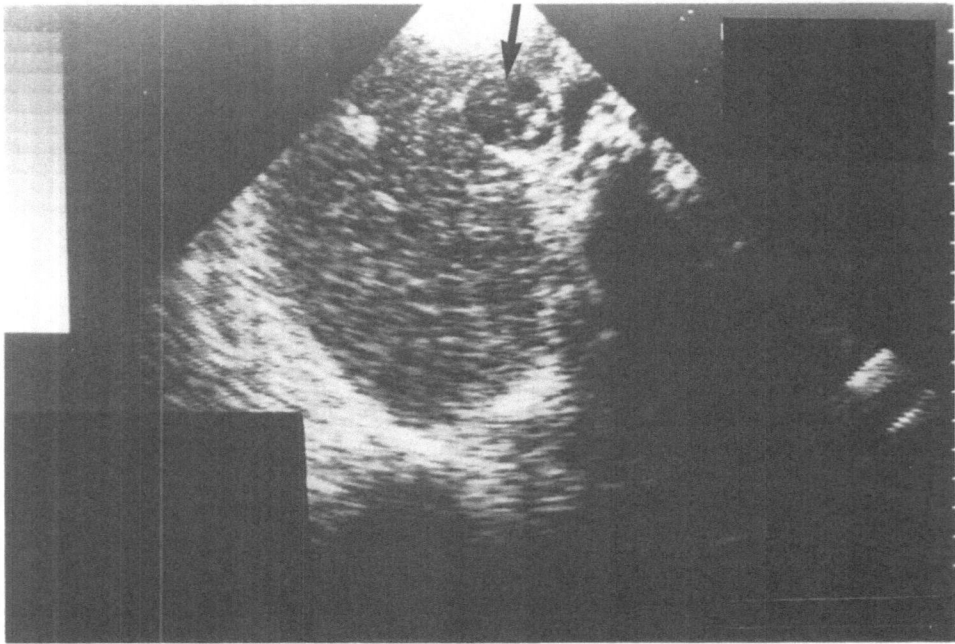

Figure 1-7. Hypoechoic mass (arrow) on right-upper-quadrant sonogram compatible with pyloric stenosis.

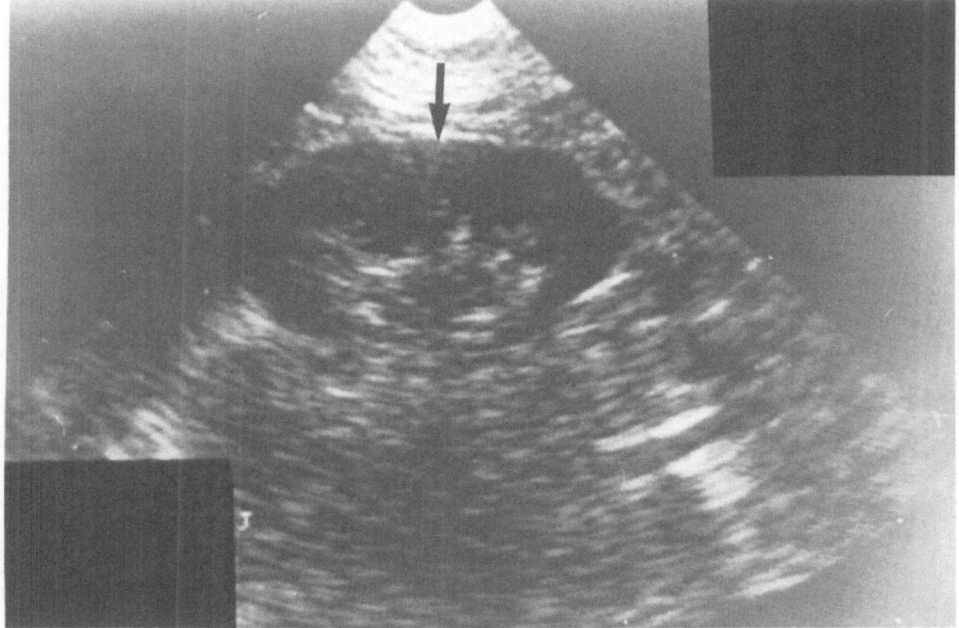

Figure 1-8. Pseudokidney sign (arrow) on upper abdominal sonogram demonstrating carcinoma of transverse colon.

1-8). Accompanying ascites will be visualized, and the possibility of retroperitoneal nodes or hepatic metastases can also be detected simultaneously.

Computerized Tomography

The primary diagnostic modality for diagnosing small and large bowel disease is the barium enema and small bowel series performed in an antegrade or retrograde fashion. These contrast examinations are limited mainly to mucosal abnormalities and changes in contour or caliber of the bowel lumen. CT is a useful supplementary examination that can document the extramucosal extension of lesions detected on the contrast study (Figs. 1-9 to 1-11). The major indication for CT is the staging of known malignancy, treatment planning, and detection or staging of postoperative tumor recurrence.[6] The response of metastases to therapy can be assessed (Figs. 1-12 to 1-14). Extraluminal lesions detected on barium studies can be evaluated. In patients with palpable masses not visualized on the contrast studies, CT is very accurate in the detection and characterization of such lesions.

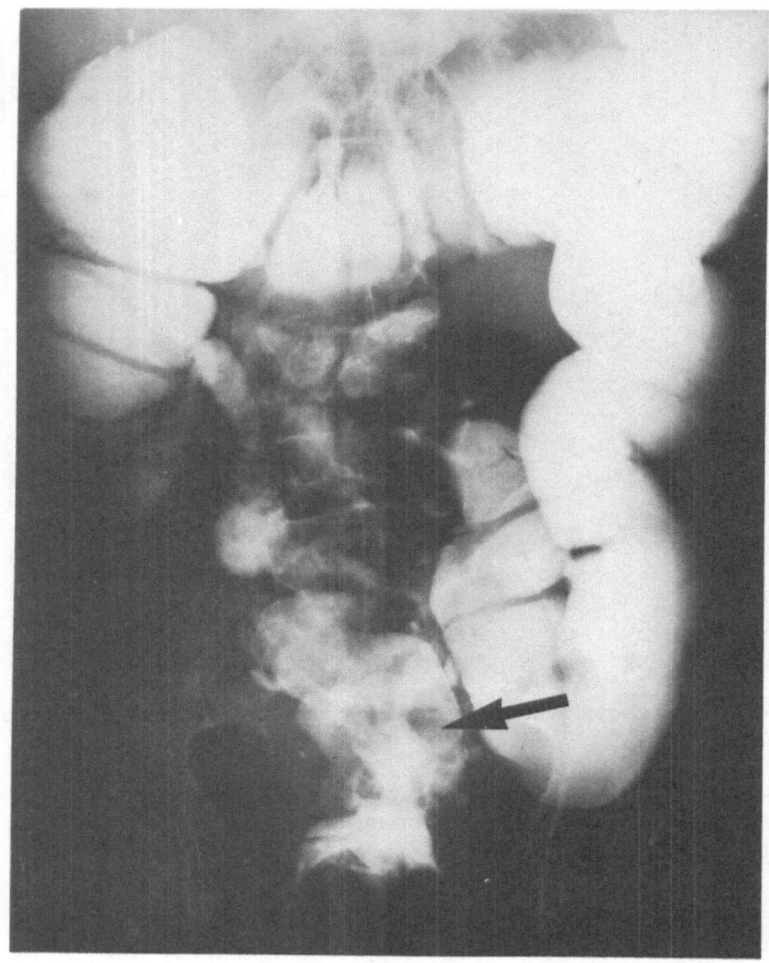

Figure 1-9. Constricting rectal carcinoma (arrow) demonstrated on barium enema.

PERITONEAL CAVITY AND ABDOMINAL WALL

Ultrasound

Ultrasound is the preferred method of localizing and directing the percutaneous aspiration of ascitic fluid. It is also useful in detecting abscesses (Figs. 1-15 and 1-16) for percutaneous drainage although artifact produced by gas from overlying bowel will limit the usefulness of the procedure. Malignancy involving the abdominal wall and peritoneal cavity may also be detected although, again, bowel gas may interfere with the examination. However, if a right-upper-quadrant or left subphrenic abscess is suspected, ultrasound is the preferred initial diagnostic study owing to

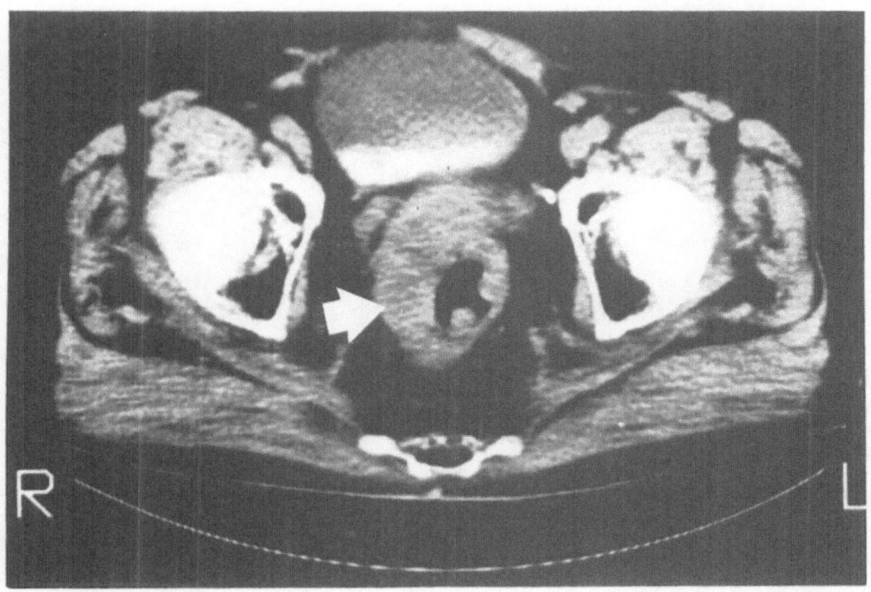

Figure 1-10. Computerized tomography demonstrates eccentric thickening of right anterior and lateral wall of rectum (arrow).

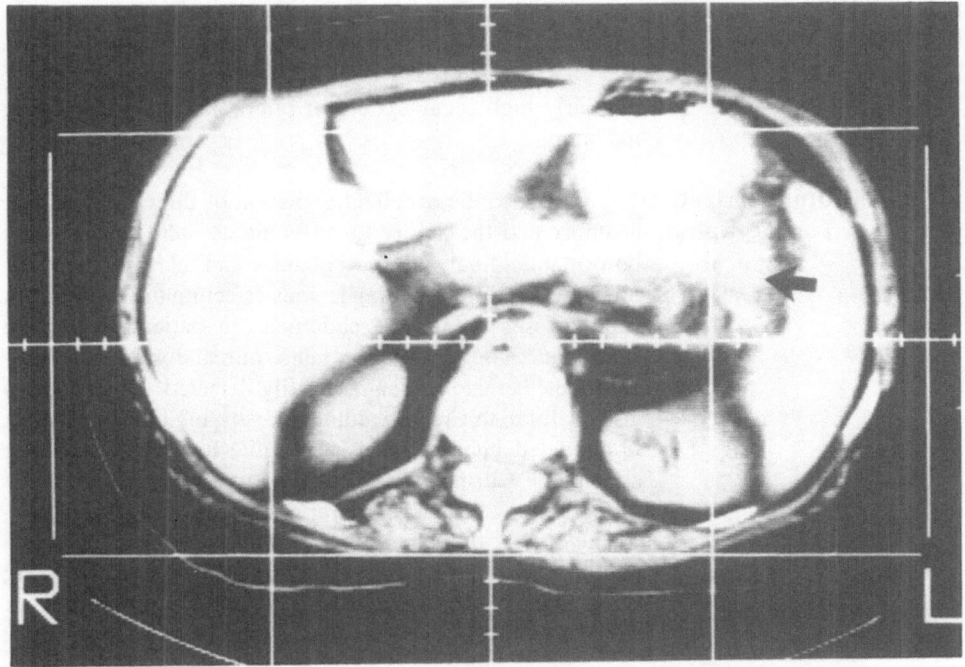

Figure 1-11. Muscular and serosal involvement of gastric tumor (arrow) demonstrated by computerized tomography.

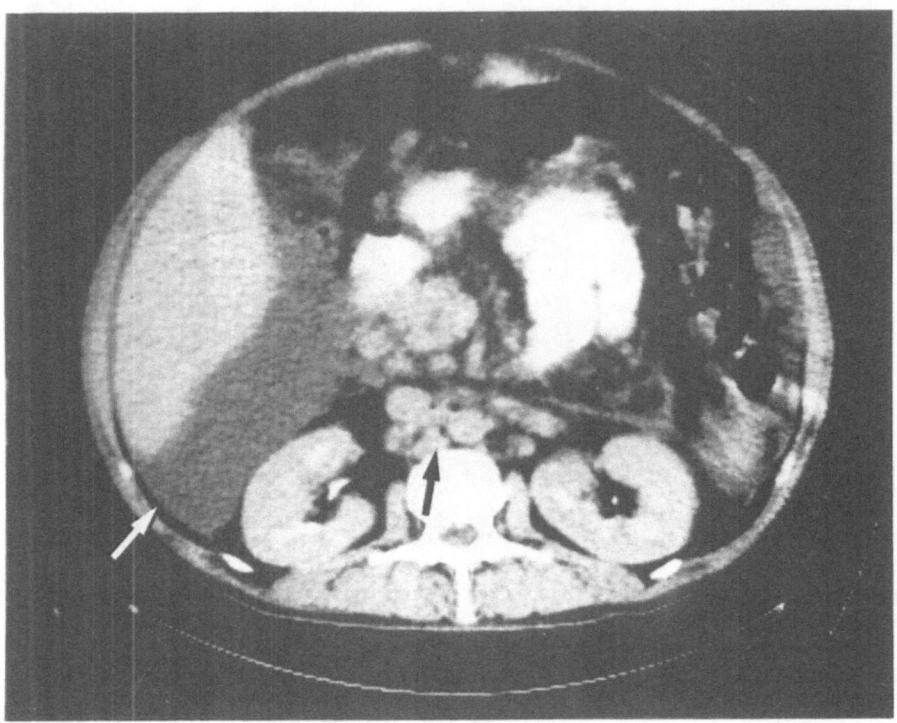

Figure 1-12. Retroperitoneal nodes (arrow), mesenteric nodes, and ascites in patient with non-Hodgkin's lymphoma.

the fairly high accuracy, lesser price, and lack of ionizing radiation.

Computerized Tomography

Owing to the excellent depiction of three-dimensional anatomy and the ability to differentiate solid organs from bowel, abdominal wall musculature, and fat, CT is the best procedure in differentiating lesions affecting the bowel from solid masses within the abdomen. In patients following acute trauma or on anticoagulants, intraabdominal or retroperitoneal hematoma can be readily detected. Ultrasound is also useful in this regard although overlying ileus will result in degraded images. CT is also quite helpful in detecting abdominal wall neoplasm and inflammatory processes and differentiating these from intraperitoneal lesions. Malignancy involving the abdominal wall, mesentery, or retroperitoneal lymph nodes can be readily detected. Utilizing CT guidance, percutaneous biopsy can be performed (Fig.

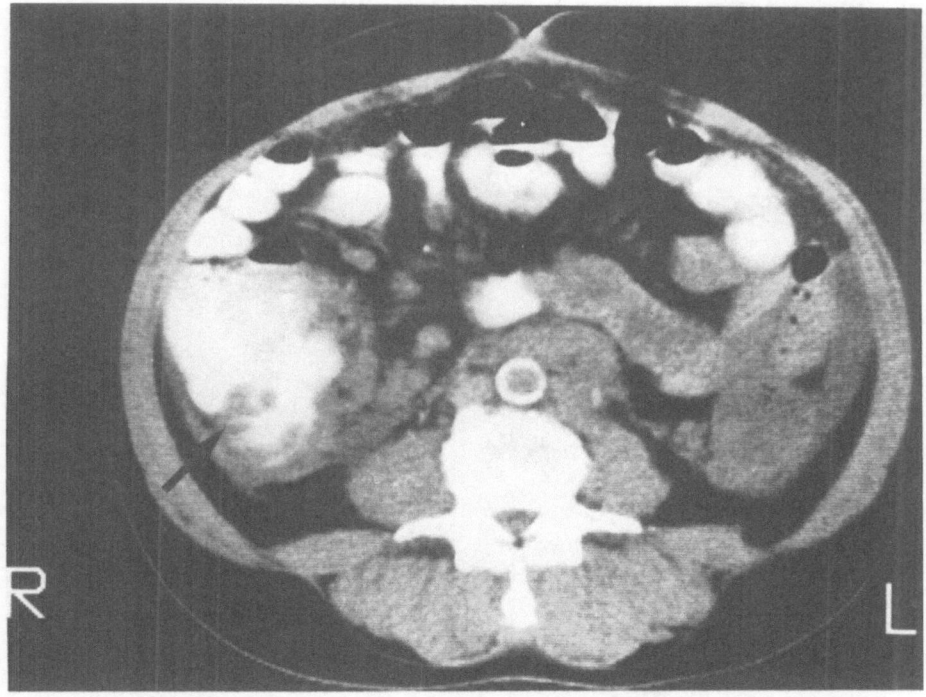

Figure 1-13. Lymphomatous involvement of cecum (arrow) as demonstrated by computerized tomography.

1-17), decreasing the need for staging laparotomy in patients with unresectable neoplasm or incurable disease. Percutaneous abscess drainage has also been performed successfully with CT guidance. Ascites is readily detected by CT, although ultrasound is the procedure of choice for ascites localization because of the lower cost and lack of ionizing radiation.

Radionuclide Scans

As stated previously, the utilization of ultrasound or CT will greatly increase the early detection of intraabdominal abscesses and certain tumors or retroperitoneal lymphadenopathy. Gallium scanning has been utilized quite frequently in the past for improved intraabdominal staging of lymphoma, particularly Hodgkin's disease, malignant melanoma, and, occasionally, lung tumors. Gallium has also been used frequently as a complementary examination with the radionuclide liver/spleen scan to help differentiate

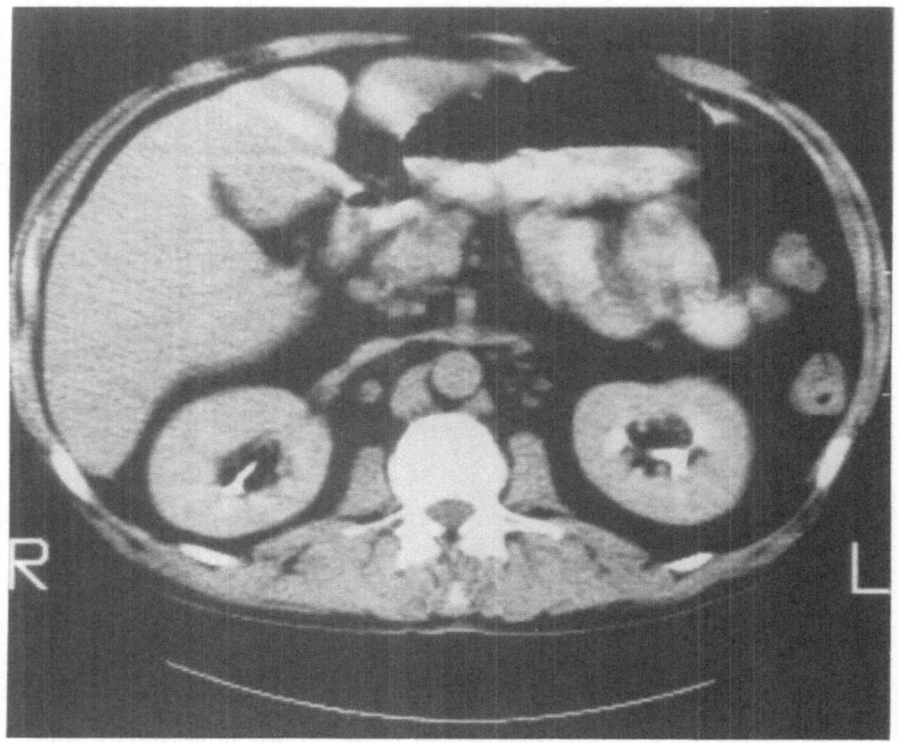

Figure 1-14. Marked regression of nodes and ascites following chemotherapy.

primary liver malignancy or hepatic abscess, which both avidly accumulate gallium, from a metastatic lesion, which will not. Gallium scanning is very useful in postoperative patients in the detection of acute inflammatory processes. The limitation of the study is that gallium will also accumulate in normal bowel, making the findings nonspecific. However, this problem can be overcome with utilization of a vigorous bowel preparation prior to the scanning. Many centers have now switched to Indium oxine tagged to leukocytes, which will also document infectious processes within the abdomen but does not accumulate within the normal bowel. In patients presenting with fever of unknown origin, gallium scanning as the primary screening modality may help localize an infectious process to either the thorax, abdomen, or pelvis, which can then be further evaluated by either CT or ultrasound for more definitive diagnosis.

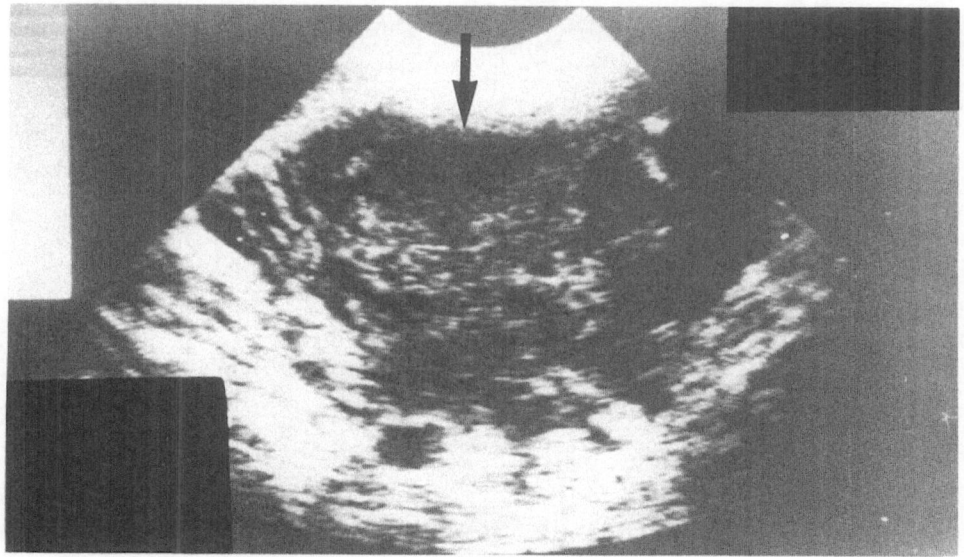

Figure 1-15. Large, complex mass (arrow) in right lower quadrant representing appendiceal abscess on sonogram.

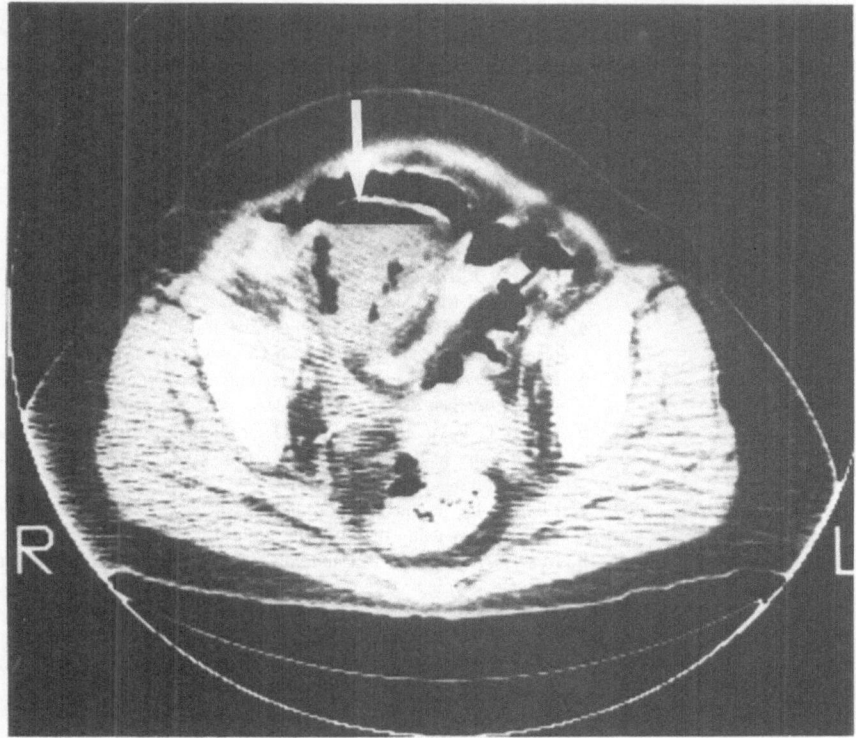

Figure 1-16. Large necrotic soft tissue mass with fluid (arrow) representing appendiceal abscess.

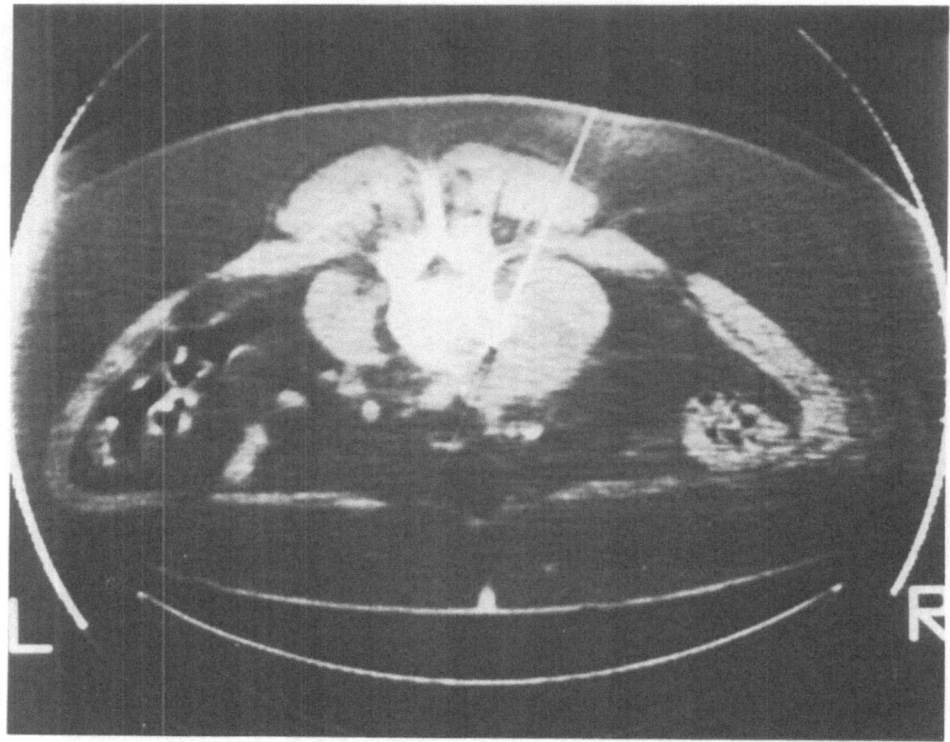

Figure 1-17. Computerized tomography-directed biopsy of enlarged iliac nodes (arrow) in patient with cervical carcinoma.

REFERENCES

1. Alavi A: Detection of gastrointestinal bleeding with 99m Tc sulfur colloid. *Sem Nucl Med* 1982;12:126–137.
2. Bluth E, Merritt C, Sullivan M: Ultrasonic evaluation of the stomach, small bowel and colon. *Radiology* 1979;133:677–680.
3. Conway J: The sensitivity, specificity, and accuracy of radionuclide imaging of Meckels diverticulum. *J Nucl Med* 1976;17:553.
4. Gordon F, Fischer NR: Diagnosis of Barrett's esophagus with radioisotopes. *Am J Roentgenol Radium Nucl Med* 1974;121:716.
5. Kazem I: A new scintigraphic technique for studying the esophagus. *Am J Roentgenol Radium Nucl Med* 1972;115:681.
6. Lee JKT, Levitt RG, Stanley RJ, et al: Utility of body computerized tomography in the clinical followup of abdominal masses. *J Comput Assist Tomogr* 1978;2:607–611.
7. Malmud LS, et al: Quantitation of gastroesophageal reflux before and after therapy using the GE scintiscan. *J Nucl Med* 1976;17:559.
8. Moss AA, Schnyder P, Candardjs G, et al: Esophageal carcinoma: Pretherapy staging by computed tomography. *Am J Roentgenol* 1981;136:1051–1056.
9. Parienty R, Lepreux J, Grissom B: Sonographic and CT features of ileocolic intussusception. *Am J Roentgenol* 1981;136:608–610.

2   Hepatobiliary System

The liver, although the largest visceral abdominal organ, has always been one of the most difficult to evaluate utilizing clinical palpation owing to its location beneath the rib cage. Radiographic evaluation of the liver prior to the era of newer imaging modalities had always utilized changes produced by the enlarged liver on the neighboring visceral organs such as the colon or right kidney. Diagnosis of hepatic disorders usually resulted in resorting to more invasive modalities such as angiography, transhepatic cholangiography, and liver biopsies. Fortunately, with the newer imaging modalities, the liver can now be directly visualized and evaluated, resulting more often in tissue-specific diagnoses without having to resort to more invasive procedures.

HEPATIC DISEASES

Liver Imaging

The radionuclide liver scan is very useful in evaluating trauma patients who present with right-sided rib fractures and falling hematocrit in which the possibility of subcapsular or intrahepatic bleed is suspected.[1] The examination, however, is limited in the sense that smaller lesions may go undetected unless they are superficial. Many institutions now advocate the use of ultrasound or computerized tomography (CT) as the primary screening procedure in patients with suspected trauma to the liver.

Trauma

Nuclear Medicine

Ultrasound

Ultrasound is a useful technique in which the presence of subcapsular or intrahepatic bleed can be readily detected. The presence of free blood within the abdomen can also be established, which is not possible with the radionuclide study. Unfortunately, however, the patient who has experienced recent trauma in many instances will have bandages, superficial wounds, or adynamic ileus, which will obscure visualization of portions of the liver parenchyma.

Computerized Tomography

Postoperative patients and those having experienced recent trauma are usually most easily and adequately evaluated with CT owing to the lack of interference from bandages and bowel gas. In addition to detection of the pres-

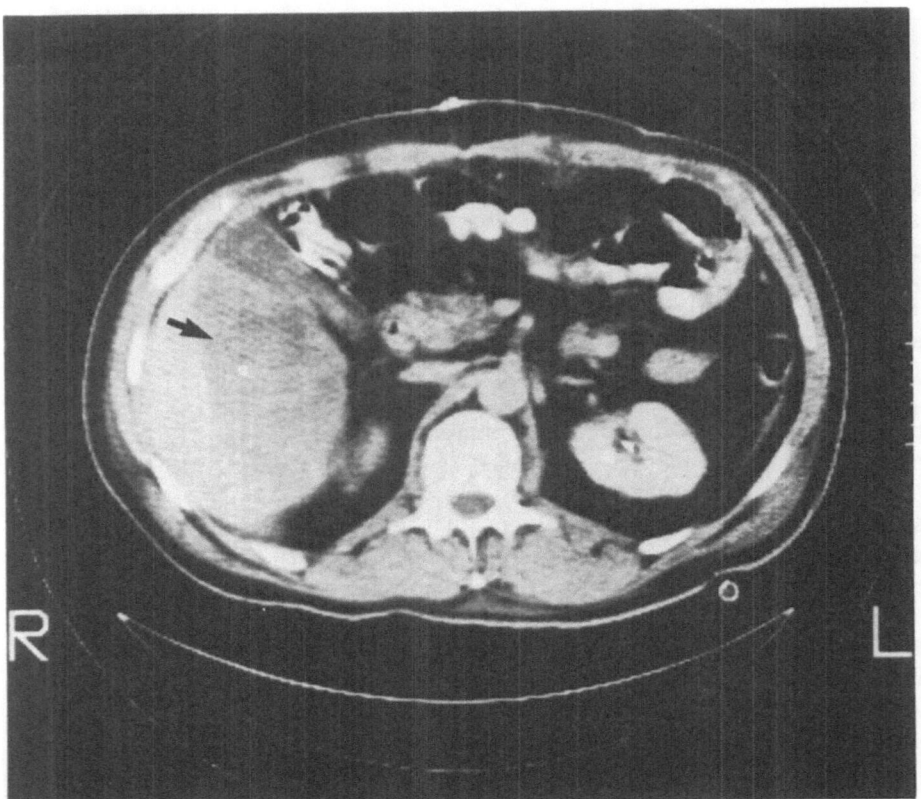

Figure 2-1. Low-density area in right lobe of liver (arrow) representing hematoma in massively traumatized patient.

ence of hepatic hematoma or laceration (Fig. 2-1), the presence of free blood within the abdomen or injuries to other organs such as the kidneys or pancreas can be readily detected owing to the excellent cross-sectional anatomic display of the abdomen. With use of a bolus technique and dynamic scanning, pseudoaneurysms or AV fistulae can be detected.[2] Many institutions now advocate CT as the initial examination of choice in acutely traumatized patients who are stable enough to undergo the procedure prior to laparotomy.[4]

The liver radionuclide exam is based on the ability of the phagocytic properties of the Kupffer cells within the liver to sequester radioactively tagged colloid materials. For purposes of interpretation, diseases resulting in enlarged liver may be divided into diffuse and focal pathologic processes. One of the more common uses of radionuclide imaging is to assess the size of the liver and the gross function as pertaining to distribution of tracer activity throughout the organ. While the findings of hepatomegaly and patchy distribution of tracer are nonspecific, the most common diseases presenting in this manner are hepatitis, cirrhosis, chronic passive congestion secondary to right heart failure and other diffuse processes such as lymphoma, leukemia, miliary metatases, infectious diseases such as mononucleosis and metabolic disorders such as Wilson's disease, amyloidosis and glycogen storage disease.[9] This scan is fairly sensitive in detecting diffuse liver processes as described above; however, the specificity is very low and correlation with clinical findings or biopsy will be necessary in many instances. The scan, however, can help discriminate between diffuse hepatic enlargement and enlargement resulting from focal lesions. Patients with known neoplasm are screened prior to undergoing therapy and following therapy for detection of metastasis. The limitation of the study is that the spatial resolution of most cameras will not detect lesions under 1.5–2 cm unless they are fairly superficial. In addition, most focal lesions appear as cold defects on the liver/spleen scan with both cystic and solid lesions having a nonspecific appearance. Ultrasound or CT can then be used to aid in differentiation. Common benign lesions of the liver include cysts, adenoma, hemangioma, and infectious processes such as abscesses and echinococcal disease.

Hepatic Enlargement (Diffuse or Focal Disease)

Nuclear Medicine

Ultrasound

Ultrasound is used mainly in patients with equivocal scintigraphic examinations or patients exhibiting normal radionuclide studies in whom the index of suspicion for liver pathology is very high. In patients with diffuse liver enlargement, ultrasound is not routinely used as a screening procedure. However, owing to the tremendous resolution of the newer ultrasound machines, the study has the ability to display internal organ structure and tissue consistency, in many instances resulting in a more specific diagnosis.[11] The hallmark of diffuse liver disease as seen on ultrasound is enlargement of the liver as manifested by bulging contours, diffusely increased parenchymal echogenicity with subsequently decreased visualization of the normal internal vascular structures and decreased through-transmission of the sound beam.[3] The other limitations of the exam are the high dependence upon operator ability and difficulty imaging portions of the organ in patients with excessive gas, overlying bandages, scars, and ribs.

Computerized Tomography

In most institutions, CT is not utilized in evaluating diffuse liver disease because of the high cost relative to radionuclide study or ultrasound examination. However, by use of contrast enhancement and dynamic scanning techniques, more tissue-specific diagnoses are possible with the utilization of CT. CT is most useful in differentiating fatty infiltration of the liver from changes seen in cirrhosis. In addition, the liver will demonstrate abnormally increased density in certain diseases such as Wilson's disease, which is a result of abnormally increased copper deposition or hemochromatosis which is manifested by abnormally increased iron deposition in the liver.[6] CT will also be useful in identifying hepatoma in patients with chronic liver disease who are at increased risk for this condition. The ascites that frequently accompanies diffuse liver disease will be demonstrated, as well as retroperitoneal or gastroesophageal varices secondary to portal hypertension (Fig. 2-2).

Liver Neoplasm (Primary or Secondary)

Nuclear Medicine

The liver/spleen scan is a fairly sensitive procedure for evaluating the presence of liver metastases, which usually appear as cold lesions within a normal-sized or enlarged liver (Fig. 2-3). However, focal lesions are nonspecific in appearance, and the studies usually have to be correlated with either ultrasound or computerized tomography to aid in differentiating between benign cysts and solid lesions. In

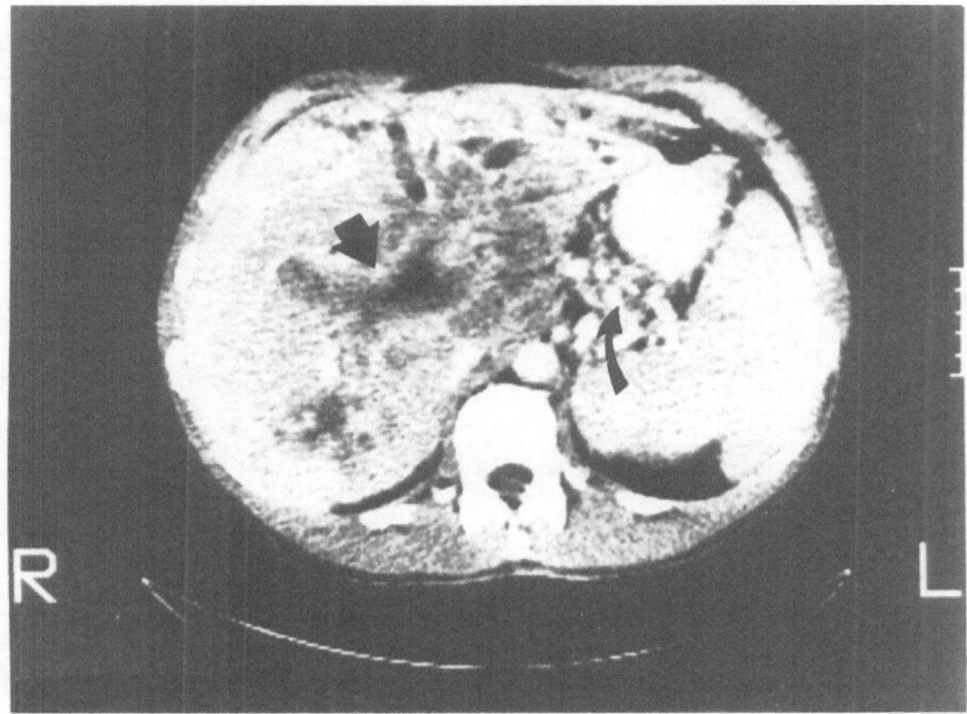

Figure 2-2. Computerized tomography of patient with pancreatic tumor with resultant dilated bile ducts (arrowhead) and gastric varices (arrow) resulting from splenic vein obstruction.

the past, the liver/spleen scan was included in the routine preoperative evaluation of carcinomas that routinely metastasize to the liver such as those of the bowel, pancreas, lung, and breast.[8] Patients were then followed postoperatively or after receiving further treatment such as chemotherapy or radiation. This, however, has become a controversial issue as many institutions now routinely stage the patients preoperatively with ultrasound or CT.

Ultrasound

As mentioned previously, ultrasound is being used in most radiology departments to better define focal lesions identified on radionuclide screening examinations and to distinguish between cystic and solid lesions (Fig. 2-4). Ultrasound is also useful in patients who have had normal scintigraphic examinations but have elevated liver enzymes and are very highly suspicious for metastatic disease.[10] In

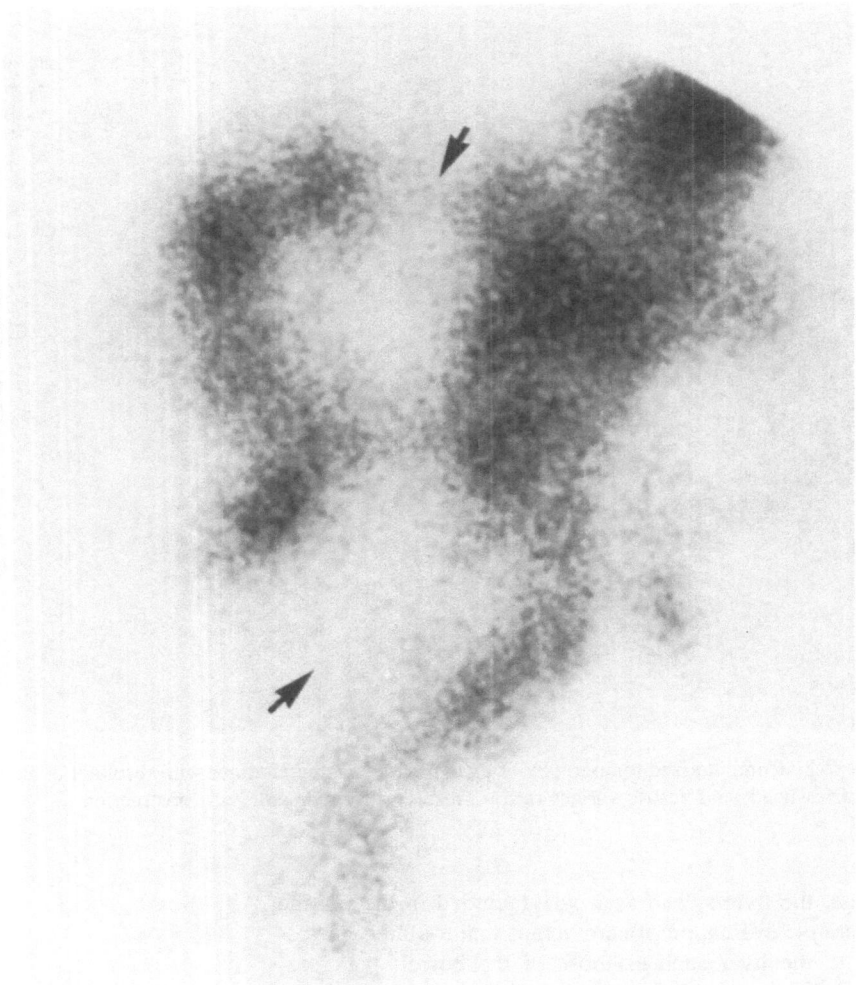

Figure 2-3. Liver spleen scan demonstrating hepatomegaly with multiple areas of decreased activity (arrows) representing metastases.

addition, when a lesion is detected on ultrasound, sonographic localization for biopsy can be performed quite readily. The other advantage of ultrasound is that the lesion can be localized to a specific lobe or lobar segment in patients in whom resection is being considered. The region of the porta hepatis is also readily visualized, and the possibility of metastasis or lymph nodes in this area can be discovered during the examination. In addition, while the abdomen is being

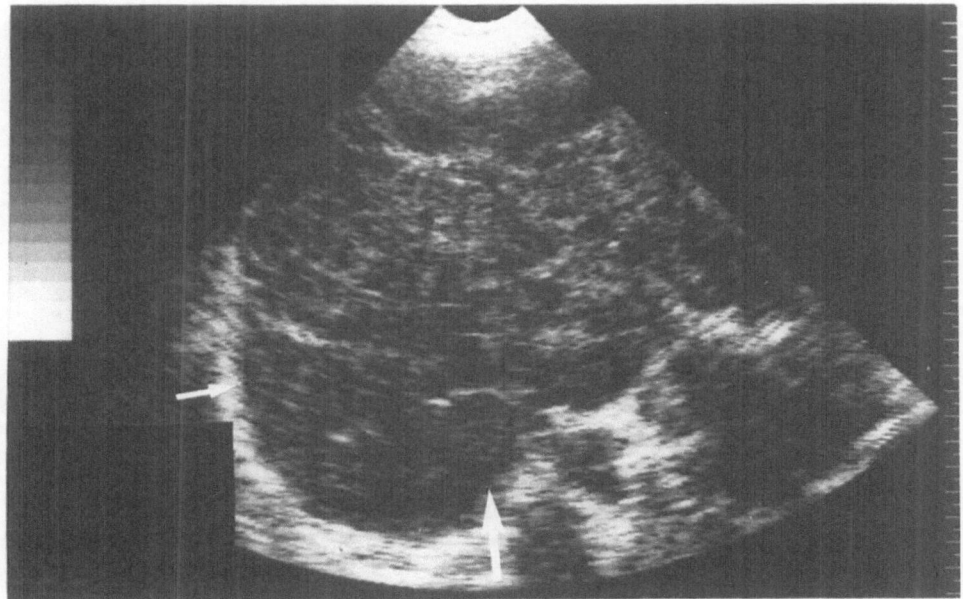

Figure 2-4. Hepatomegaly with multiple focal areas of irregular echoes (arrows) representing lung metastases.

scanned, the possibility of retroperitoneal lymphadenopathy can also be evaluated. Many institutions utilize ultrasound as the initial screening procedure of choice to detect hepatic metastasis and follow the patients after therapy.

CT and ultrasound have similar capabilities in detecting focal lesions within the liver, although by use of contrast enhancement and dynamic scanning techniques, more tissue-specific diagnoses can be made with CT.[12] For instance, a benign lesion such as cavernous hemangioma (Figs. 2-5 to 2-7) will show increasing temporal enhancement as opposed to a malignant lesion, which will not.[5] The major advantage of CT in evaluating patients before and after therapy for malignancy is visualization of the entire abdominal cross-sectional anatomy. This will facilitate biopsies that can be performed utilizing CT guidance. In addition, metastasis to other organs or lymph nodes and other incidental lesions can be routinely identified. Also, in postoperative patients the abdomen is usually better evaluated with CT because of the lack of interference from surgical clips, bandages, and bowel gas, which may obscure the

Computerized Tomography

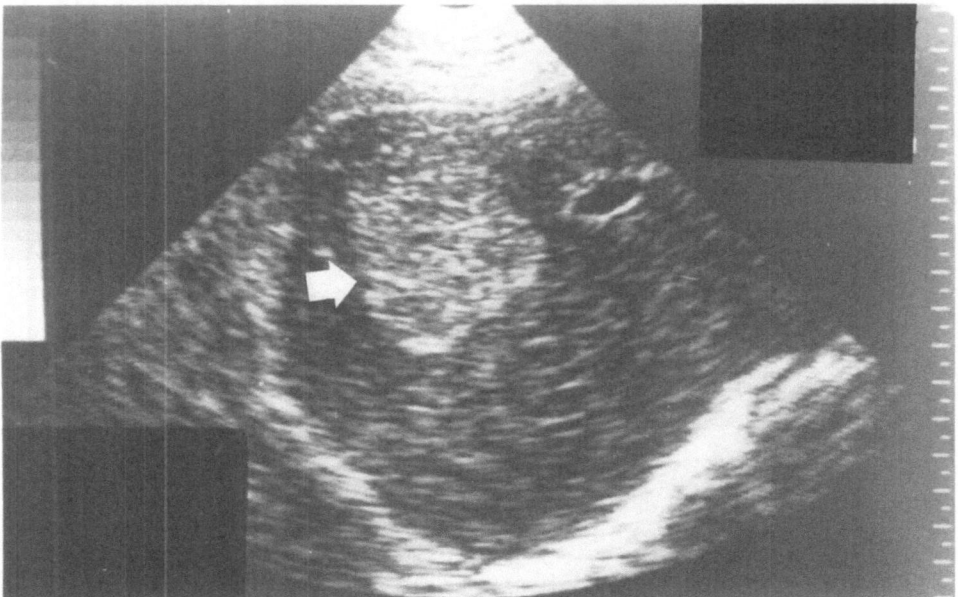

Figure 2-5. Large, solid mass in right lobe of liver (arrow) discovered incidentally during gall bladder sonogram.

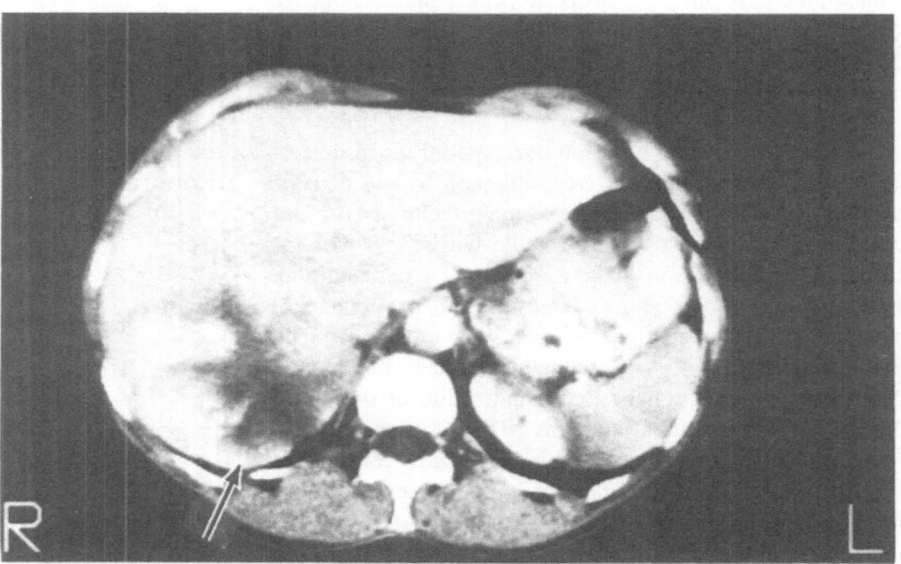

Figure 2-6. Computerized tomography scan demonstrating large, peripherally enhancing mass (arrow) in right lobe of liver representing hemangioma.

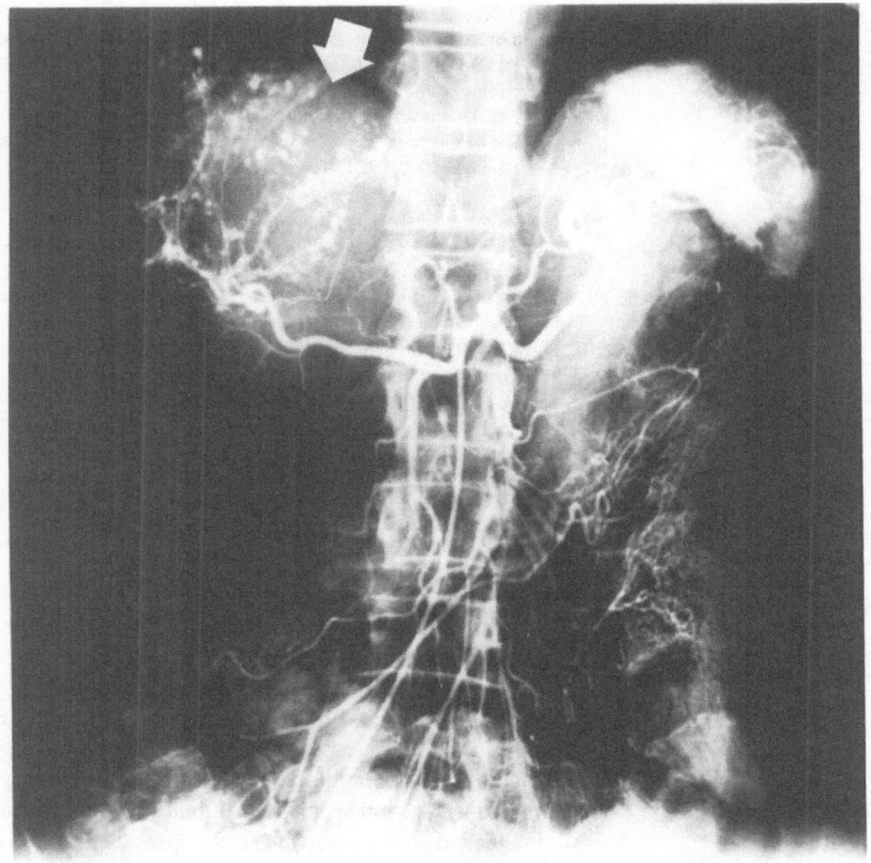

Figure 2-7. Angiography confirming presence of highly vascular hepatic hemangioma (arrow).

anatomy during an ultrasound examination. CT has also been used to measure liver volume and tumor volume both pre- and posttherapy.[7] Radiation ports can be constructed utilizing CT guidance, as well as detection of radiation-induced damage to the liver in certain instances.

REFERENCES

1. Aronsen KF, et al: Evaluation of hepatic regeneration by scintillation scanning, cholangiography and angiography in man. *Ann Surg* 1970;171:567.
2. Axel L, Mbss AA, Berninger W: Dynamic computed tomography demonstration of hepatic arteriovenous fistula. *J Comput Assist Tomogr* 1981;5:95–98.
3. Birnholz J: Diffuse liver disease. *Clin Diagnostic Ultrasound* 1979;1:35–37.

4. Federle MP, Goldberg HI, Kaiser JA, et al: Evaluation of abdominal trauma by computed tomography. *Radiology* 1981;138:637–644.
5. Itai Y, Furui S, Araki T, et al: Computed tomography of cavernous hemangioma of the liver. *Radiology* 1980;137:149–155.
6. Mills SR, Doppman JL, Neinhus AW: Computed tomography in the diagnosis of disorders of excessive iron storage in the liver. *J Comput Assist Tomogr* 1977;1:101–104.
7. Moss AA, Cann CE, Friedman MA, et al: Volumetric analysis of hepatic tumors. *J Comput Assist Tomogr* 1981;3:714–718.
8. Drum DE, Beard JM: Scintographic criteria for hepatic metastases from cancer of the colon and breast. *J Nucl Med* 1976;17:677.
9. Rocha AFG, Harbert JC: *Textbook of Nuclear Medicine: Clinical applications.* 1979;166.
10. Snow JH, Goldstein HM, Wallace S: Comparison of scintigraphy, sonography and computed tomography in the evaluation of hepatic neoplasms. *Am J Roentgenol* 1979;132:915–918.
11. Taylor KJW, Gorelick FS, Rosenfield AT, et al: Ultrasonography of alcoholic liver disease with histological correlation. *Radiology* 1981;141:157–161.
12. Wooten WB, Bernardino ML, Goldstein HM: Computed tomography of necrotic metastases. *Am J Roentgenol* 1978;131:839–842.

BILIARY SYSTEM

The bilary system is composed of the gall bladder and bile ducts, which are both intrahepatic and extrahepatic in location. In previous years, the gold standard imaging procedure for gall bladder disease was the oral cholecystogram, which was supplemented by the intravenous cholangiogram and transhepatic cholangiogram. The oral cholecystogram is a very sensitive and specific examination for detection of gall bladder disease. However, the presence of a nonvisualized gall bladder on the oral cholecystogram may at times be representative of other disease states rather than simply reflecting gall bladder pathology. For instance, intestinal malabsorption of the orally administered contrast material may present as a false-positive or nonvisualized gall bladder. The intravenous cholangiogram has also been limited in use owing to a relatively high morbidity and mortality rate related to the intravenous contrast reactions. These studies have since been supplemented and in many instances replaced by radionuclide biliary imaging procedures and ultrasound of the gall bladder and bile ducts.

Inflammatory Disease of the Gall Bladder

Nuclear Medicine

Biliary scanning is a fairly recent procedure utilizing technetium–IDA agents, which are derivatives of amino acetanilid compound. This compound, in contradistinction to sulfur colloid, is an agent directly handled by hepatocytes in a manner similar to bilirubin, thus making the scan a physiologic study of liver function with visualization of the bile ducts and filling of the normal gall bladder. This study is most commonly used to exclude the presence of cystic duct obstruction resulting in acute cholecystitis (Fig. 2-8). Delayed filling of the gall bladder in many instances is a sign of chronic cholecystitis and will confidently exclude the diagnosis of acute cholecystitis in most cases.[5] Owing to fairly good visualization of the main intrahepatic and extrahepatic ducts, the scan can also be utilized to evaluate the possibility of biliary ductal obstruction. Since the tracer clearance, tracer time, and biliary anatomy can be evaluated, other diffuse diseases of the liver resulting in intrahepatic cholestasis can also be diagnosed utilizing this examination.

Ultrasound

Ultrasound of the gall bladder in many institutions is now the preferred examination to exclude the presence of cholelithiasis (Fig. 2-9). It compares favorably with the oral cholecystogram in accuracy but does not require oral contrast or a relatively normal functioning digestive tract nor involve radiation to get comparable results. It is most useful in patients with nonvisualized gall bladders on the oral cholecystogram, pregnant patients, and young patients to whom radiation exposure should be limited. In some institutions, favorable results have been reported utilizing ultrasound to detect acute cholecystitis and to distinguish the condition from chronic cholecystitis in conjunction with the presence of stones. Complications of acute cholecystitis such as hydrops of the gall bladder or perforation with pericholecystic abscess formation can also be more readily detected.[1]

Computerized Tomography

CT has very limited utilization in the evaluation of inflammatory disease of the gall bladder, although occasionally stones or complications secondary to acute cholecystitis such as gall bladder perforation can be visualized with CT.

Jaundice— Obstructive versus Nonobstructive

Nuclear Medicine

At this time, controversy rages over which imaging modality is the preferred method to evaluate dilated bile ducts. The radionuclide scan is fairly sensitive in depicting the presence of dilated ducts; however, the etiology of the dilatation is difficult to determine utilizing this scan alone, making it necessary to correlate with ultrasound or CT examination.

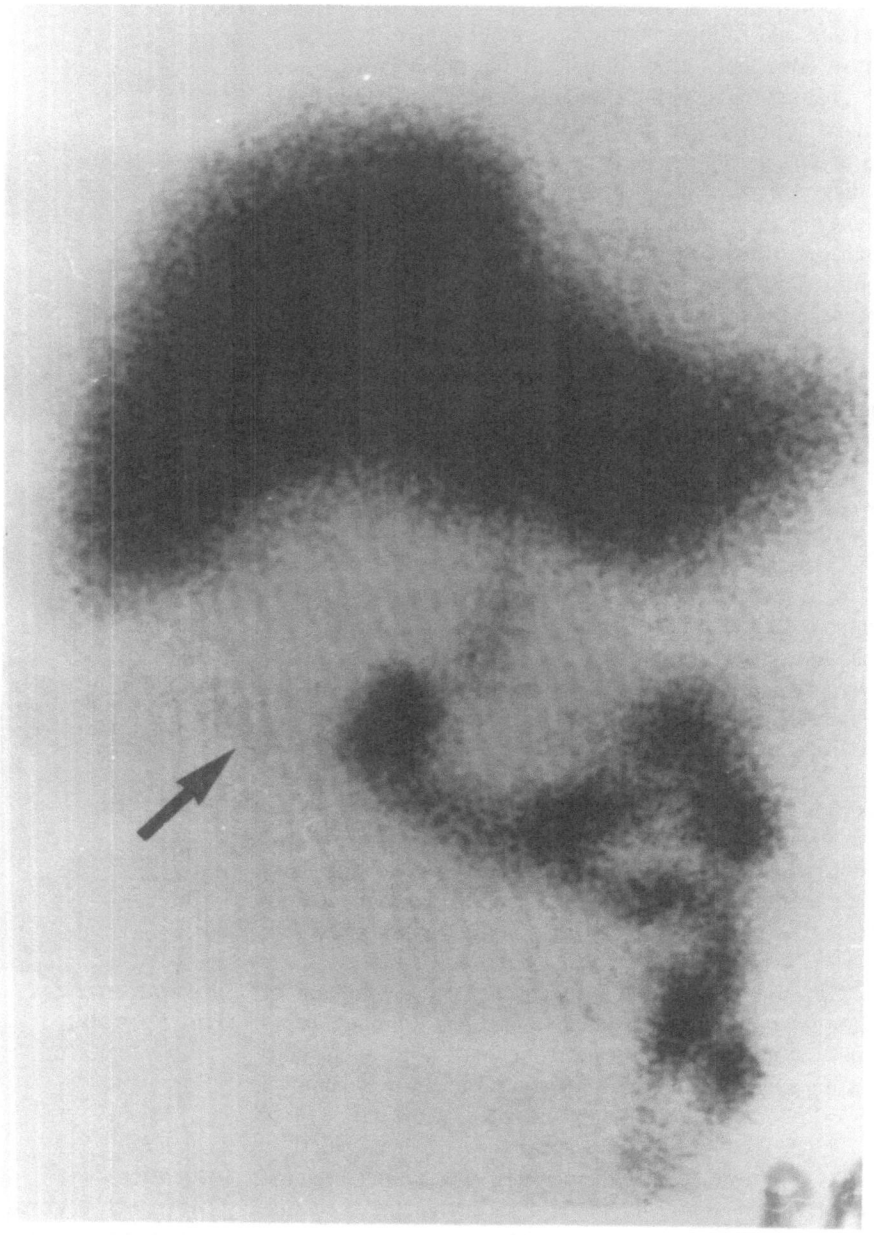

Figure 2-8. Large photon-deficient area (arrow) representing distended gall bladder secondary to acute cystic duct obstruction and subsequent acute cholecystitis.

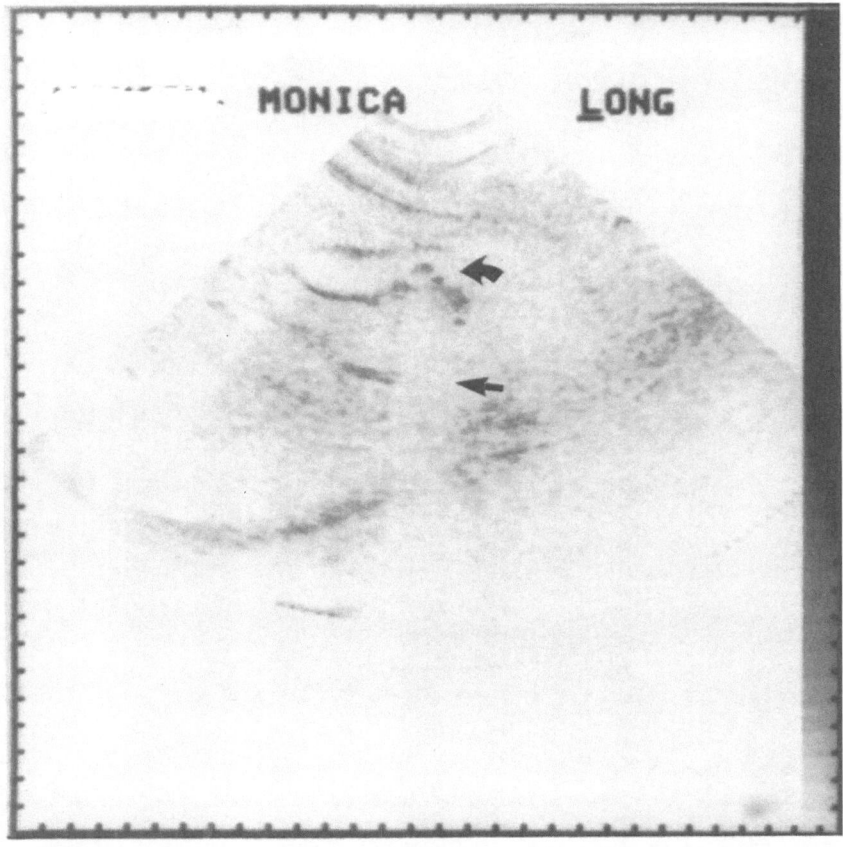

Figure 2-9. Single gallstone (curved arrow) in gall bladder with characteristic acoustic shadowing (straight arrow).

Ultrasound

Most medical centers now favor the use of ultrasound as the screening modality of choice in evaluating the cause of jaundice. Spatial resolution of the newer machines readily demonstrates the presence of dilated intrahepatic or common hepatic ducts. (Fig. 2-10) In many instances, the etiology, whether it be choledocholithiasis, pancreatic tumor, or pancreatitis, can be also demonstrated.[3] In some instances, however, the level of obstruction can be revealed but not the etiology and transhepatic cholangiogram, or endoscopic retrograde cholangiopancreatography (ERCP) will be needed for better anatomic delineation of the intrahepatic ducts and the obstructing lesion.

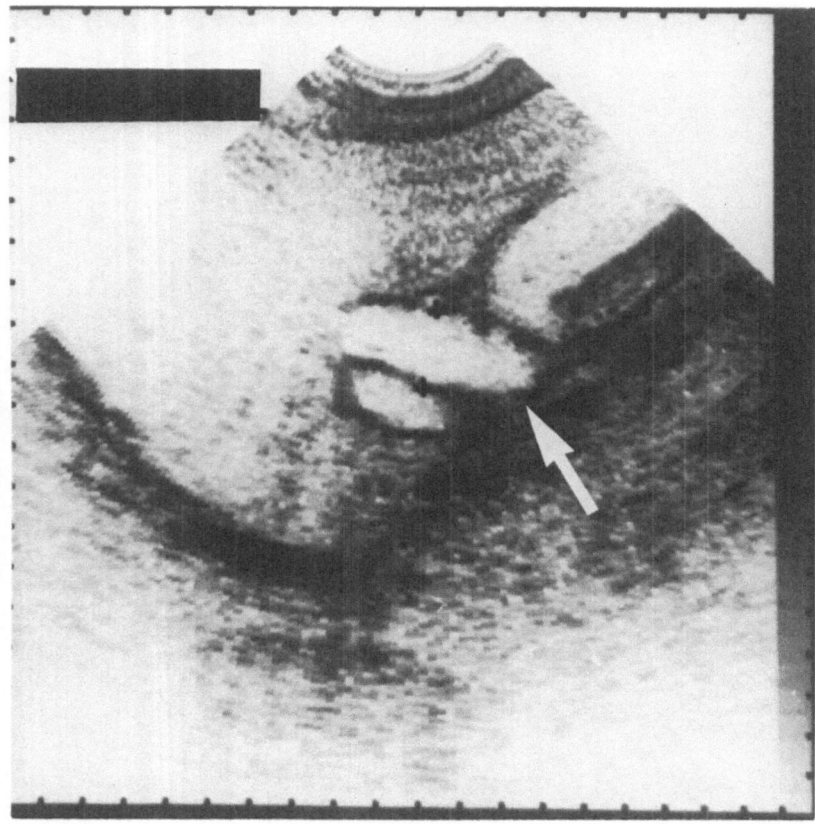

Figure 2-10. Dilated bile duct (arrow) secondary to pancreatic neoplasm.

Computerized Tomography

Other institutions favor the use of CT as the primary mode of investigation of biliary ductal dilatation. Utilizing high-resolution, thin-sliced tomography, the level and etiology of biliary ductal obstruction have been determined in almost 90% of cases.[2] The disadvantages of this procedure, however, are the increased radiation dose to the patient and increased cost. Again, it should be noted that although the level of obstruction can be determined in many patients, the etiology still cannot be seen, such as in patients with strictures or small intraductal lesions, which still necessitate the performance of some other, more invasive procedure such as ERCP or transhepatic cholangiogram.

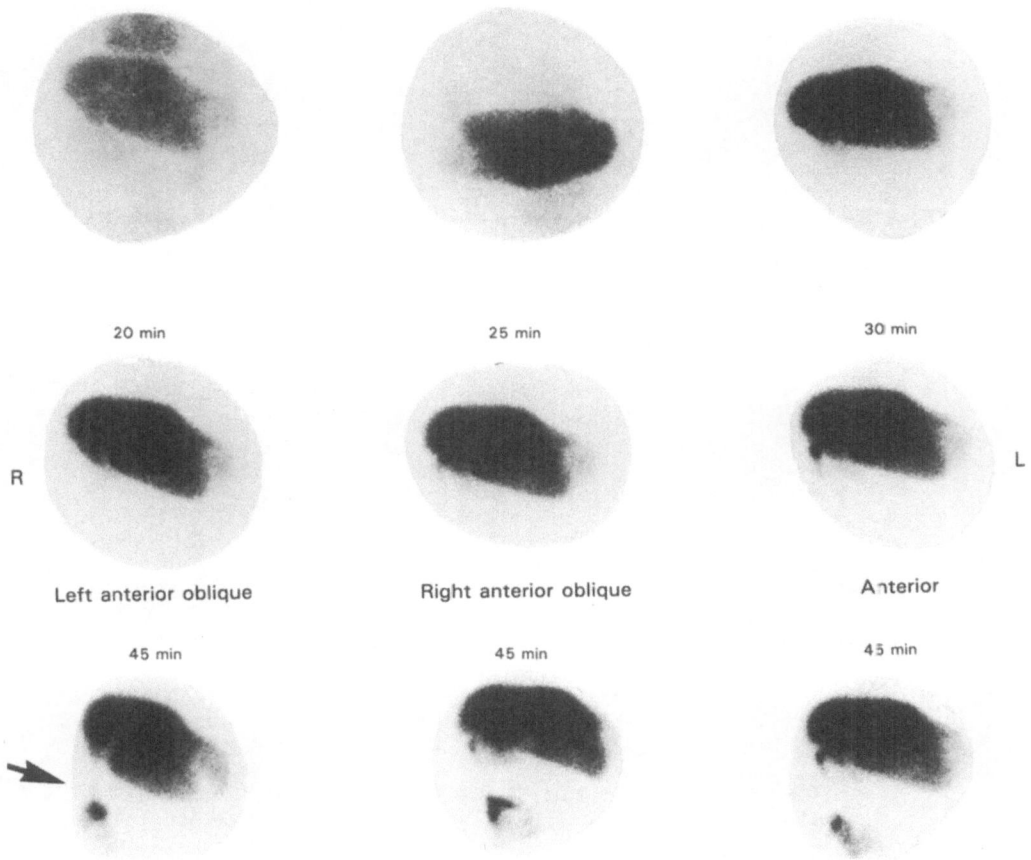

20 min	25 min	30 min
Left anterior oblique	Right anterior oblique	Anterior
45 min	45 min	45 min

R

L

Figure 2-11. Demonstration of patent biliary ductal anastomosis to small bowel (arrow) in patient with right hepatic lobectomy and cholecystectomy.

The physiologic basis of the radionuclide scan with high-contrast and spatial resolution makes this study ideal for bile leak detection and evaluation of patients with surgically altered biliary systems (Fig. 2-11) such as intestinal biliary tract anastomosis and T-tube diversions.[5] Post-traumatic bilomas or biliary fistulae (Fig. 2-12) can also be easily demonstrated as a site of extravasation of tracer activity from either the bile ducts or the gall bladder.

Trauma and Postoperative Complications

Nuclear Medicine

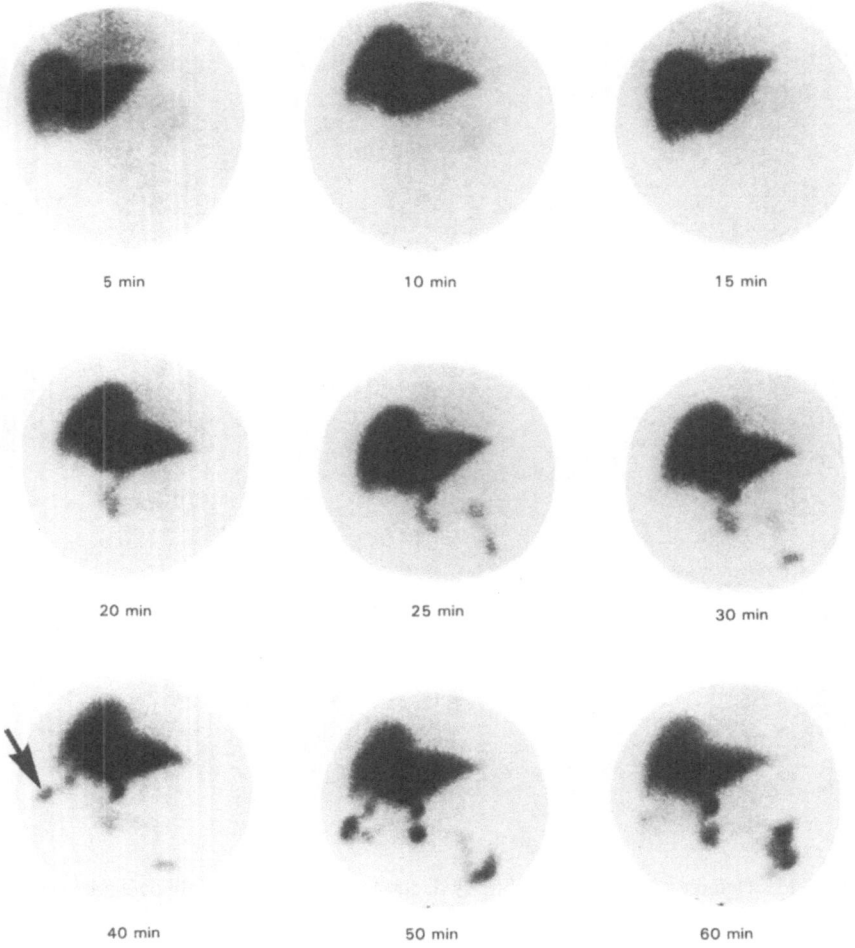

5 min   10 min   15 min

20 min   25 min   30 min

40 min   50 min   60 min

Figure 2-12. Pipida scan demonstrates cholecystocolonic fistula (arrow) as demonstrated by activity leaking from gall bladder into colon.

Ultrasound

Ultrasound may be useful in patients who have had cholecystectomy to rule out the possibility of postoperative complications such as hematoma, abscess, retained stones in the biliary system, or postoperative biloma.[3] However, this study is somewhat limited owing to the presence of artifact created by postoperative scars and surgical clips. Posttraumatic complications involving the gall bladder and

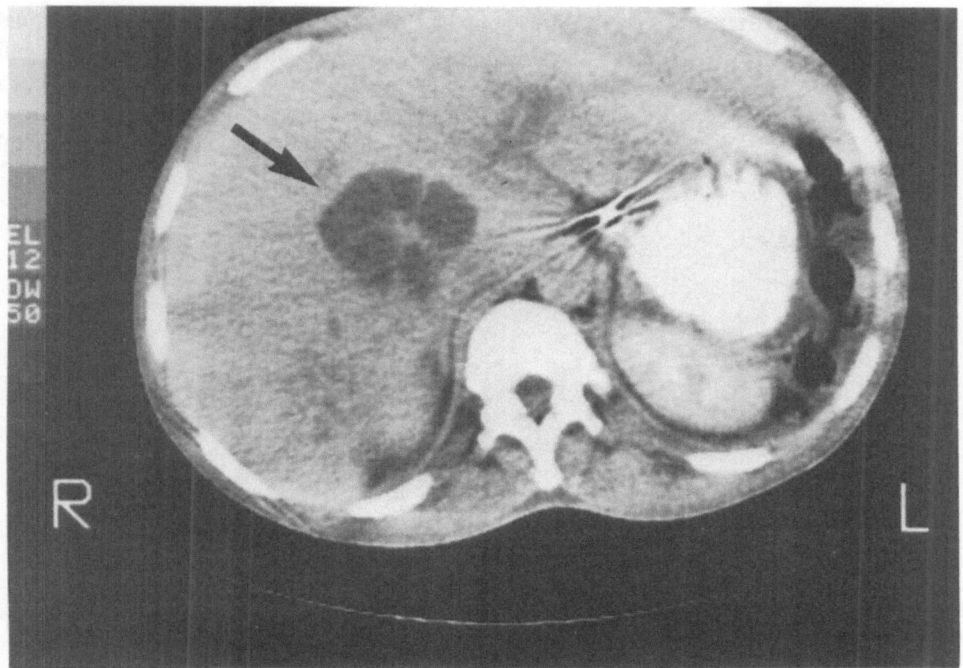

Figure 2-13. Intrahepatic abscess (arrow) following cholecystectomy.

bile ducts may also be visualized as pericholecystic or subhepatic fluid collections, which may represent either bile or blood.

Computerized Tomography

CT is a very useful procedure in the detection of possible postoperative complications in patients with previous surgery involving the biliary system (Fig. 2-13) and is useful in patients with suspected trauma to the biliary system. The advantages of CT over ultrasound are mainly related to the excellent cross-sectional anatomic display of the normal and abnormal structures as well as lack of interference from overlying bowel gas, surgical clips, or subcutaneous bandages.

Malignancy of the Biliary Tract

Nuclear Medicine

Malignancy of the biliary tract involving either the gall bladder or bile ducts is virtually undiagnosable utilizing the radionuclide scan although the presence of intrahepatic biliary ductal dilatation may be the first indication of a cholangiocarcinoma involving the bile ducts.

Ultrasound   Ultrasound has been useful in detecting intraluminal gall bladder polyps (Fig. 2-14) and carcinomas of the gall bladder. Metastatic disease to the gall bladder has been detected although the appearance is indistinguishable from that of other intraluminal lesions. Resultant biliary ductal

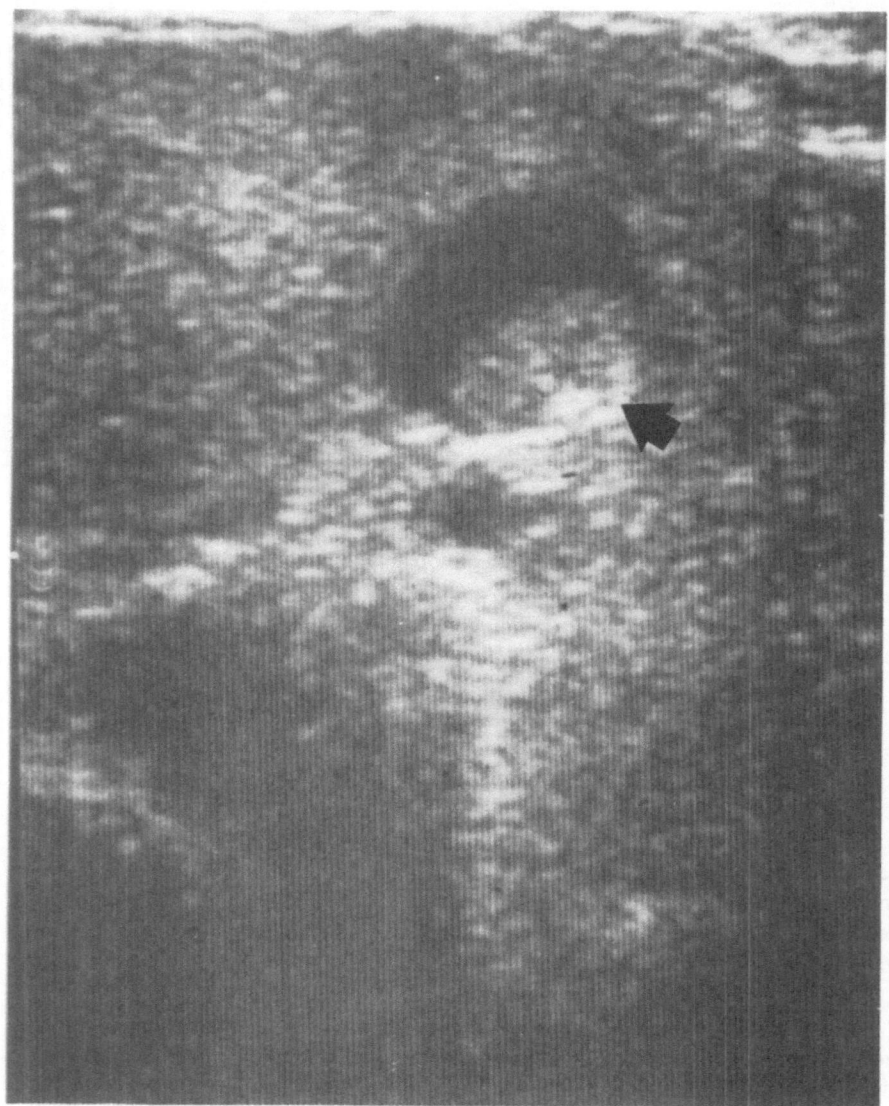

Figure 2-14. Single gall bladder polyp (arrow) without shadowing expected from stone.

dilatation is readily detected, as is metastatic disease to the surrounding liver parenchyma or porta hepatis. Preliminary staging of tumor and serial scans following therapy can be obtained. An occasional case report of biliary ductal polyp or malignancy detected on ultrasound has been reported in the literature; however, the usual manifestation of such disease may merely be dilatation of the intrahepatic ducts proximal to the lesion, and the actual offending lesion is usually not seen until either a percutaneous cholangiogram or ERCP has been performed.

CT of biliary malignancy is helpful in the detection of the level of obstruction in the biliary ducts but, in many instances, will not demonstrate the ductal lesion. Gall bladder tumors can be visualized, and the local extent and intrahepatic metastatic spread can be evaluated both prior to and following therapy.[2]

Computerized Tomography

Owing to the low radiation dose received from the physiologic agent utilized in the biliary scan, this study has been very useful in neonates to exclude the presence of congenital malformations such as choledochal cysts and help distinguish between biliary atresia and neonatal hepatitis. In the past, this procedure involved the use of radioiodinated rose bengal; however, this compound has recently been replaced by the technetium-labeled compound, which produces a much lower radiation dose to the patient.[4,5]

Jaundice in the Newborn
Nuclear Medicine

REFERENCES

1. Kazam E, Schneider M, Rubenstein WA: (1980). The role of ultrasound and CT in imaging the gall bladder and biliary tract, in Alavi A, Arger P (eds): *Multiple Imaging Procedures: Abdomen.* New York, Grune & Stratton Inc, 1980, pp 233–310.
2. Koehler RE, Stanley RJ: Computed tomography of the gall bladder and bile ducts, in Berk RN, Ferruci JT, Leopold GR (eds): *Radiology of the Gall Bladder and Bile Ducts,* Philadelphia, WB Saunders Co, 1983, pp 239–259.
3. Leopold GR: Biliary ultrasonography, in Berk RN, Ferruci JT, Leopold GR (eds): Philadelphia, WB Saunders Co, 1983, pp 201–238.
4. Thaler MM, Gellis SS: Studies in neonatal hepatitis and biliary atresia. Diagnosis. *Am J Dis Child* 1965;116:280.
5. Weissman HS, Sugarman LA, Freeman LM: The clinical role of technetium 99m iminodiacetic acid in cholescintigraphy, in Freeman LM, Weissman HS (eds): *Nuclear Medicine Annual,* New York, Raven Press, 1981, pp 35–89.

3   Pancreas, Spleen, and Reticuloendothelial System

The pancreas is a mixed exocrine–endocrine organ that is almost impossible to evaluate during a physical examination owing to its retroperitoneal location. Previous evaluation of the pancreas had relied on the availability of laboratory screening tests such as amylase and lipase levels, which when abnormal are relatively nonspecific. Until approximately 10 years ago, the pancreas had been difficult to evaluate radiographically as well, with the diagnosis relying on direct pressure effects exerted on adjacent organs such as the stomach and small bowel produced by pancreatic masses. Occasionally, calcifications of chronic pancreatitis were detected on plain films. Unfortunately, malignant disease at the time of detection utilizing these modalities was usually far advanced and most often incurable. The other diagnostic modalities available were angiography and endoscopic retrograde cholangiopancreatography (ERCP), both of which are more invasive and could not be used as screening procedures.

The prototype noninvasing imaging procedure for the pancreas consisted of nuclear studies based on pancreatic function. Radioactive selenium tagged to methionine was discovered to be utilized by the pancreas to form enzymes in a manner similar to normal proteins. Scintigraphic images

PANCREAS

Inflammatory Disease of the Pancreas

Nuclear Medicine

of the pancreas could be obtained following intravenous injection of the radioactively tagged methionine.[1] The test was useful in detecting focal pancreatic masses as well as diagnosing pancreatitis by nonvisualization of the entire pancreas, which was due to the decreased function and hence diminished enzyme production. However, unfortunately, the findings were nonspecific because of the similar appearance of both malignant and benign disease. There were also many false-positive studies due to the study requiring that the patient have normal secretion of hydrochloric acid and other gastric enzymes as well as pancreozymin from the duodenum.

Ultrasound

Ultrasound is an accurate and sensitive technique in detecting pancreatic disease. Acute pancreatitis and complications resulting from the disease such as pseudocyst (Fig. 3-1), abscess, or phlegmon can be detected and followed on serial examinations both pre- and posttherapy.[3]

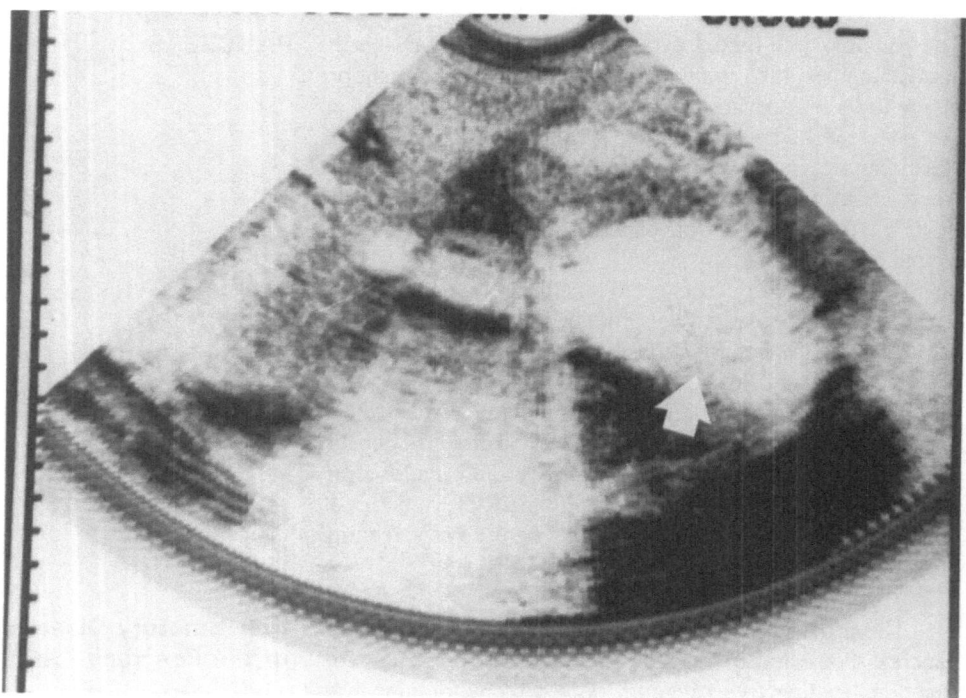

Figure 3-1. Large pseudocyst (arrow) in tail of pancreas in 42-year-old male with left-upper-quadrant pain.

The major advantages of this examination are the low cost and the lack of ionizing radiation, which makes this the screening procedure of choice in children and pregnant women. Unfortunately, imaging of the pancreas is limited in patients who have had previous surgery with resultant scars and overlying bandages. In addition, many patients acutely ill with pancreatitis will have an ileus and poor visualization of the pancreas due to bowel gas artifact production. The examination is also dependent on the expertise of the technologist in delineating the anatomy, although with real-time ultrasound, the sensitivity of the examination has been markedly improved.

Computerized Tomography

Computerized tomography (CT) of the pancreas is most useful in patients with pancreatitis because of the lack of degradation of the image by bowel gas. Pancreatic masses can be readily identified by differences in parenchymal texture.[4] Occasionally, peripancreatic fluid collections prior to the actual pseudocyst formation can be detected (Fig. 3-2). In addition, areas of increased attenuation within the fluid may represent acute hemorrhagic pancreatitis. Gas bubbles within the peripancreatic fluid collections can represent abscess formation although occasional spontaneous drainage into the bowel may also result in gas bubbles within the fluid.[5] Many institutions now use CT as the primary procedure in the initial evaluation of acute pancreatitis; however, ultrasound may be utilized for follow-up serial examinations because of the lack of radiation and the lesser cost of the study.

Pancreatic Neoplasm

Nuclear Medicine

In the past, utilizing selenium-tagged methionine, focal cold lesions within the pancreas resulted in the localization of pancreatic tumors. However, owing to the limited sensitivity and specificity of the examination, the study is no longer utilized.

Ultrasound

Ultrasound is a very accurate and sensitive means of detecting pancreatic masses. The typical pancreatic tumor will present either as an area of focal enlargement of the pancreatic gland or perhaps as a focal area of decreased echogenicity within the substance of the pancreatic tissue[2] (Fig. 3-3). However, in addition to actual detection of tumors, ancillary findings such as dilated bile ducts (Fig. 3-3), vessel encasement, liver metastases, and portal or

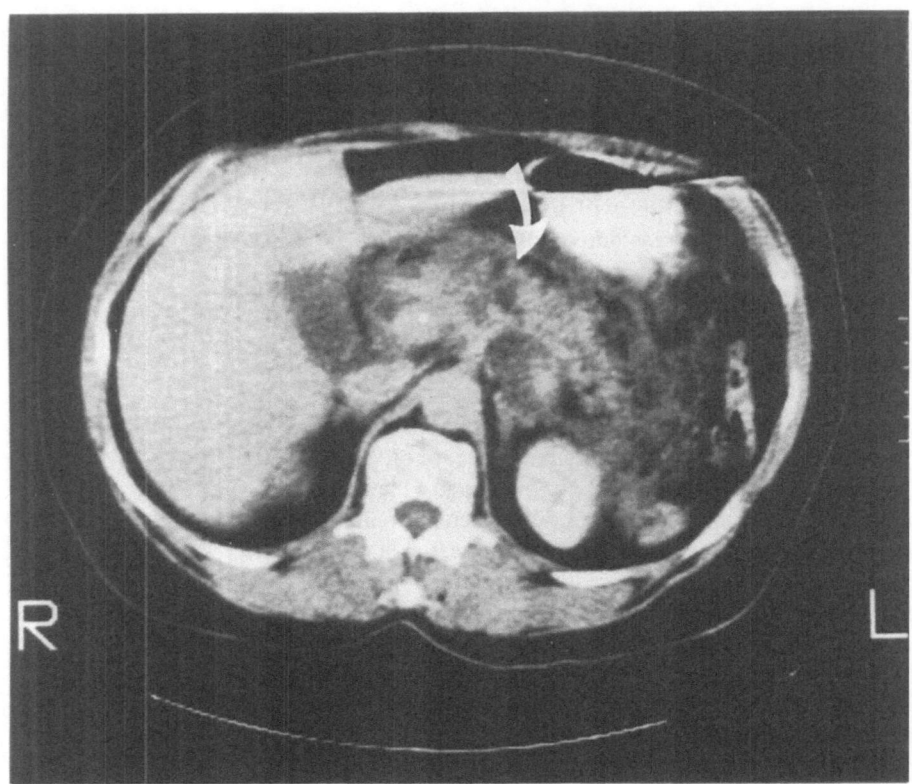

Figure 3-2. Diffusely enlarged edematous pancreas (arrow) with small collections of fluid representing early pseudocyst formation.

retroperitoneal lymphadenopathy are in many instances demonstrated. Unfortunately, occasionally focal areas of chronic pancreatitis can simulate a neoplastic mass on the ultrasound examination, but with sonographic guidance, percutaneous biopsy of the mass can be performed enabling pathologic diagnosis to be made and thus eliminating the need for surgery of unresectable lesions. Ultrasound is also useful in evaluating the progress of pancreatic lesions or metastases following a regimen of therapy.

Computerized Tomography

High-resolution, contrast-enhanced CT of the pancreas is probably the most sensitive means of diagnosis of pancreatic neoplasm at its earliest stage. Unfortunately, in most

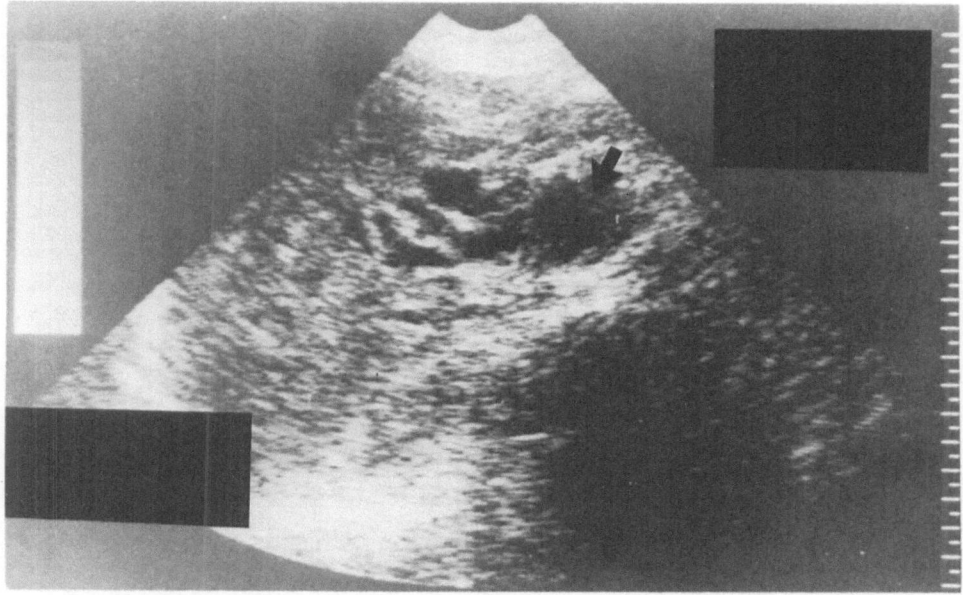

Figure 3-3. Solid mass in head of pancreas (arrow) with dilatation of common bile duct (arrow).

instances the patients will present when clinical symptoms manifest themselves at which time the tumor is usually beyond resection or cure. Initial staging and evaluation of neoplasm is easily performed with CT owing to the excellent cross-sectional anatomy resulting in accurate visualization of tumor, neighboring bowel, liver metastasis, dilated ducts (Figs. 3-4 and 3-5), or nodes in the porta hepatis and retroperitoneum. Indeterminate masses involving the pancreas may be biopsied percutaneously utilizing CT guidance.[7] In addition, CT will make it possible to detect focal invasion of the lesion into adjacent bowel, which cannot be determined utilizing ultrasound. Patients can be followed with serial studies postoperatively. Perhaps the most single important advantage of CT when compared to ultrasound is the detection of lesions at a smaller stage as well as the ability to be able to differentiate between tumors of different cell types utilizing the enhanced CT characteristics of different lesions. Adenocarcinoma will typically show little enhancement, whereas the opposite is true of islet cell tumors.

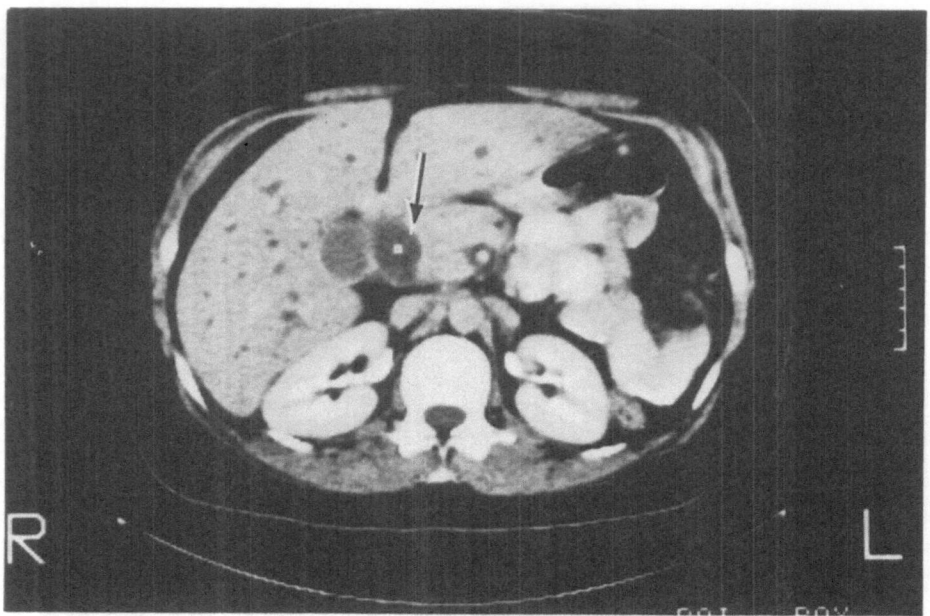

Figure 3-4. Computerized tomography demonstrating common bile duct dilatation (arrow) within pancreatic head due to neoplasm.

Trauma

Ultrasound

There is little use for ultrasound in the evaluation of pancreatic trauma owing to the almost certain presence of gastric distention or small bowel ileus, which obscures visualization of the pancreas during the study. If the pancreatic duct has been severed, however, ultrasound may be able to detect a collection of fluid in the region of the pancreas.

Computerized Tomography

CT of the upper abdomen is the procedure of choice in suspected injury to the pancreas. The pancreas is usually well delineated, as is the pancreatic duct, and a number of cases have been reported in which a severed pancreatic duct has been seen utilizing CT.[6] In addition, adjacent hematoma in the retroperitoneum or intramural duodenal hematoma can be detected simultaneously. Peripancreatic fluid collections will also be readily seen and anatomically localized utilizing CT following pancreatic injury.

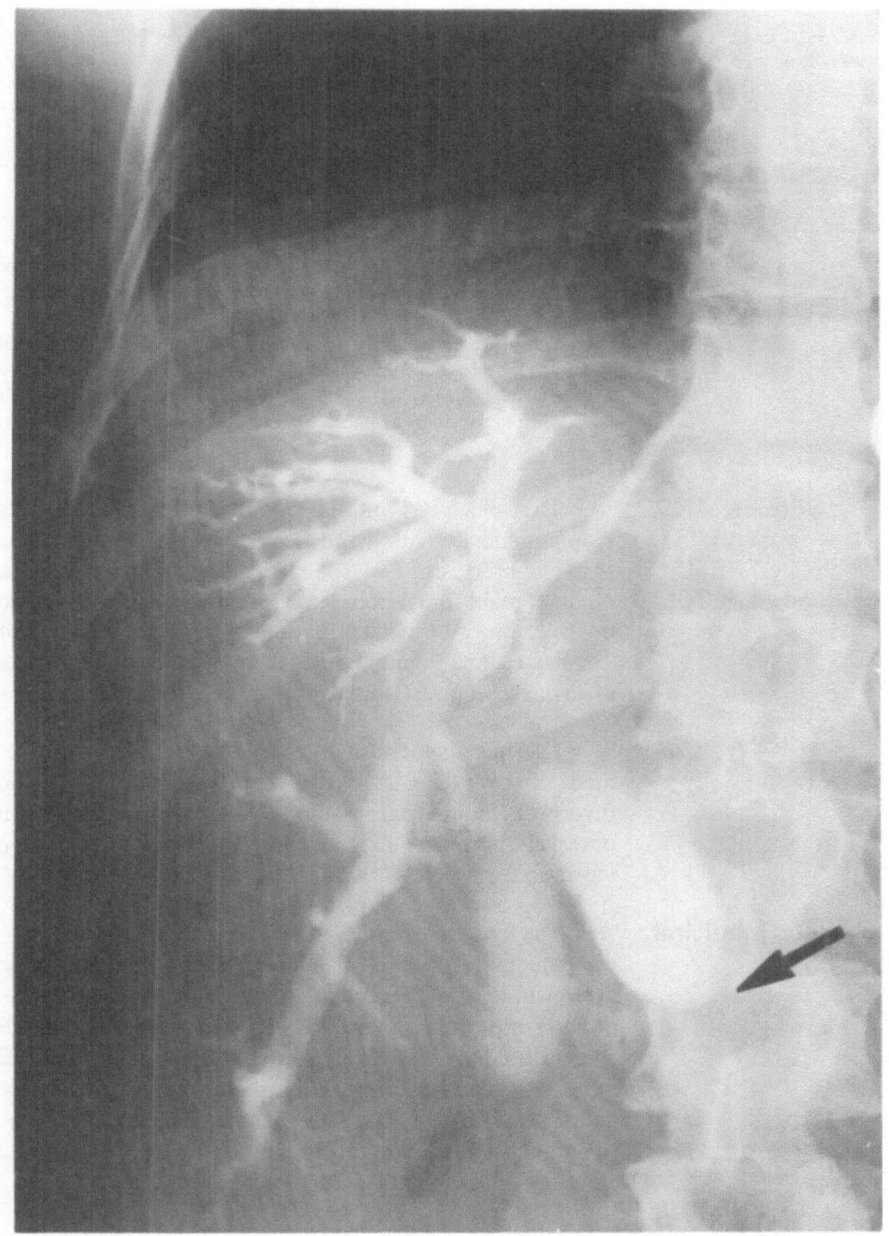

Figure 3-5. Endoscopic retrograde cholangiopancreatography confirms dilatation of intrahepatic bile ducts with abrupt termination of common bile duct secondary to pancreatic tumor (arrow).

REFERENCES

1. Agnew JE, Maze M, Mitchell CJ: Pancreatic scanning. *Br J Radiol* 1976;49:979.
2. Carroll BA, Sample WF: Pancreatic cystadenocarcinoma: CT body scan and grey scale ultrasound appearance. *Am J Roentgenol* 1978;131:339–341.
3. Doust BD, Pearce JD. Grey scale ultrasonic properties of the normal and inflamed pancreas. *Radiology* 1976;120:653–657.
4. Kreel L: Computerized tomography of the pancreas. *Computed Axial Tomögr* 1977;1:287–297.
5. Mendez G, Isikoff MB: Significance of intrapancreatic gas demonstrated by CT: A review of nine cases. *Am J Roentgenol* 1979;132:59–62.
6. Toombs BD, Lester RG, Ben Manchem Y, Sandler CM: Computed tomography in blunt trauma. *Radiol Clin North Am* 1981;19:17–35.
7. Weyman PJ, Stanley RJ, Levitt RG: Computed tomography in evaluation of the pancreas. *Semin Roentgenol* 1981;16:301–311.

SPLEEN AND RETICULO-ENDOTHELIAL SYSTEM

The spleen has long been a difficult organ to evaluate radiographically with diagnoses previously being made utilizing indirect signs of splenic enlargement noted on abdominal plain films, upper-gastrointestinal series, and more invasive procedures such as angiography or venography. The newer imaging modalities have decreased the necessity of invasive contrast studies to evaluate the spleen.

Trauma

The management of splenic injuries has changed dramatically over the past several years with many centers now favoring a more conservative course of management and observation rather than routine splenectomy for splenic laceration.

Nuclear Medicine

The liver/spleen scan is the cheapest and fastest way to evaluate the presence of splenic trauma. The study will demonstrate a cold defect either within the spleen (Fig. 3-6) or as a crescentic area of decreased activity around the splenic border.[5] However, the study is limited in spatial resolution and restricted to abnormalities involving the liver and spleen. In the massively traumatized patient, there is often multiorgan involvement, and ultrasound or CT will be able to evaluate the other organs as well.

Ultrasound

Ultrasound is a relatively inexpensive means of visualizing splenic and perisplenic hemorrhage in either the acute of subacute stage. The advantage of sonography is the lack of ionizing radiation and the detection of other associated traumatic injuries to the left upper quadrant such as

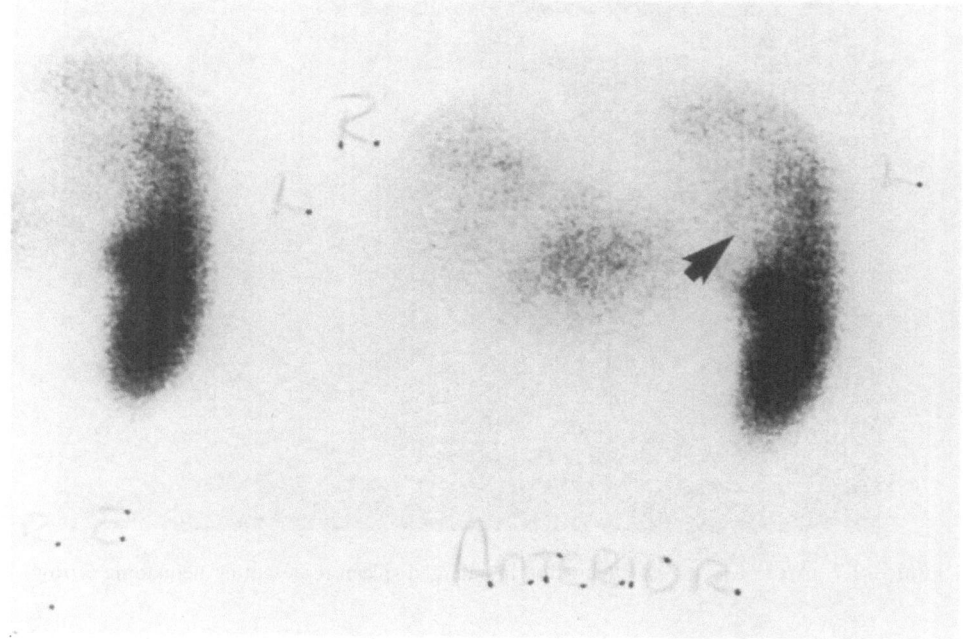

Figure 3-6. Focal area of decreased activity (arrow) in spleen representing hematoma following trauma.

unsuspected renal injury, pancreatic injury, or blood within the subphrenic space.[2] If a laceration or hemorrhage has been detected, the progress of the lesion can be followed on serial studies. The major disadvantage of the study is limited visualization of the organ because of its location in the left upper quadrant beneath the ribs and the frequent presence of ileus or gastric distention with resultant production of artifact.

Computerized Tomography

Splenic and perisplenic injury can be easily detected utilizing CT in either the acute, subacute, or chronic stage (Fig. 3-7). The resolution of the hemorrhage can be evaluated utilizing serial scans although this is more expensive than utilizing sonography. A complicating splenic abscess will be easily visualized (Fig. 3-8). Patients who have had splenectomy or splenorrhaphy can be evaluated for possible postoperative complications, such as subphrenic abscess, utilizing CT.[3] The evaluation of postoperative complica-

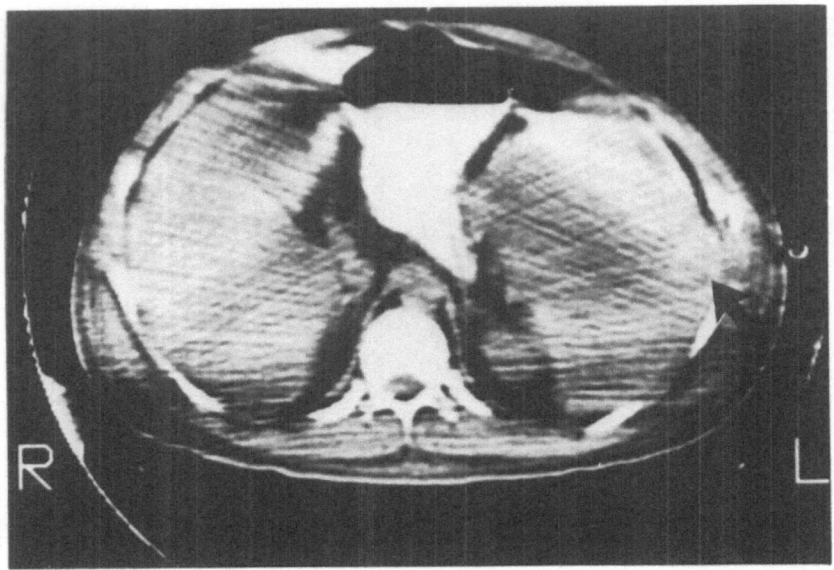

Figure 3-7. Area of increased attenuation in enlarged spleen representing hematoma (arrow).

tions would be more difficult with ultrasound because of the presence of overlying bandages and surgical clips at the surgical site.

Splenic Enlargement

Splenic enlargement can be evaluated clinically although this is somewhat difficult because of the overlying rib cage. In the past, a flat plate of the abdomen was the most readily available means of evaluation of splenic enlargement noted by displacement of the gastric air bubble toward the midline or splenic flexure of the colon toward the pelvis. The value of the newer imaging modalities is the increased ability now to diagnose diffuse splenic disease as opposed to focal enlargement.

Nuclear Medicine

Splenomegaly with increased tracer activity may be representative of any of a number of liver diseases with resultant portal hypertension. This may be seen in patients with cirrhosis, diffuse metastatic disease, or metabolic disorders involving the liver. Splenic enlargement may also result from hematologic disorders such as leukemia, lymphoma, or hemolytic disorders such as idiopathic thrombocytopenic purpura (ITP). A similar appearance can also be created by certain infectious diseases such as mono-

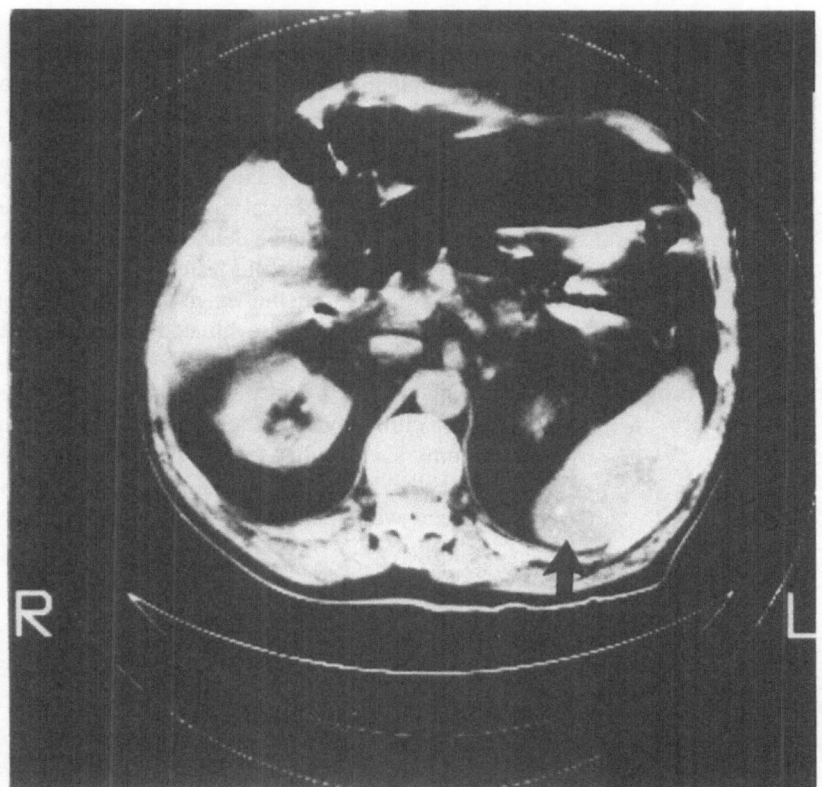

Figure 3-8. Low attenuation mass (arrow) in splenic tip seen on computerized tomography representing abscess.

nucleosis and Weil's disease. Focal cold lesions in the enlarged spleen may be seen in patients with metastasis from certain primary tumors such as breast, lung, and melanoma. Splenic abscesses and other benign lesions such as congenital cysts can also have a similar appearance, which necessitates correlation with either ultrasound or CT examination. Cold lesions in a normal-sized spleen may also be secondary to splenic infarcts or hemorrhage in the recently traumatized patient.

Ultrasound

With the use of sonographic criteria, splenomegaly can be detected and the presence or absence of focal lesions can be determined. In many instances, splenic ultrasound is the study performed following the liver/spleen scan to evaluate the cystic or solid nature of lesions detected on the radionuclide exam (Figs. 3-9 and 3-10). Ultrasound is a very sensitive examination in determining the presence of focal lesions although it does lack somewhat in specificity.

Computerized Tomography

CT has been determined to be a very sensitive indicator of splenic enlargement. Focal involvement by leukemia or lymphoma (Fig. 3-11) can be determined in a large percentage of cases.[1] Cystic and solid lesions can be easily differentiated. Posttraumatic hemorrhage and inflammatory processes can be localized and evaluated on serial studies.

Functional Asplenia

The radionuclide liver/spleen scan has proven useful in patients with clinically suspected splenic dysfunction or autosplenectomy such as that seen in patients with sickle cell disease or celiac disease.[6] Occasionally, patients with infarcted spleen will demonstrate bone tracer activity (Fig. 3-12).

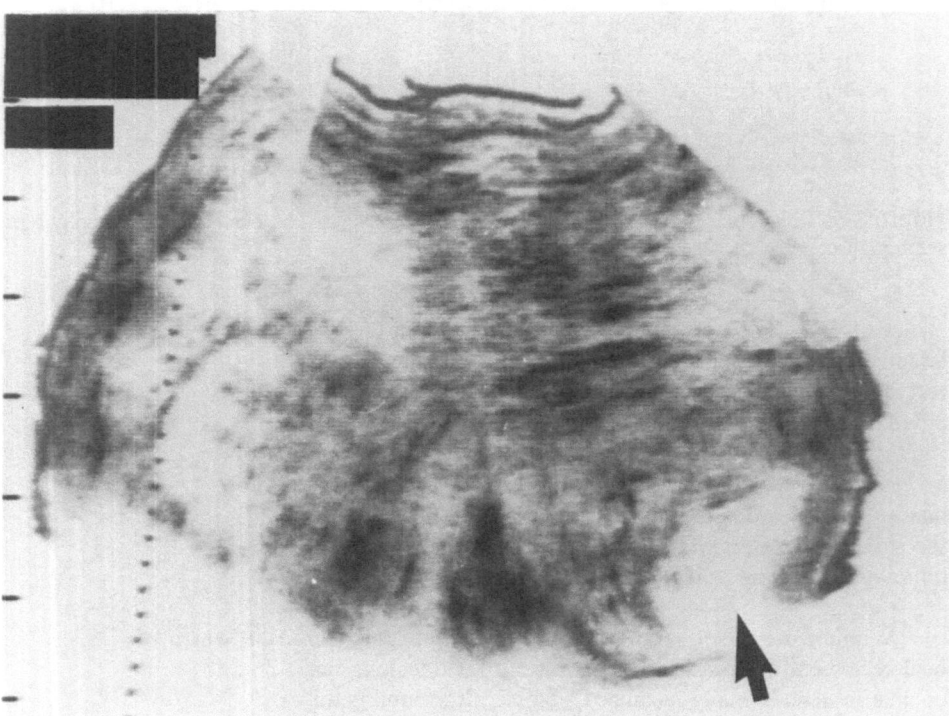

Figure 3-9. Sonolucent mass (arrow) in left upper quadrant representing splenic abscess.

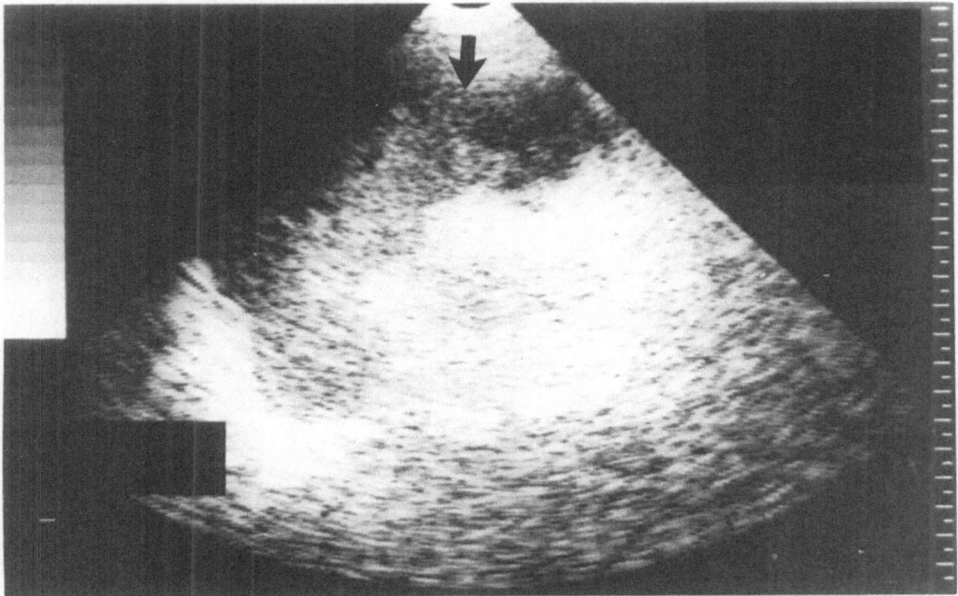

Figure 3-10. Area of diminished echoes (arrow) in spleen representing infarct in patient with sickle cell anemia.

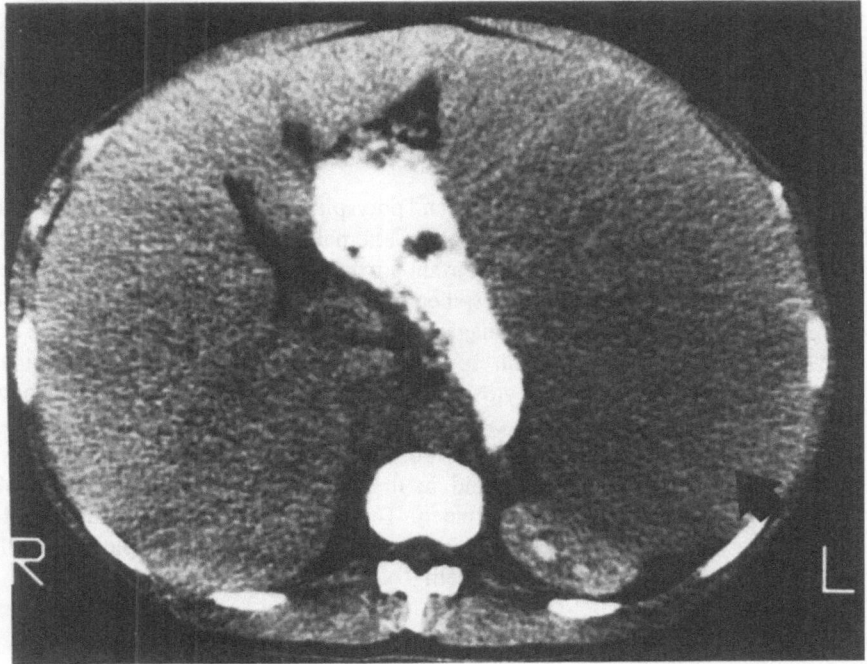

Figure 3-11. Massive splenic (arrow) and hepatic enlargement in patient with lymphoma.

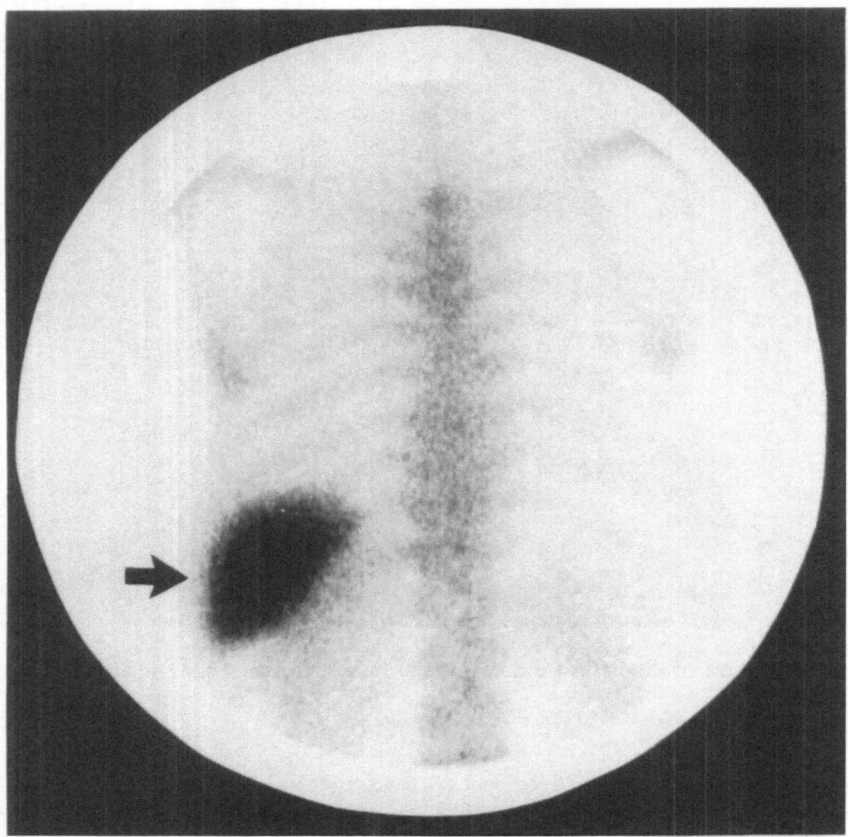

Figure 3-12. Increased activity of bone tracer in spleen (arrow) due to autosplenectomy resulting from sickle cell disease.

Asplenia, Polysplenia, and Accessory Spleen

Asplenia and polysplenia are associated with significant cardiac and other anomalies making recognition of these entities important in the clinical management of patients. Accessory spleen or splenosis following splenectomy is crucial to management of patients with certain hemolytic disorders such as ITP or other hematologic disorders such as spherocytosis[4] that result in the destruction of erythrocytes. In these cases spleen scans are usually performed with tagged red blood cells rather than sulfur colloid since uptake of sulfur colloid in the liver may mask the presence of an accessory spleen. Technetium bound to heat-damaged red blood cells will localize specifically in the spleen and alleviate this problem.

REFERENCES

1. Alcorn FS, Mategrano VC, Petasnick JP, et al: Contributions of computed tomography in the staging and management of malignant lymphoma. *Radiology* 1977;125:717–723.
2. Asher WM, Parvin S, Virgilio B, et al: Echographic evaluation of splenic injury after blunt trauma. *Radiology* 1976;118:411–415.
3. Giuliano AE, Lim RC: Is splenic salvage safe in the traumatized patient? *Arch Surg* 1981;116:651–656.
4. Hamilton RG, et al: Splenic imaging with 99m Tc labelled erythrocytes: A comparative study of cell damaging methods. *J Nucl Med* 1976;17:1038.
5. Nebesar RA, Rabinov KR, Potsaud MA: Radionuclide imaging of the spleen in suspected splenic injury. *Radiology* 1974;110:609–614.
6. Pearson, HA, Spencer RP, Cornelius EA: Functional asplenia in sickle cell anemia. *N Engl J Med* 1969;281:923.

4   Genitourinary Tract

The "bread-and-butter" radiographic procedure for visualizing urinary tract pathology has been the abdominal film and intravenous urogram. These studies have been supplemented by the cystogram, retrograde pyelogram, and urethrogram performed in either a retrograde or antegrade fashion. More invasive procedures such as angiography, venography, and retroperitoneal pneumography have also been involved in the radiologic workup of urinary tract pathology. The first nonradiographic procedures utilized in genitourinary tract imaging were the radionuclide renal scans. Within the past 10 years, ultrasound and computerized tomography (CT) have also complemented, and in some circumstances replaced, the aforementioned contrast radiographic studies.

The radionuclide renal scan is a very valuable procedure in the detection of renal vascular hypertension and can be used in several different ways depending on the isotopes utilized. The radionuclide flow study has been found to be more sensitive than the intravenous urogram in detecting renal vascular disease (Figs. 4-1 and 4-2). In addition, the function of both kidneys can be compared utilizing the radioiodide Hippuran renogram to aid in the determina-

RENAL VASCULAR HYPERTENSION

Radionuclide Studies

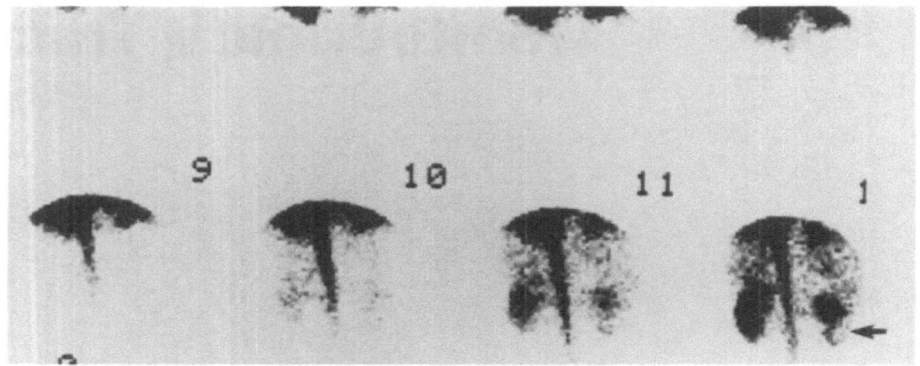

Figure 4-1. Dynamic renal flow study reveals decreased and delayed perfusion to lower pole of right kidney (arrow) secondary to localized infarct.

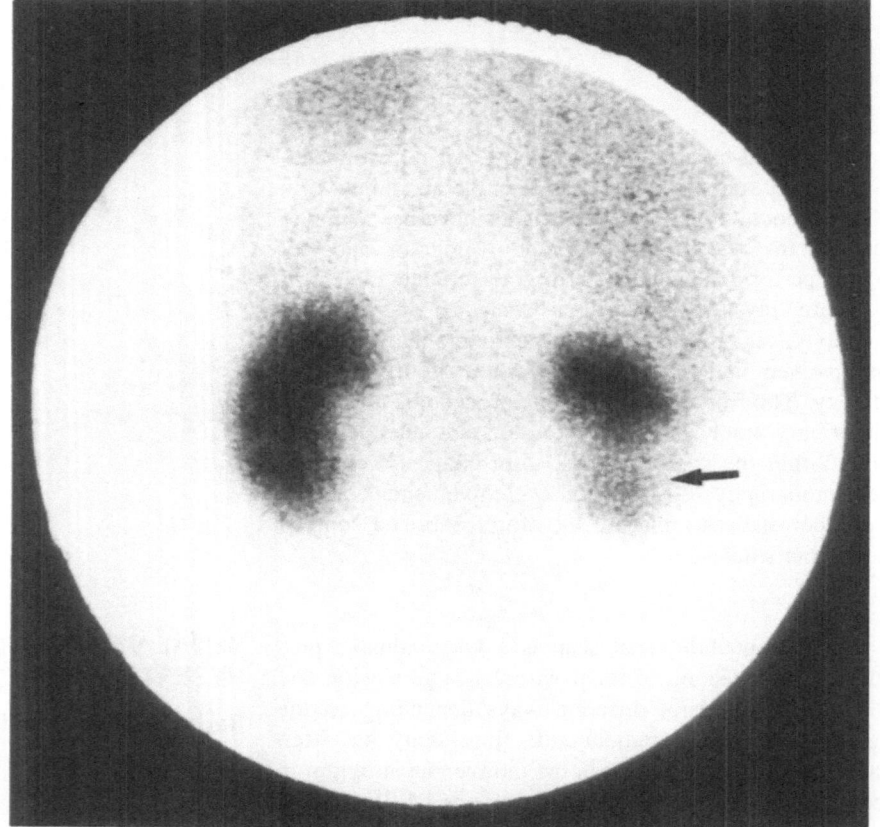

Figure 4-2. Static renal scan reveals localized infarct (arrow) in lower pole of right kidney.

tion of both effective renal plasma flow (ERPF) and glomerular filtration rate (GFR). Control of hypertension without antirenin therapy and a normal flow study in most instances will effectively exclude renal vascular disease as the etiology of hypertension. If the perfusion study is suggestive of renal vascular disease, i.e., decreased perfusion of one kidney relative to the other, the next step is renal vein renins and renal angiography or digital subtraction angiography utilizing intravenous contrast. This procedure will better define the offending vascular lesion, which can then be dilated utilizing a balloon catheter following routine angiography.

Ultrasound

Sonography of the kidneys may be useful in the evaluation of patients with renal vascular hypertension by demonstrating a discrepancy in the relative size of both kidneys and by detecting the presence or absence of chronic renal parenchymal disease (Fig. 4-3) in patients who have had chronic renal insufficiency secondary to renal vascular disease. The study is somewhat limited, however, in that the findings are nonspecific in many instances. Occasionally, an unsuspected renal or adrenal neoplasm may be found. The chief advantage of utilizing ultrasound as a primary study is the ability to visualize the kidneys without having to resort to intravenous contrast administration in patients whose renal function is already impaired. Unsuspected hydronephrosis may also be detected.

Computerized Tomography

Although CT can detect the presence of small kidneys or localize renal infarcts,[9] the fact that contrast administration is necessary limits the utility of this examination as a screening procedure in patients with compromised renal function. Extensive renal arterial calcification may be seen although the spatial resolution of the images is not optimal for actual visualization of renal artery stenosis.

TRAUMA

Radionuclide Scan

In patients with suspected trauma, the renal scan can be a very useful procedure. The study can be utilized to evaluate the relative perfusion of each kidney and relative function especially in patients allergic to iodinated contrast medium. The possibility of obstruction can be excluded as well as extravasation of radionuclide from either the kidney or the ureters. Parenchymal hematoma or laceration can be

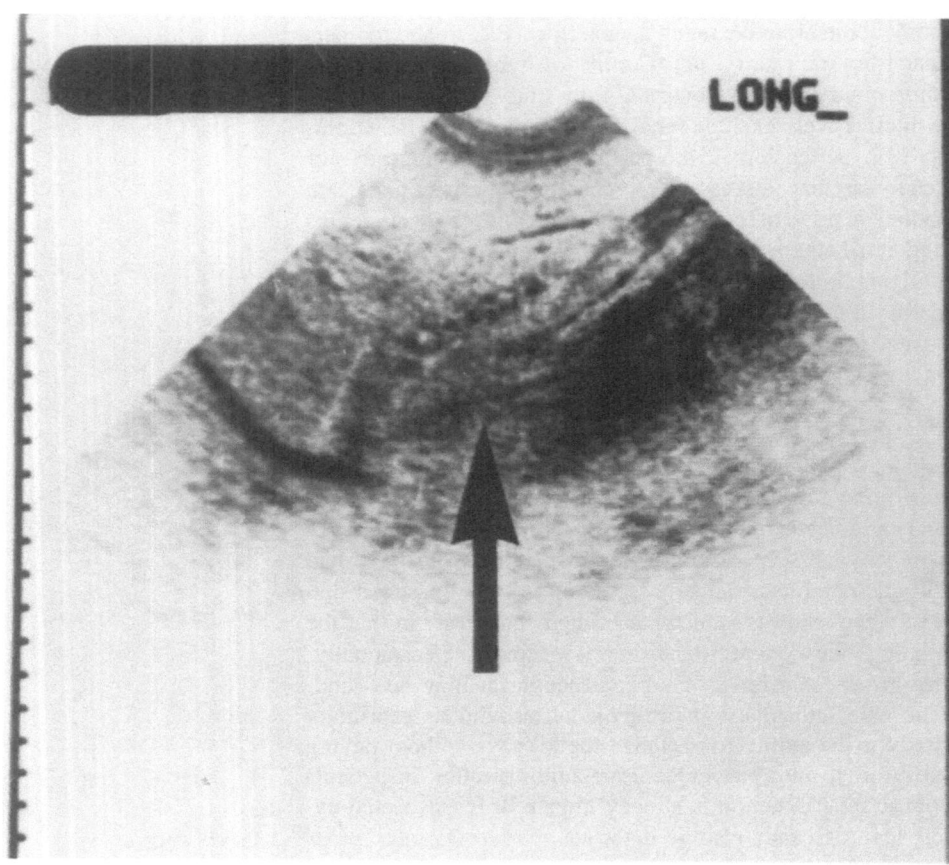

Figure 4-3. Sonography reveals echogenic kidney (arrow) due to chronic diabetic nephropathy.

detected in addition to the possible extravasation of tracer. However, the study is usually limited by the decreased spatial resolution of the camera limited to visualization of lesions no smaller than 1–2 cm. Another disadvantage is that only the kidneys, ureters, and bladder can be evaluated. Trauma to adjacent organs can only be inferred at best.

Ultrasound   Ultrasound has better spatial resolution than the radionuclide study and will detect smaller renal and perirenal hematomas. It may also detect the presence of renal obstruction and in some instances can diagnose renal vein thrombosis in the acute stage.[10] This procedure is especially advantageous in pregnant women or children because of the lack of ionizing radiation. Other retroperitoneal pathology such as psoas hematoma or urinoma may also be detected. One disadvantage of ultrasound is the seemingly omnipresent ileus in most severely traumatized patients. Another disadvantage is its lack of capability to assess renal function. However, in patients with minor renal injuries, ultrasound is a fairly sensitive, inexpensive method for both diagnosis and subsequent observation of patients who are being managed conservatively.

CT has become the procedure of choice to evaluate renal trauma in many institutions. It is more sensitive than ultrasound or the renal scan in detecting renal lacerations and subcapsular and perinephric hematomas (Fig.4-4).[3]

Computerized Tomography

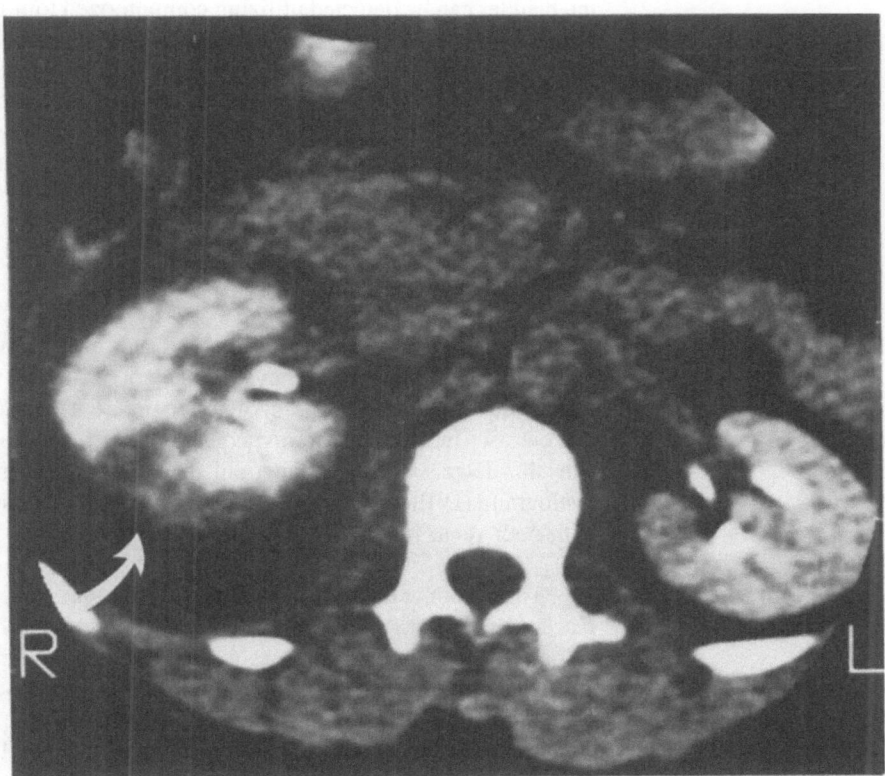

Figure 4-4. Abdominal computerized tomography scan reveals wedge-shaped and crescentic areas (arrows) of decreased attenuation representing renal laceration and subcapsular hematoma.

Owing to the improved three-dimensional display of the anatomy of the abdomen, early detection of posttraumatic lesions involving other neighboring retroperitoneal organs can also be determined, such as posttraumatic pancreatitis or psoas hemorrhage. The major disadvantages of computerized tomography are the increased cost and radiation exposure to the patient.

BLADDER AND URETHRAL TRAUMA

In patients with pelvic fractures and suspected urethral or bladder injuries, the radionuclide examination may demonstrate evidence of extravasation of tracer from either the urethra or bladder although the actual site of leakage may not be evident. Ultrasound can also demonstrate the presence of pelvic urinoma or hematoma, as can CT. Intraperitoneal or extraperitoneal extravasation of contrast from the bladder can be detected utilizing computerized tomography (Figs. 4-5 and 4-6). However, again, the exact site of injury may not be adequately demonstrated. The presence of clot within the bladder can also be determined utilizing cross-sectional imaging techniques. In most cases, however, the radiographic cystogram or urethrogram will be necessary to demonstrate posttraumatic rupture of the bladder or urethra to localize the actual site of injury and extravasation.

RENAL FAILURE

Patients in renal failure used to present a dilemma to radiologists, in that the kidneys would not visualize well during the intravenous urogram owing to poor concentration of contrast. In addition, intravenous contrast may exacerbate the decreasing renal function. Thus, the intravenous pyelogram (IVP) is now infrequently utilized in patients with poor renal function.

Nuclear Medicine

The radionuclide flow study and renogram have replaced the IVP in the evaluation of renal function and have helped to determine the cause as well as severity of impairment. The radionuclide Hippuran renogram is a method by which the total ERPF and GFR can be determined and compared for both kidneys.[2] The perfusion study will be useful in determining the presence of renal vascular lesions, while the static images are useful in excluding the presence of hydronephrosis. Unfortunately, in some instances, the

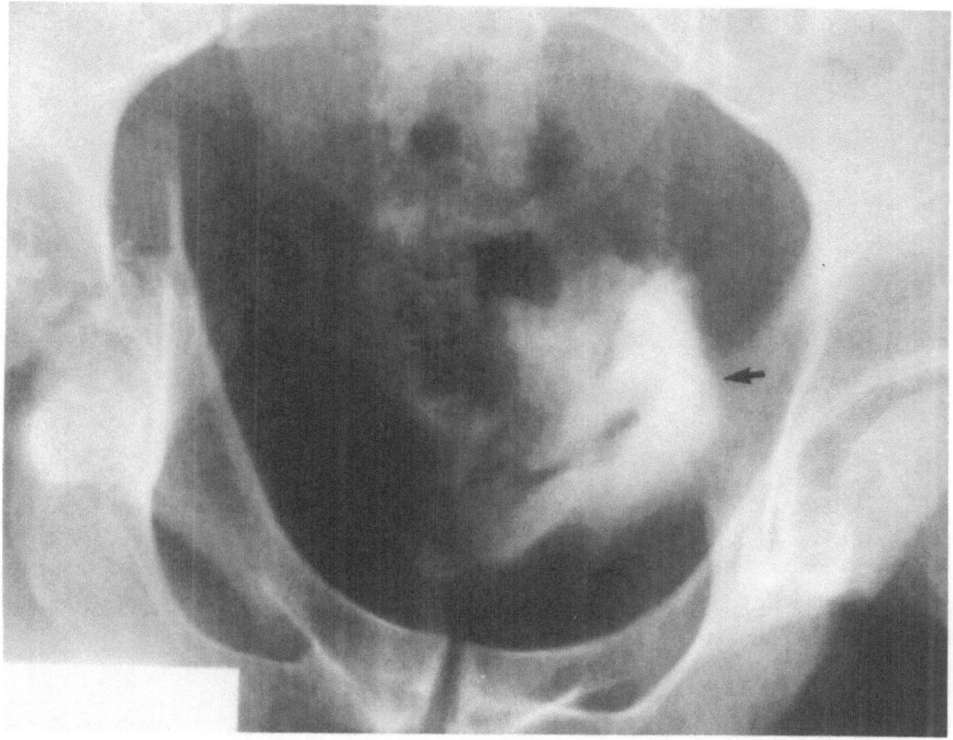

Figure 4-5. Conventional cystogram demonstrates extraperitoneal rupture of bladder with contrast extravasation (arrow).

similar findings make it impossible to separate the poorly functioning kidneys secondary to chronic parenchymal disease from those which are severely obstructed. In equivocal cases of possible renal obstruction, the diuretic renogram is useful to help differentiate between obstruction and urinary stasis such as that which may be caused by an extrarenal pelvis or overhydration.[6]

Ultrasound

In many institutions, the procedure of choice in patients with renal failure is sonography to exclude the presence of hydronephrosis (Fig. 4-7). This is also an accurate means by which to measure renal size, evaluate the parenchyma, and possibly guide percutaneous renal biopsy for more specific tissue diagnosis. This is also the preferred procedure in pregnant women and children because of the

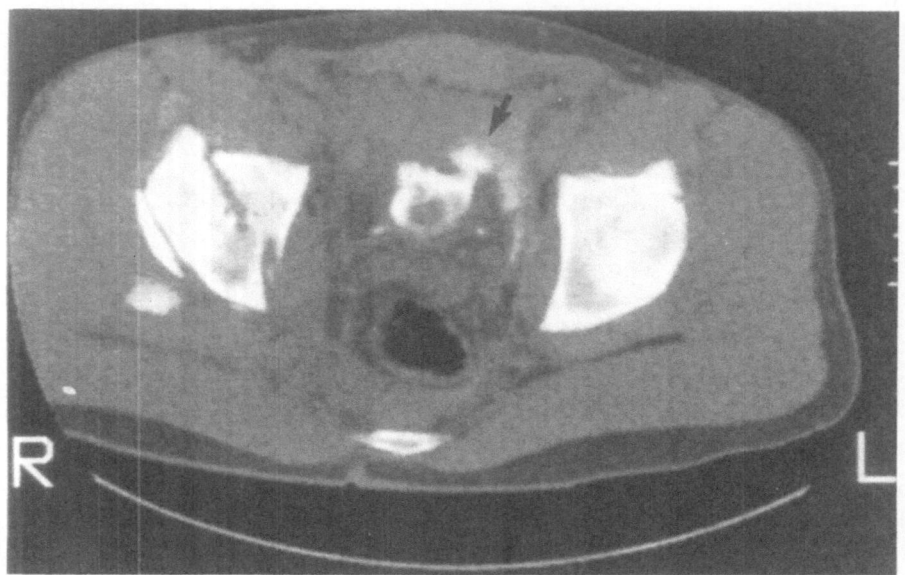

Figure 4-6. Computerized tomography reveals extraperitoneal extravasation of contrast (arrow) due to bladder rupture resulting from multiple pelvic fractures.

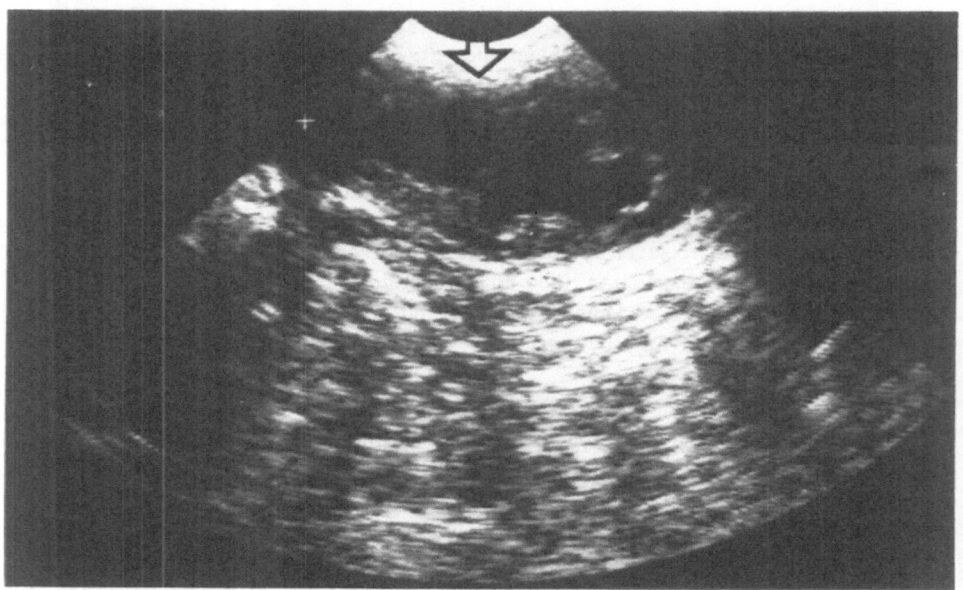

Figure 4-7. Severe hydronephrosis (arrow) secondary to bladder outlet obstruction.

lack of ionizing radiation. Unfortunately, while hydronephrosis may be determined, the source of obstruction in many instances may not be seen. Occasionally a pelvic ultrasound will reveal the cause of bladder outlet obstruction such as an enlarged prostate, pelvic tumor, posterior urethral valves, or ureterocele.[8]

Computerized Tomography

CT is most useful in evaluating the source of an obstruction when it is caused by a lesion extrinsic to the ureter, kidney, or bladder such as that which may be caused by retroperitoneal lymphadenopathy or retroperitoneal fibrosis (Figs. 4-8 and 4-9). Pelvic masses resulting in bladder outlet obstruction or distal ureteral obstruction may be detected, such as prostatic lesions, lymphadenopathy, or even ureteroceles (Fig. 4-10). Intrinsic ureteral lesions, however, may require antegrade or retrograde pyelography for better definition of the lesions. Bladder outlet obstruction, however, will commonly necessitate the use of a voiding cystourethrogram for more definitive evaluation of the urethra.

RENAL MASS OR ENLARGED KIDNEY

Patients presenting with palpable renal masses or masses found incidentally on intravenous urograms previously were evaluated utilizing renal angiography or venography. With the introduction of modern imaging procedures, angiography is no longer a necessity for the diagnostic workup of renal masses, although intraarterial occlusion of renal vessels in vascular tumors or AV malformations may now be performed preoperatively or instead of surgery.

Renal Scan

The nuclear renal scan is nonspecific and cannot determine the cystic or solid nature of a mass lesion. It is insensitive in that lesions under 2 cm may be missed unless they are superficial. However, in patients with a questionable lobular cortical mass detected on IVP or ultrasound, the renal scan can help distinguish between the functioning column of Bertin or a nonfunctioning, space-occupying lesion of other etiology.

Ultrasound

The diagnostic evaluation of renal masses in many instances will begin with the ultrasound examination and terminate at this point. If the mass is determined to be a

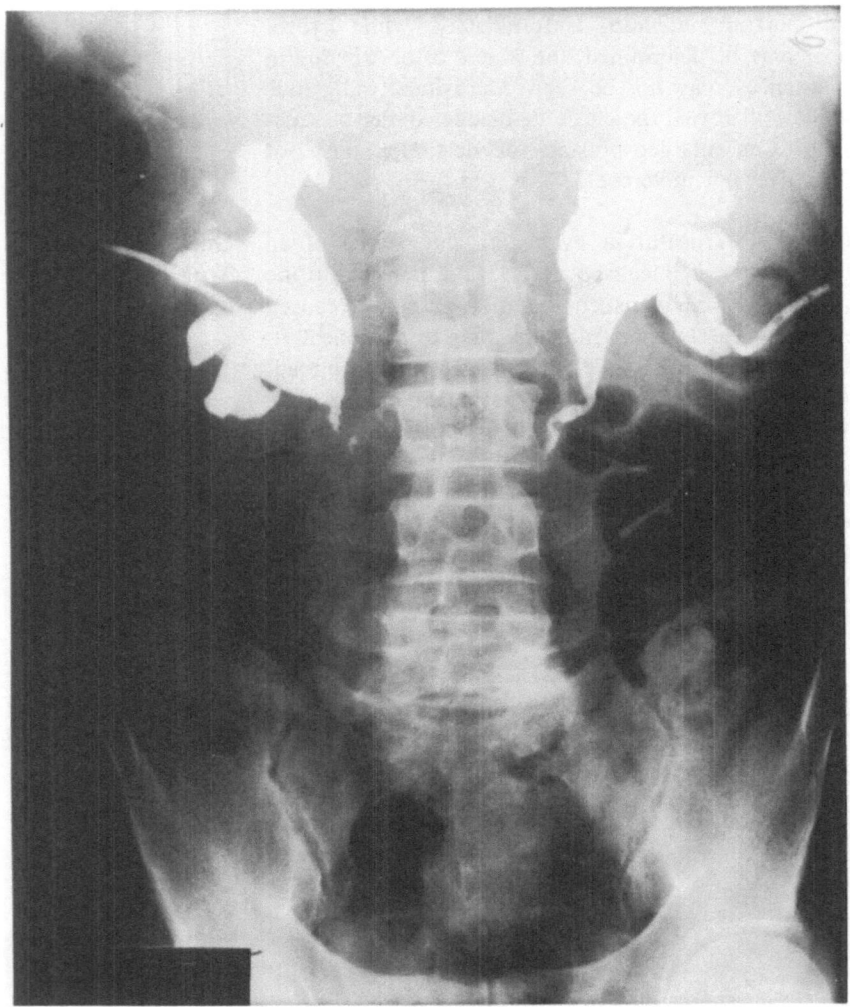

Figure 4-8. Percutaneous nephrostogram demonstrates severe bilateral hydronephrosis (arrow).

simple cyst (Fig. 4-11), utilizing sonographic criteria, usually no further studies are indicated. If the cyst is somewhat irregular or very large and interfering with renal function, such as producing localized obstruction, aspiration of the cyst can be performed utilizing sonographic guidance. If the mass is determined to be solid, the extent of tumor or inferior vena cava involvement can be detected in some cases (Fig. 4-12). The possibility of hepatic metastasis or retro-

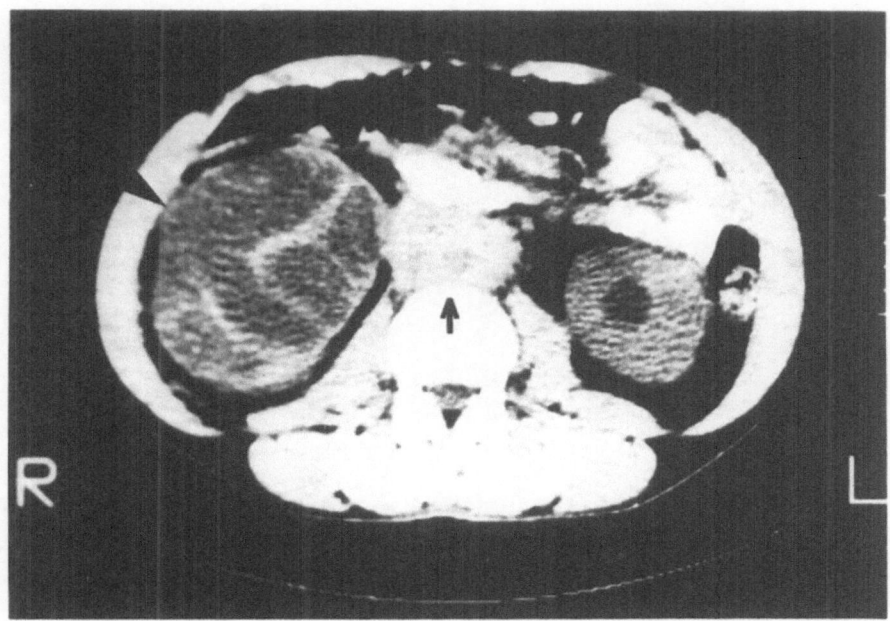

Figure 4-9. Severe bilateral hydronephrosis due to retroperitoneal (arrow) fibrosis (arrowhead) demonstrated by computerized tomography.

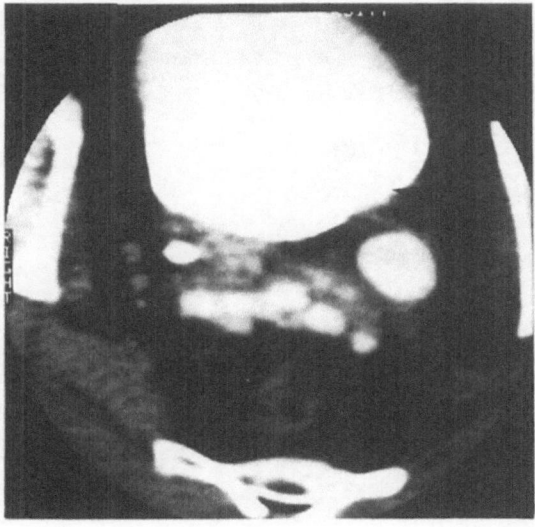

Figure 4-10. Fluid-filled mass at the base of the bladder representing urine-filled ureterocele (arrow).

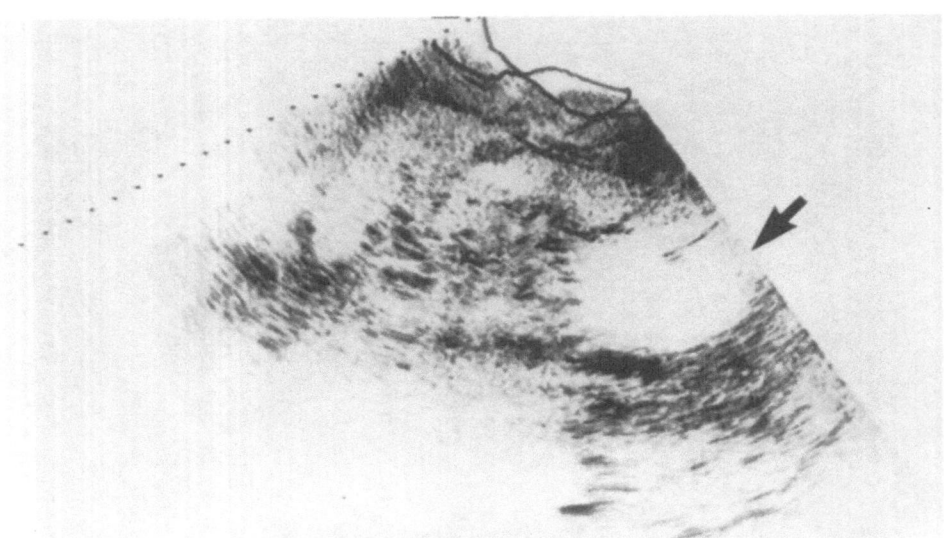

Figure 4-11. Sonolucent mass (arrow) in kidney representing simple cyst.

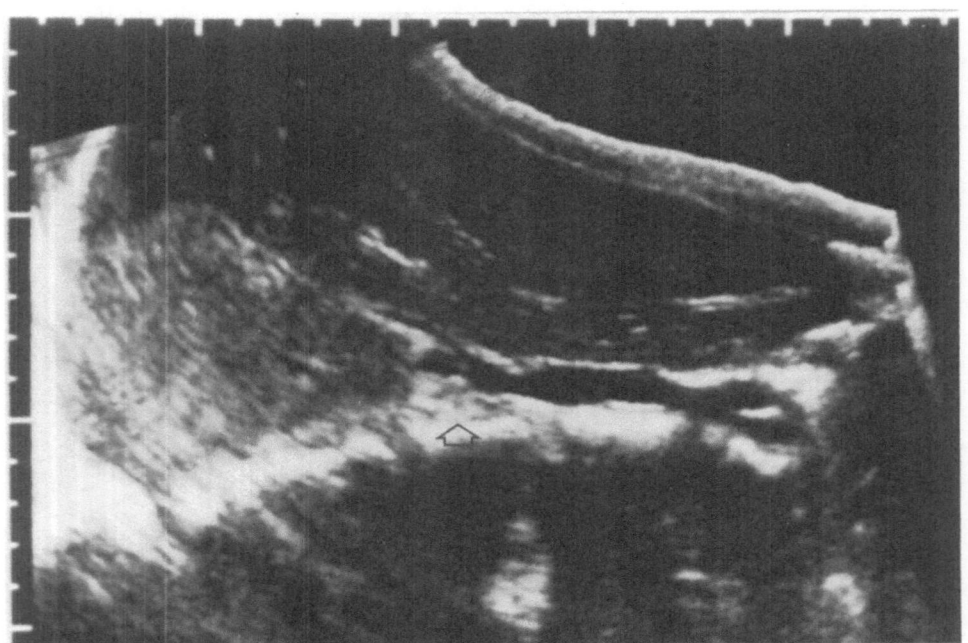

Figure 4-12. Large echogenic mass representing hypernephroma (arrow) filling inferior vena cava.

peritoneal lymphadenopathy can also be determined during the examination. Sonography is also a useful method for screening young patients with a family history of polycystic kidney disease.

Although CT cannot always categorize a mass as benign or malignant, the presence of fat in the lesion indicates the presence of benign angiomyolipoma.[5] Polycystic kidney disease may be detected (Fig. 4-13), as may the possible complicating hemorrhagic or infected cyst. The malignant nature of a mass may be determined when discrete invasion of other organs such as the liver or metastasis to the lymph nodes (Fig. 4-14) is present. In addition, CT is a useful means of staging renal malignancy preoperatively, enabling the determination of local extension and possible tumor invasion into either the renal vein or inferior vena cava.[11] Percutaneous biopsies may spare patients with unresectable lesions the need for surgical exploration. Renal

Computerized Tomography

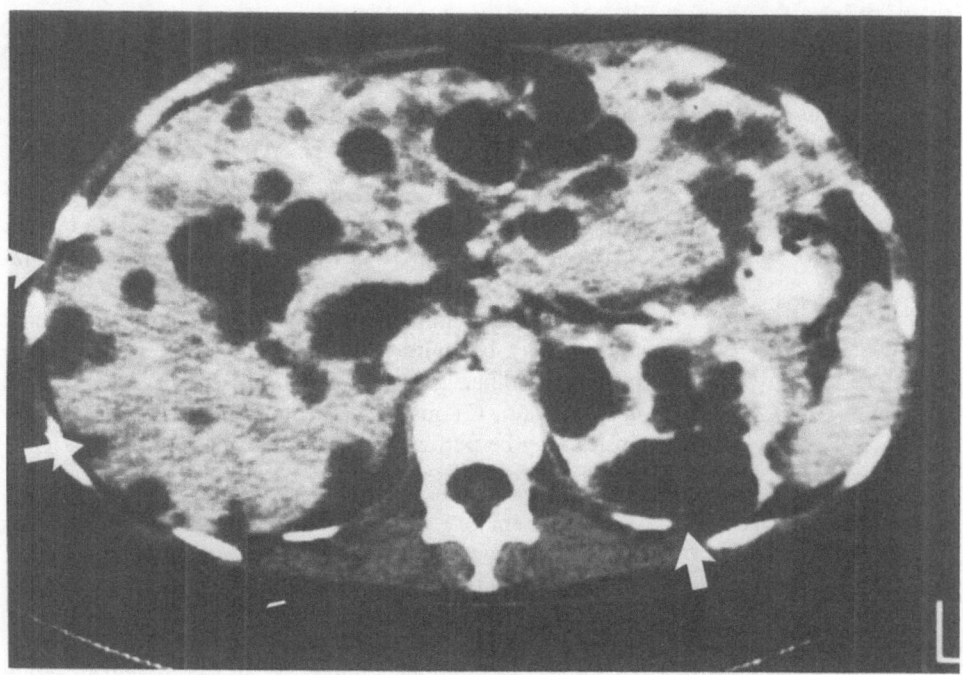

Figure 4-13. Large cystic masses in liver and left kidney (arrows) secondary to polycystic kidney disease.

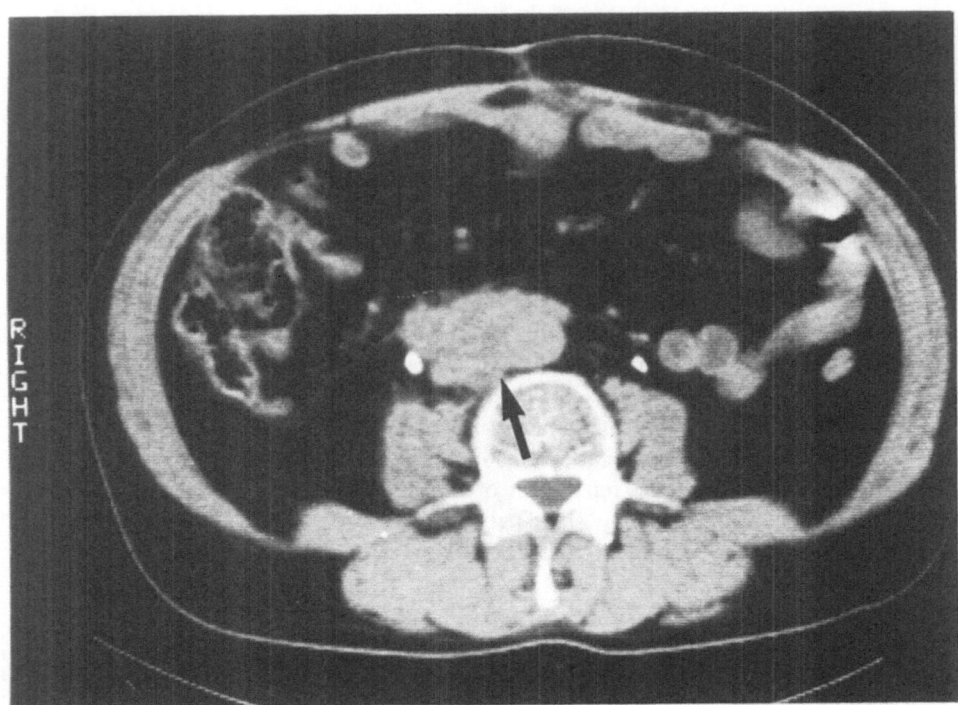

Figure 4-14. Metastases to lymph nodes (arrow) from hypernephroma.

angiography is now infrequently utilized for diagnostic staging although it may still be helpful for detecting lesions that are equivocal on CT as well as preoperatively embolizing vascular but otherwise resectable tumors. Owing to the excellent visualization of all retroperitoneal structures, renal masses may be quite readily differentiated from adrenal lesions or other retroperitoneal masses (Figs. 4-15 and 4-16). Again, CT-guided, percutaneous, skinny-needle biopsies may be performed for diagnostic purposes.

INFECTION AND REFLUX

Inflammatory disease of the kidneys and bladder as well as vesicoureteral reflux have been grouped together since reflux in many instances is the cause of chronic infections, especially in children.

Radionuclide Study

When the clinical diagnosis of pyelonephritis is in doubt, gallium imaging may be useful in detecting active inflammation of sequelae thereof such as renal or per-

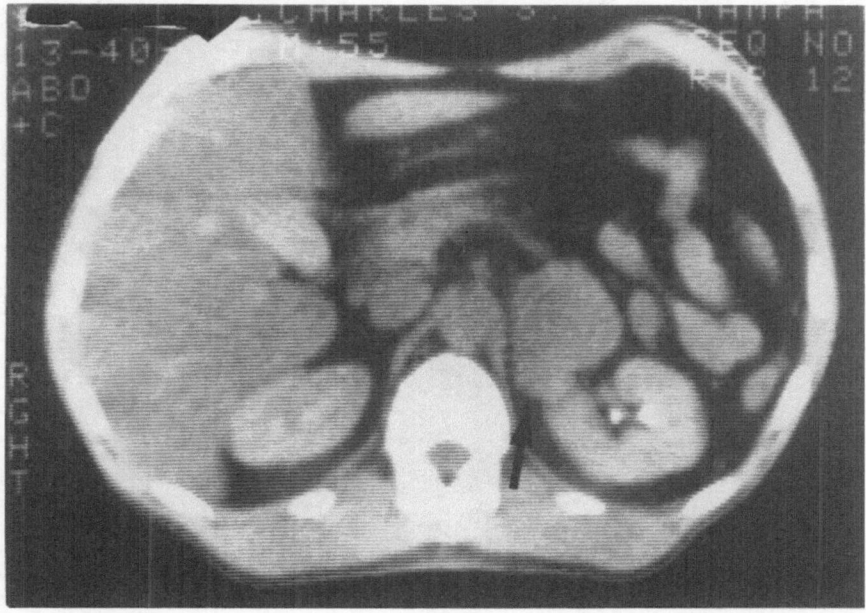

Figure 4-15. Large left adrenal mass (arrow) representing pheochromocytoma.

inephric abscess. When a patient has been known to have had chronic pyelonephritis, the radionuclide Hippuran study can be useful in evaluating renal function of both kidneys especially if a nephrectomy is being considered as a therapeutic option. The radionuclide voiding cystourethrogram is a much more sensitive study than the radiographic voiding cystourethrogram in which vesicoureteral reflux may be both detected and quantitated.[1] Owing to the lesser degree of ionizing radiation, this is the procedure of choice in children at this time.

Ultrasound

Sonography may be useful in diagnosing acute pyelonephritis. However, it is more useful in evaluating complications of inflammatory disease such as detecting renal carbuncles, abscesses, or perirenal abscesses. Patients being treated with antibiotics can be followed up with serial scans.[4] Chronic pyelonephritis is usually evident as small, scarred kidneys. In addition, the presence of large calculi within the collecting system may signify the presence of xanthogranulomatous pyelonephritis.

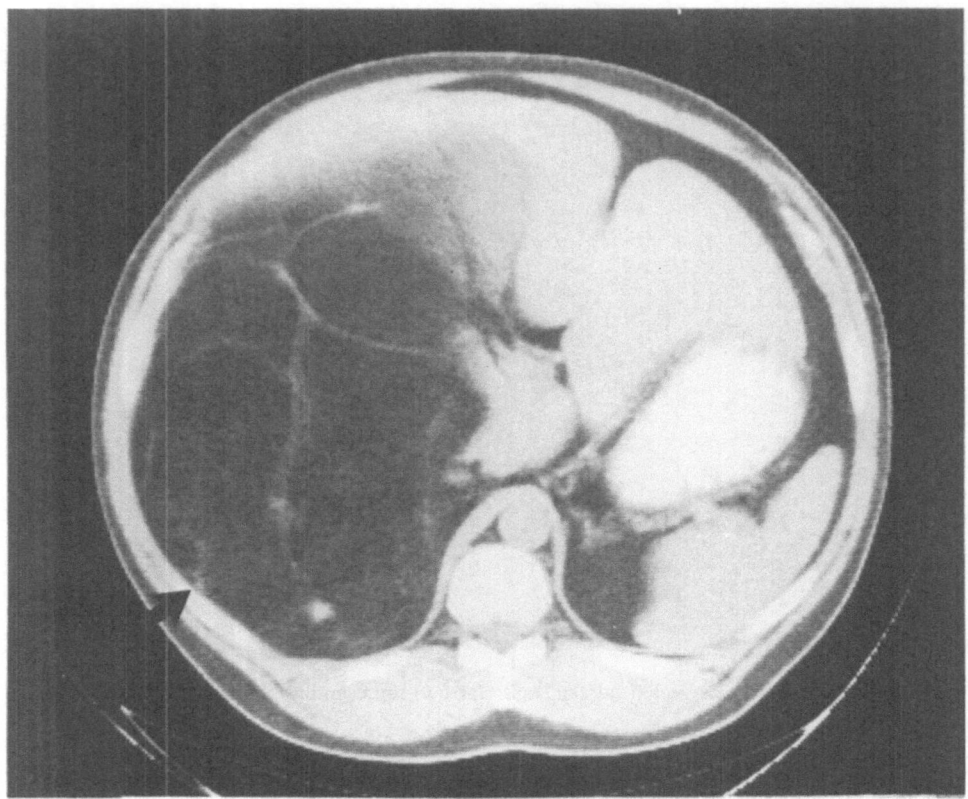

Figure 4-16. Large retroperitoneal liposarcoma (arrow) displacing liver anteriorly.

Computerized Tomography   CT is most useful in detecting renal inflammatory disease and, in many instances, may be able to differentiate abscesses from malignancy. The anatomic extent of an abscess may be evaluated (Figs. 4-17 and 4-18) as well as progression or regression of inflammatory processes following surgical or antibiotic therapy. Percutaneous drainage can be performed utilizing CT guidance if clinically desirable in patients who are not responding to antibiotics and are poor surgical risks owing to other debilitating conditions.

RENAL TRANSPLANT

Nuclear Medicine   Radionuclide studies have been utilized to evaluate renal function following transplant to detect early signs of rejection or acute tubular necrosis or to demonstrate ureteral leaks and identify sites of ureteral obstruction.

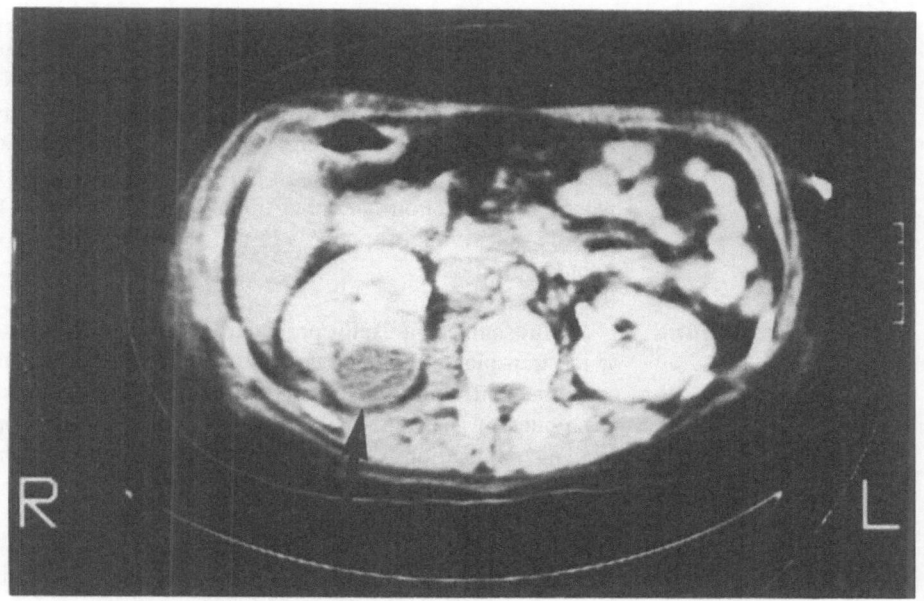

Figure 4-17. Large, low-density mass (arrow) in right kidney due to infected hematoma.

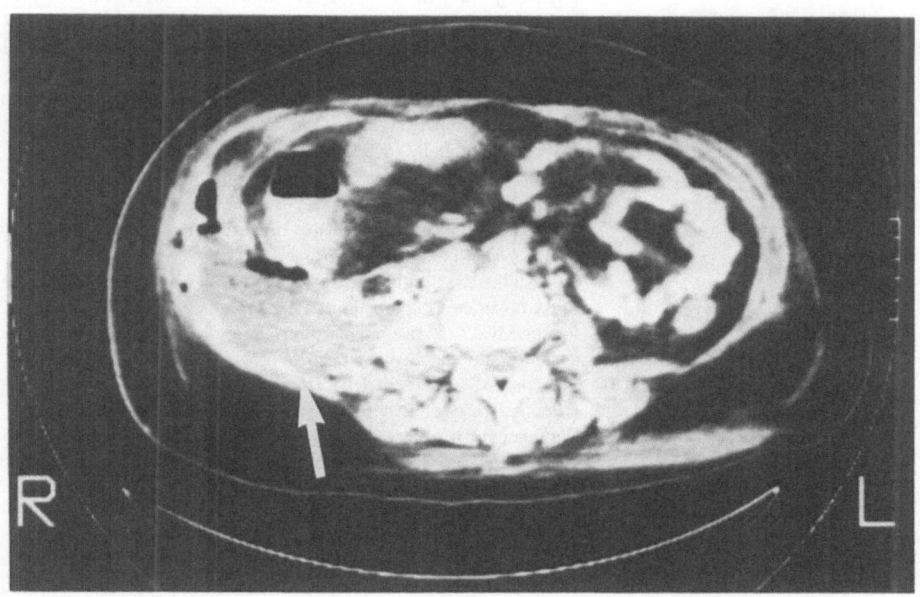

Figure 4-18. Retroperitoneal abscess (arrow) secondary to ruptured cecum.

Decreasing renal function early in the posttransplant period may be secondary to acute tubular necrosis (ATN), acute rejection, arterial occlusion, or venous thrombosis. The flow study may be useful to detect the presence of arterial occlusion. The Hippuran renogram is also useful in quantitating function and can monitor the response to steroids or immunosuppressives in patients with documented rejection.

Ultrasound

Ultrasound is a useful procedure to detect obstruction of the transplanted kidney as obstruction and rejection are sometimes difficult to distinguish utilizing the radionuclide techniques. It is also a sensitive means of detecting postoperative complications, such as hematoma, urinoma, or lymphocele, which may result in obstruction.

REFERENCES

1. Conway JJ, Belman AB, King LR: Direct and indirect radionuclide cystography. *Semin Nucl Med* 1974;41:197.
2. Dubovsky EV, Bueschen AJ, Tabin M, et al: A comprehensive computer assisted renal function study: A routine procedure in clinical practice, in Hollenberg NK, Lange S (eds): *Radionuclides in Nephrology*. New York, Thieme-Stratton, 1980, pp 52–58.
3. Federle MP, Goldberg HI, Kaiser L, et al: Evaluation of abdominal trauma by computer tomography. *Radiology* 1981;138:637–644.
4. Goldman SM, Minkin SD, Naravol DC, et al: Renal carbuncle: The use of ultrasound in its diagnosis and treatment. *J Urol* 1977;118:525–528.
5. Hansen GC, Hoffman RB, Sample WF, et al: Computed tomography diagnosis of renal angiomyolipoma. *Radiology* 1978;128:789–791.
6. Koff SA, Thrall JM, Keyes JW: Diuretic radionuclide urography: A non-invasive method for evaluating nephroureteral dilatation. *J Urol* 1979;122:451–454.
7. Kontzen F, et al: Comprehensive renal function studies:Technical aspects. *J Nucl Med Tech* 1977;5:81.
8. Mascatello VJ, Smith EH, Ceurrerra GF, et al: Ultrasonic evaluation of the obstructed duplex kidney. *Am J Roentgenol* 1977;129:113–120.
9. Parker MD: Acute segmental renal infarction:Difficulty in diagnosis despite multimodality approach. *Urology* 1981;18:523–526.
10. Pollack HM, Goldberg BB: The Kidney, in *Abdominal Gray Scale Ultrasonography*. New York, John Wiley & Sons, 1977.
11. Weyman PJ, McClenan BL, Stanley RL, et al: Comparison of computed tomography and angiography in the evaluation of renal cell carcinoma. *Radiology* 1980;137:417–424.

5   Male Pelvis and Scrotum

Prostatitis is a fairly common disorder that is easily diagnosed clinically. If an abscess of the prostate is suspected, ultrasound or computerized tomography (CT) would be equally effective documenting the presence of a prostatic mass although differentiation from other causes of enlargement would be difficult.

MALE PELVIS

Inflammatory Disease

The introduction of transrectal sonographic probes for the evaluation of prostatic enlargement has resulted in increased efficiency in differentiating benign from malignant prostatic disease.[6] In addition, local extent of malignancy, such as bladder invasion (Fig. 5-1) or pelvic lymphadenopathy, can be detected. Rectal involvement is more difficult to detect because of the presence of artifact producing gas within the rectum. Distal ureteral obstruction secondary to prostatic disease can also be evaluated sonographically.

Prostatic Enlargement

Ultrasound

In patients with documented prostatic malignancy, CT at this time is the procedure of choice for local staging of tumor prior to therapy and following treatment.[4] Invasion of adjacent organs or spread to pelvic or abdominal lymph nodes can be easily detected (Fig. 5-2). CT is also well suited for postoperative evaluation and planning of radiotherapy. The seminal vesicles are very clearly defined utilizing high-

Computerized
Tomography

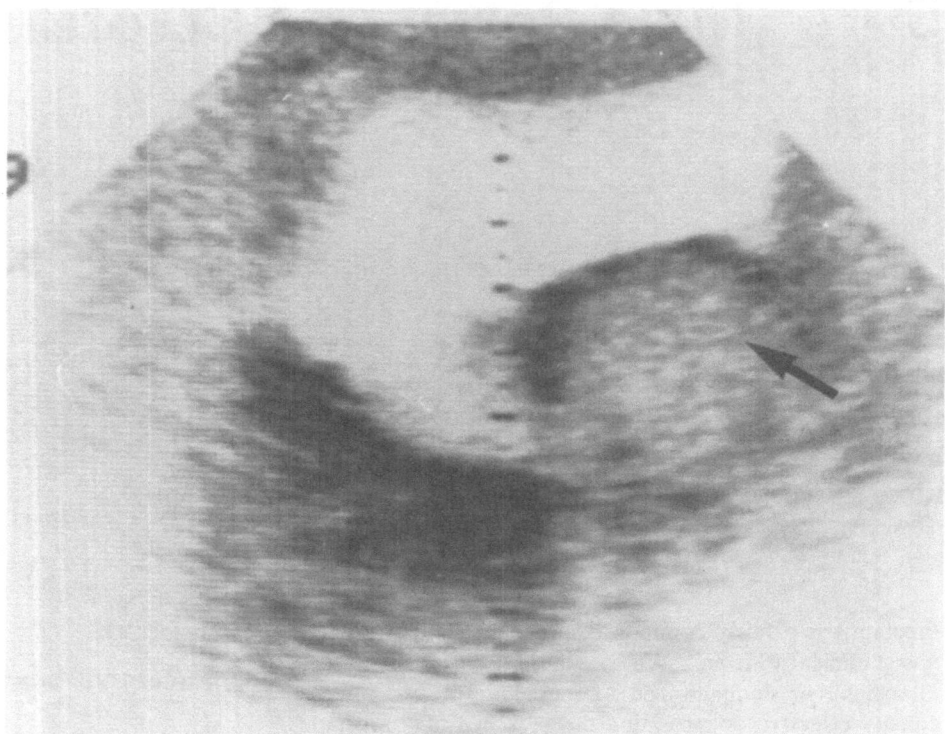

Figure 5-1. Pelvic sonogram demonstrates large prostatic mass (arrow) invading the bladder.

resolution scans and can also be evaluated regarding the possible spread of bladder or prostate malignancy. It is believed, however, that magnetic resonance imaging will eventually replace CT in the staging of pelvic malignancy.

SCROTUM   The common pathologic processes affecting the scrotum include inflammatory changes secondary to torsion or infection, scrotal masses, neoplasm, trauma, and scrotal hernias. Prior to the advent of newer imaging procedures, the clinical presentation and physical findings were the primary means of diagnosis except in the cases of scrotal hernia, which occasionally could be detected by the presence of bowel gas in the scrotal sac seen on plain radiographs of the pelvis.

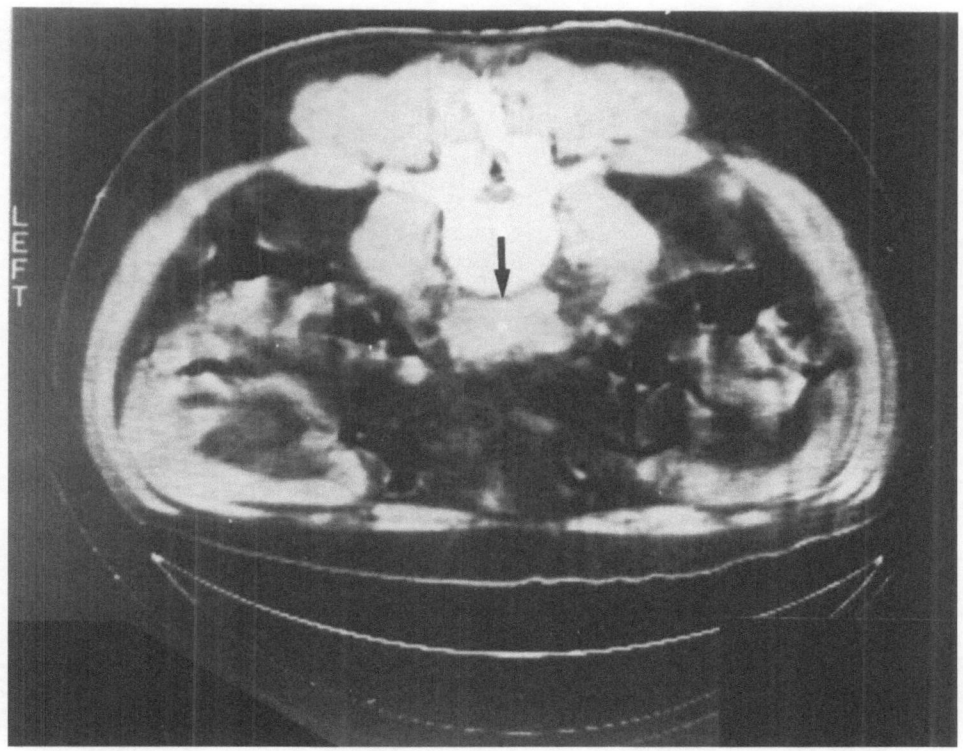

Figure 5-2. Retroperitoneal adenopathy (arrows) secondary to prostatic tumor.

Inflammatory Disease versus Torsion of the Testicle

Radionuclide Study

The radionuclide testicular flow study and static scans will, in most instances, readily distinguish between the hyperemic inflammatory changes of epididymoorchitis (Figs. 5-3 and 5-4) versus the lack of perfusion and nonvisualization of the testicle that has undergone torsion.[1] Equivocal cases can be referred to ultrasound, which will usually show a relatively normal-appearing ischemic testicle in the early stages with areas of necrosis seen at a later stage. Epididymoorchitis will present as an enlarged, edematous, inhomogeneous testicle with associated inflammation of the epididymis and occasionally a reactive hydrocele.

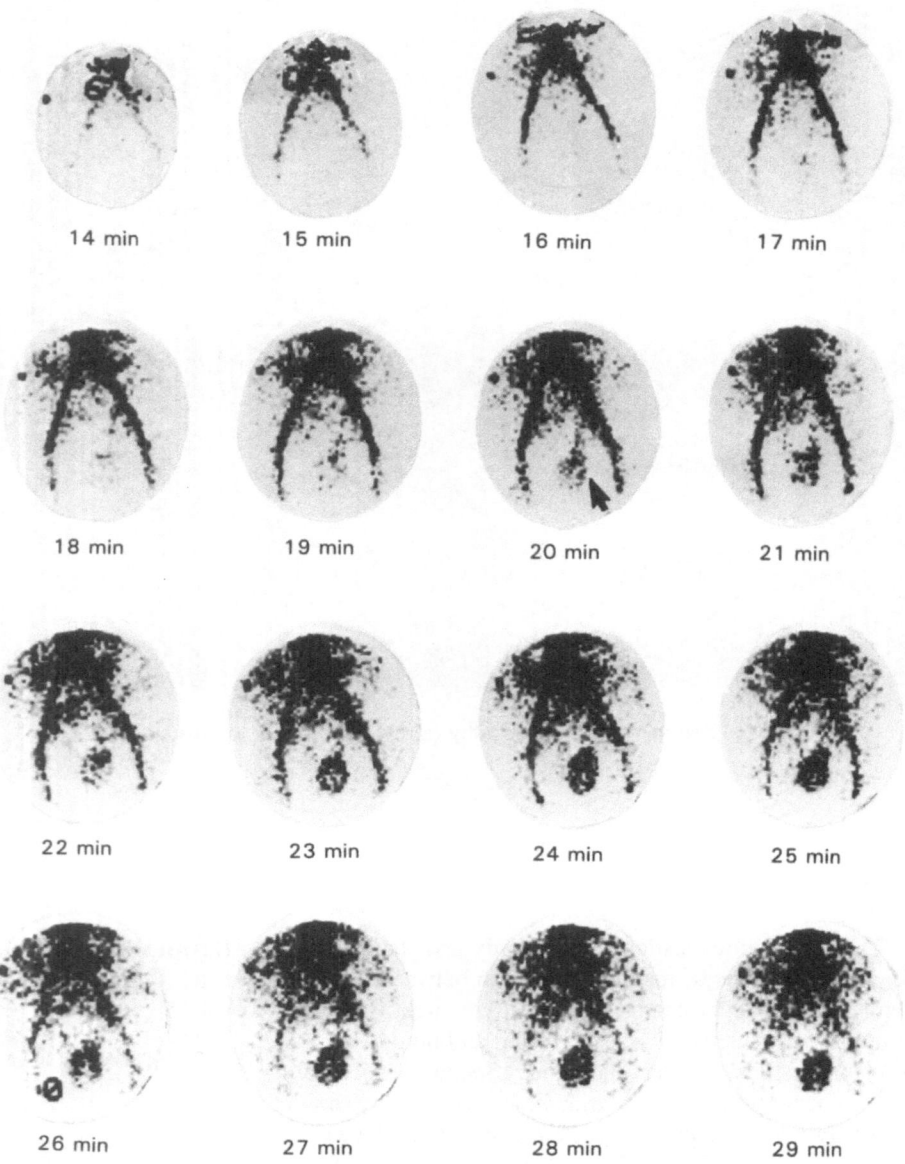

Figure 5-3. Dynamic testicular scan shows markedly increased flow to left testicle (arrow).

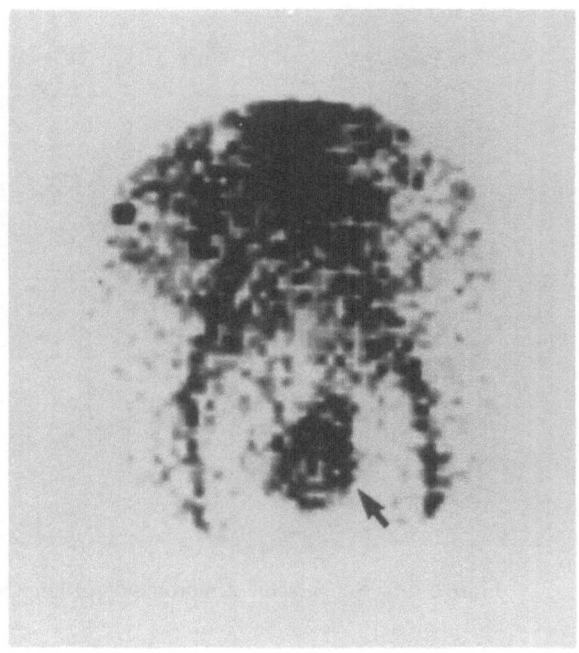

Figure 5-4. Delayed image shows
hyperemic left testicle (arrow) secondary to epididymoorchitis.

Nuclear imaging is not useful in evaluation of the enlarged scrotum except for cases in which a chronic indolent
testicular abscess or occasional tumor may accumulate gallium. However, gallium has also been reported in normal
bowel within scrotal hernias.

The procedure of choice in evaluating the enlarged
testicle is ultrasound. The procedure is sensitive in identifying testicular masses secondary to trauma, neoplasm, or
inflammation.[5] In many cases, the finding is nonspecific
and clinical correlation is mandatory. Fluid collections such
as hydroceles are readily identified (Fig. 5-5), as are fluid-
filled loops of bowel within the scrotal hernia. Proven cases
of varicoceles and epididymitis have also been reported.

Ultrasound

The utilization of CT related to diseases affecting the
scrotum is limited to staging known testicular neoplasms
regarding the presence and localization of metastasis or
lymphadenopathy involving the retroperitoneal nodes. The
progression or regression of disease can be evaluated utilizing serial scans.

Computerized
Tomography

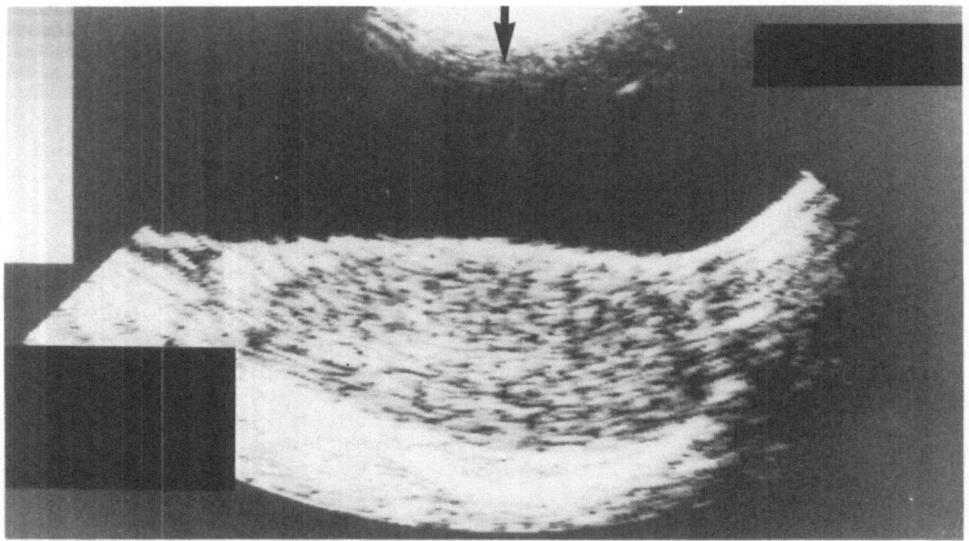

Figure 5-5. Sonographic demonstration of large hydrocele (arrow) anterior to testicle.

Undescended Testes

Failure of the testes to descend into the scrotal sac is associated with a fairly high incidence of testicular malignancy, making localization of the testes and prophylactic orchiopexy necessary. Preoperative localization of testes often helps in planning the surgical approach and shortens anesthesia time. Formerly, the only radiologic procedures available were angiography and venography, both of which were invasive, painful, and utilized ionizing radiation. Occasionally, ultrasound has been useful in detection of undescended testes[3]; however, since the testes are usually located in the inguinal canal or lower pelvis, CT is the better imaging modality for detection owing to lack of interference from overlying bowel[2] and other soft tissue structures.

REFERENCES

1. Holder LE, Martire JR, Holmes ER, et al: Testicular radionuclide angiography and static imaging: Anatomy, scintigraphic interpretation and clinical indications. *Radiology* 1977;125:739–752.
2. Lee JK, McClennan BL, Stanley RJ, et al: Utility of computed tomography in the localization of the undescended testis. *Radiology* 1980;135:121–125.
3. Madrazo BL, Klugo RC, Parks JA, et al: Ultrasonographic demonstration of the undescended testis. *Radiology* 1979;133:181–183.

4. Price JM, Davidson AJ: Computed tomography in the evaluation of the suspected carcinomatous prostate. *Urol Radiol* 1979;1:38–42.
5. Sample WF, Goltesman JE, Skinner DG, et al: Gray scale ultrasound of the scrotum. *Radiology* 1978;127:225–228.
6. Watanabe H, Igari D, Tanahaski Y, et al: Transrectal ultrasonography of the prostate. *J Urol* 1975;114:734–739.

6

Female Pelvis (Obstetrics/Gynecology)

Prior to the widespread utilization of ultrasound in the management of obstetric patients, there was little need for radiography in clinical obstetric care. The studies were limited primarily to radiographic pelvimetry and the more invasive procedure of aminography. Ultrasound currently occupies a very important role in the routine prenatal care of obstetric patients because of lack of ionizing radiation. The indications for obstetric ultrasound can be further subdivided into maternal and fetal indications.

Ultrasound is commonly used in early pregnancy both to confirm the presence of an intrauterine pregnancy as well as to exclude common complications of early pregnancy such as blighted ovum, incomplete abortion, missed abortion, molar pregnancy[1] (Figs. 6-1 and 6-2), or evaluation of adnexal masses such as ectopic pregnancy (Fig. 6-3) or corpus luteum cyst. Other problems related to early pregnancy may be the coexistent presence of an intrauterine device or the presence of a uterine leiomyoma, which may undergo degeneration or necrosis. The presence of a cervical myoma will alert the obstetrician to the need for cesarean section.

In many instances, knowledge of fetal gestational age is critical in the management of complicated pregnancies.

OBSTETRICS

Maternal Indications

First Trimester

Defining Gestational Age

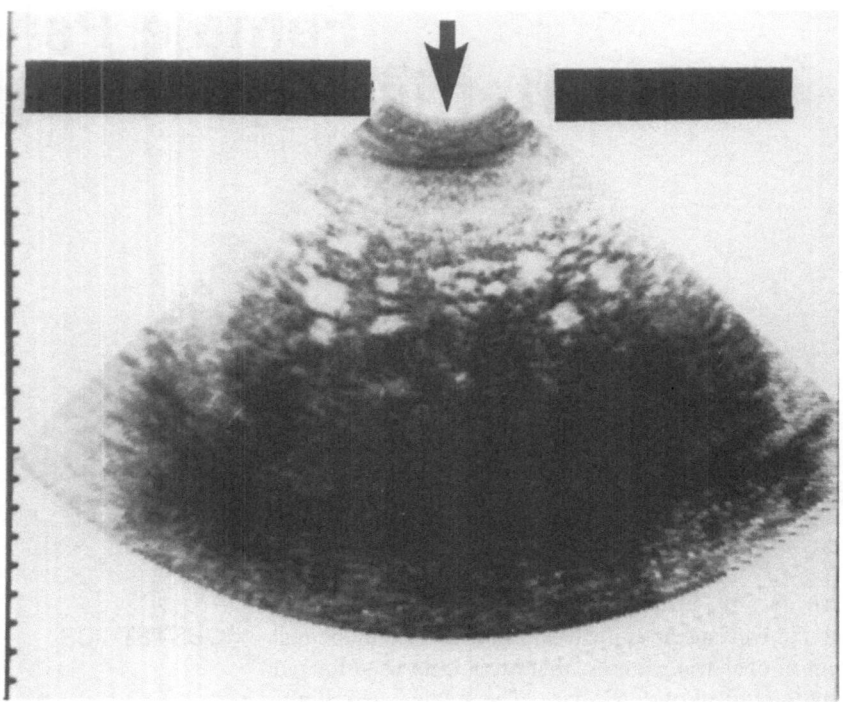

Figure 6-1. Pelvic sonogram reveals intrauterine mass with cystic areas (arrow) compatible with hydatidiform molar pregnancy.

The gestational age may be determined in various ways. In the first trimester, the crown–rump length is the most accurate measurement. During the later stages of pregnancy, i.e., second and third trimesters, the biparietal diameter measurement (Fig. 6-4) is an accurate means of assessing gestational age although this method of staging is not as accurate during the lattermost portion of the third trimester. Other methods have been devised to calculate the age of a fetus such as measuring femoral length, binocular distance, or head-to-abdominal-circumference ratio. The latter method is especially useful when trying to determine the possibility of intrauterine growth retardation.

In patients with preeclampsia, diabetes, or other systemic illness that can result in fetal distress or in intrauterine growth retardation,[6] it is important to accurately date the fetus to determine when pregnancy can be safely terminated from both maternal and fetal standpoints.

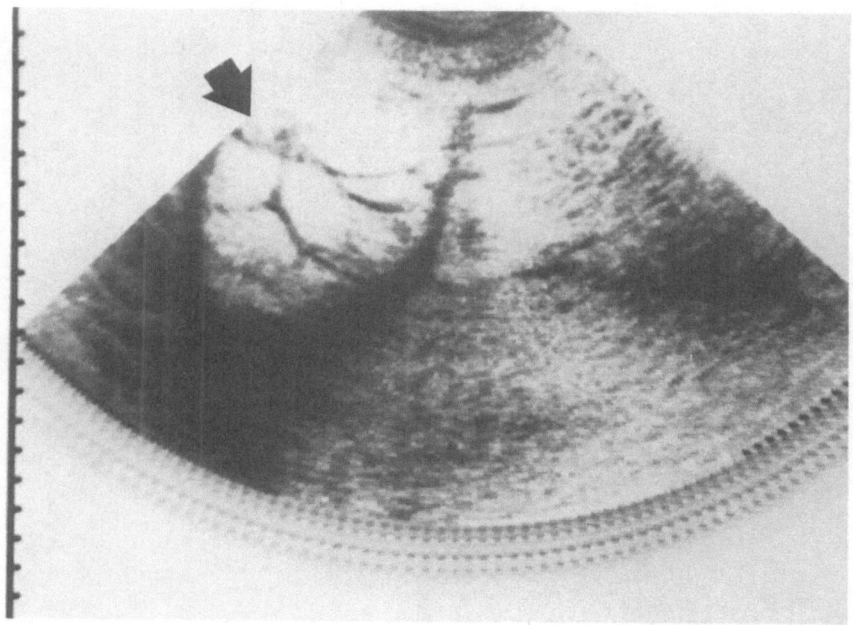

Figure 6-2. Large, multiloculated thecal luteum cyst (arrow) coexistent with molar pregnancy.

Placenta

The placenta can be easily localized for purposes of amniocentesis as well as detecting placenta previa[7] or, less frequently, abruptio placentae in patients with third-trimester bleeding. With current high-resolution, gray-scale ultrasound equipment, subtle textural changes in the placenta can be detected, which will enable the obstetrician to predict functional maturity of the placenta and similarly maturation of the fetal lungs.[2] Occasionally, placental anomalies such as vascular tumors may be detected as incidental findings.

Fetal Indications

Multiple Gestations

The most common cause of a "large-for-date" pregnancy is multiple gestations (Fig. 6-5). This has become more commonplace in recent years with the increasing utilization of the so-called "fertility drugs." It is common and convenient to follow twin gestation throughout pregnancy utilizing serial scans to assess both growth and development of the individual fetuses as well as excluding the presence of congenital anomalies. Ultrasound is essential in situations where it may be necessary to perform amniocentesis on each individual amniotic sac.

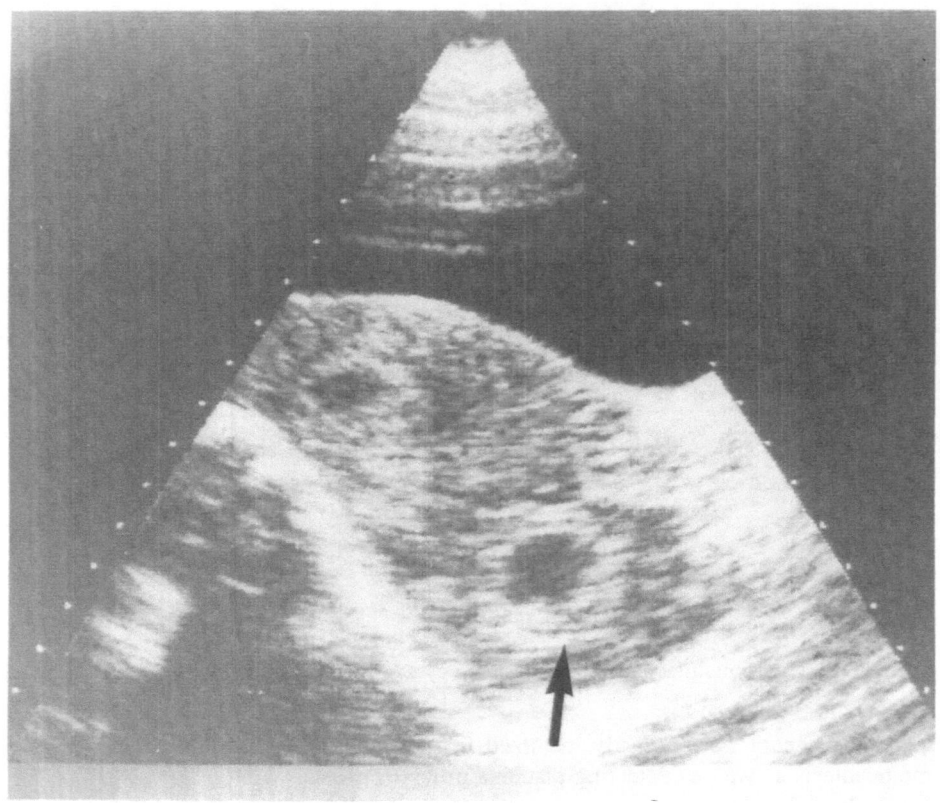

Figure 6-3. Intrauterine decidual cast with ectopic pregnancy (arrow) in cul-de-sac.

Congenital Fetal Anomalies

Many patients who have already delivered a fetus with a deformity or are experiencing pregnancies with complicating conditions known to be associated with fetal anomalies are being scanned routinely to evaluate the fetus for possible anomalies. Abnormalities involving almost every organ system have been detected *in utero*. These range from central nervous system problems such as hydrocephalus, anencephaly, microcephaly, and meningoceles to simple neural tube defects.[4] Gastrointestinal tract anomalies such as gastroschisis, omphaloceles, intestinal obstructing lesions, and duodenal atresia can result in polyhydramnios. Genitourinary tract anomalies with associated oligohydramnios may be detected, such as renal agenesis, polycystic kidneys, or hydronephrosis with varying levels of obstruction. Certain deleterious conditions, such as Turner's syndrome with asso-

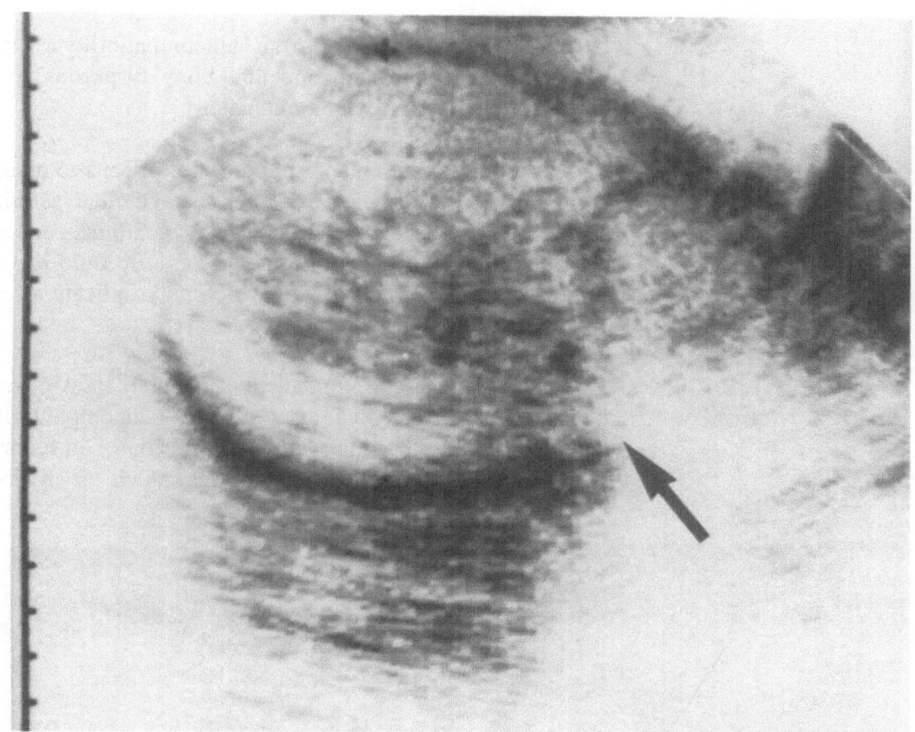

Figure 6-4. Cross-section of fetal skull (arrow) utilized in determining fetal age.

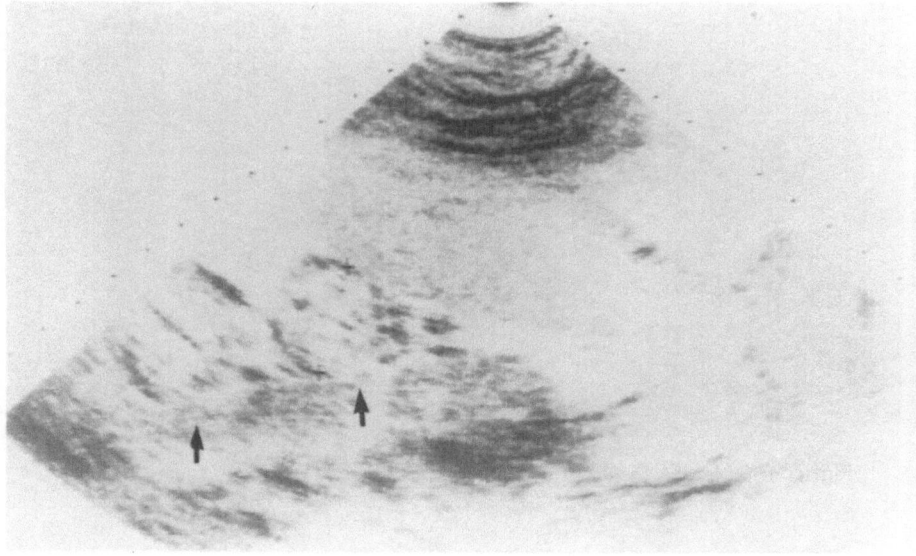

Figure 6-5. Sonogram of patient with "large-for-date" gestation reveals twin fetuses (arrows).

ciated cystic hygroma (Fig. 6-6), RH incompatibility associated with fetal ascites, and congenital bony dysplasias, may also be frequently discovered antenatally.[3]

Fetal Viability

Ultrasound is the quickest and easiest means to assess the viability and well-being of a fetus. Fetal cardiac activity can be directly visualized, as can fetal breathing patterns such as prolonged periods of apnea. Amniotic fluid meconium can also be demonstrated, which may indicate a less than optimal prognosis.

Interventional Techniques

With sonographic guidance, antenatal transfusions have been performed in fetuses with RH incompatibility syndrome, while other interventional procedures in fetuses with surgically correctable conditions, such as hydro-

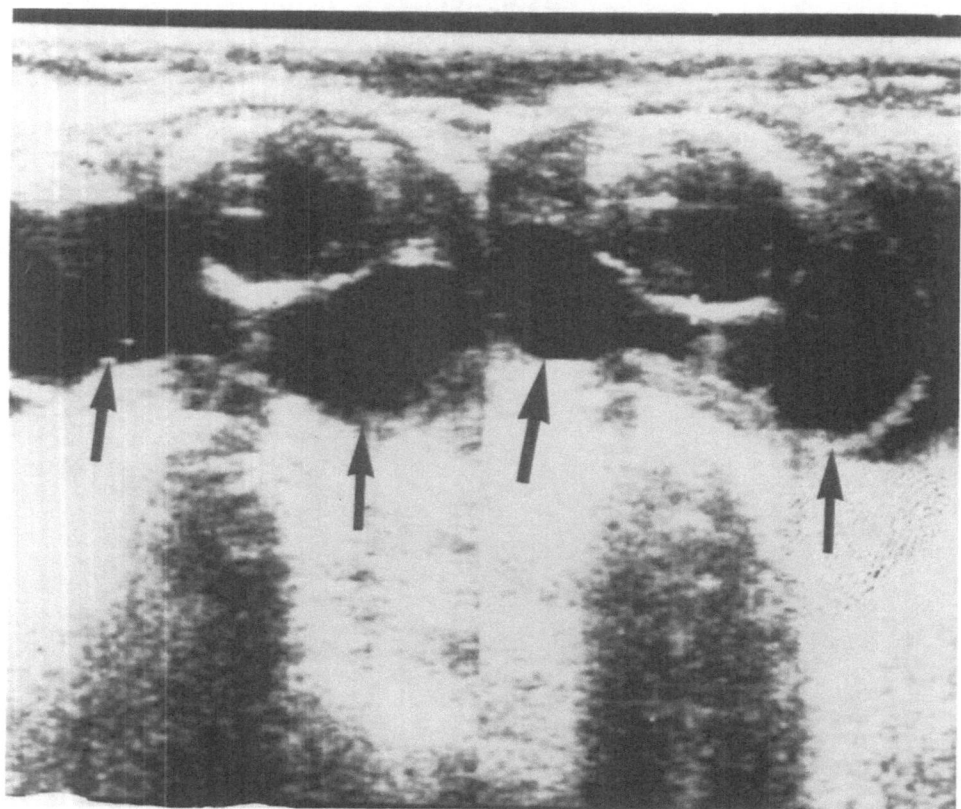

Figure 6-6. Large, loculated cystic hygroma (arrows) adjacent to fetal skull.

nephrosis and hydrocephalus, have also been performed *in utero*.

1. Fleischer AC, James AE Jr, Krause DA, et al: Sonographic patterns in trophoblastic diseases. *Radiology* 1978;126:215–220.
2. Grannum PAT, Hobbins JC: The ultrasonic changes in the maturing placenta and their relation to fetal pulmonic maturity. *Am J Obstet Gynecol* 1979; 133:8, 915–922.
3. Hobbins JC, Mahoney MJ: The diagnosis of skeletal dysplasias with ultrasound, In Sanders R, James AE (eds): *Ultrasonography in Obstetrics and Gynecology*. New York, Appleton-Century-Crofts, 1979, pp 191–197.
4. Hobbins JC, Mahoney MJ, Berkowitz RE, et al: Use of ultrasound in diagnosing congenital anomalies. *Am J Obstet Gynecol* 1979;135:331–346.
5. Maklad NF, Wright CH: Gray-scale ultrasonography in the diagnosis of ectopic pregnancy. *Radiology* 1978;126:221–225.
6. Sabbagha RE: Intrauterine growth retardation. *Obstet Gynecol* 1978;52:252.
7. Williamson D, Bjorgen J, Barer B, et al: Ultrasonic diagnosis of placenta previa-value of post void scan. *J Clin Ultrasound;*6:1,58.

GYNECOLOGY

Pelvic Masses

Prior to the introduction of ultrasound and computerized tomography (CT), the only diagnostic radiologic techniques available to assess pelvic pathology were the intravenous pyelogram and barium enema, both of which confirmed the presence of masses extrinsic to the bowel or bladder but occasionally were able to document invasion of lesions into these organs.

Ultrasound

Ultrasound is a fairly simple, expedient means of evaluating the organ of origin of pelvic masses without resorting to ionizing radiation or more invasive techniques. Other than routine pregnancies, the most common pelvic mass in the adult female is the fibroid uterus (Fig. 6-7). Classic sonographic presentation is often an enlarged uterus with focal collections of irregular echoes. These lesions may be calcified or demonstrate cystic degeneration.[4] Cervical tumors may occasionally be staged locally detecting bladder invasion, obstruction of the distal ureters, or pelvic lymphadenopathy. Other pelvic masses that may be seen are nonuterine in origin, involving either the ovaries or neighboring organs such as the bowel. The most common ovarian lesion is the follicular ovarian cyst. Cystic neoplasms, which may

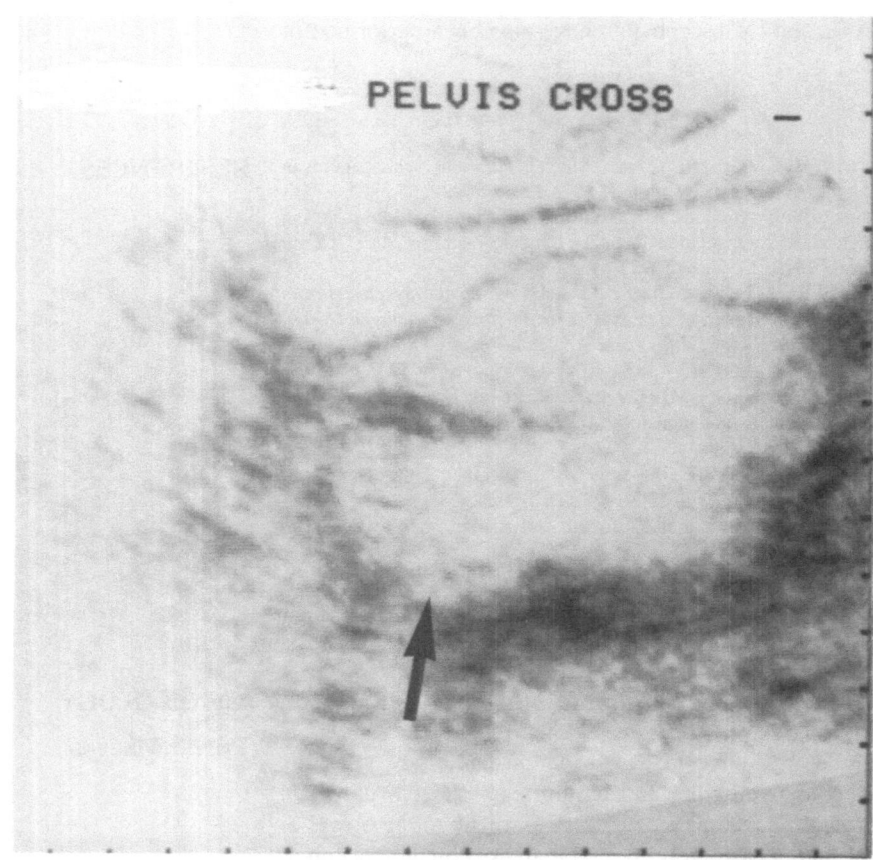

Figure 6-7. Lobulated uterine fibroid (arrow) compressing the bladder.

be benign (Fig. 6-8) or malignant (Fig. 6-9), can be detected. Complex ovarian masses such as tubal ovarian abscesses, teratomas, endometriomas (Fig. 6-10), or ectopic pregnancy may be diagnosed. These lesions, however, may be difficult to distinguish sonographically without an adequate clinical history. Positive pregnancy tests are strongly suggestive of ectopic pregnancy, whereas fever and leukocytosis will be more compatible with pelvic inflammatory disease or bowel abscess, which may result from appendicitis, diverticulitis, or postoperative infection. The presence of dense fat within a lesion in a young female is compatible with a benign teratoma (Fig. 6-11).[1] The presence of ascites and a coexist-

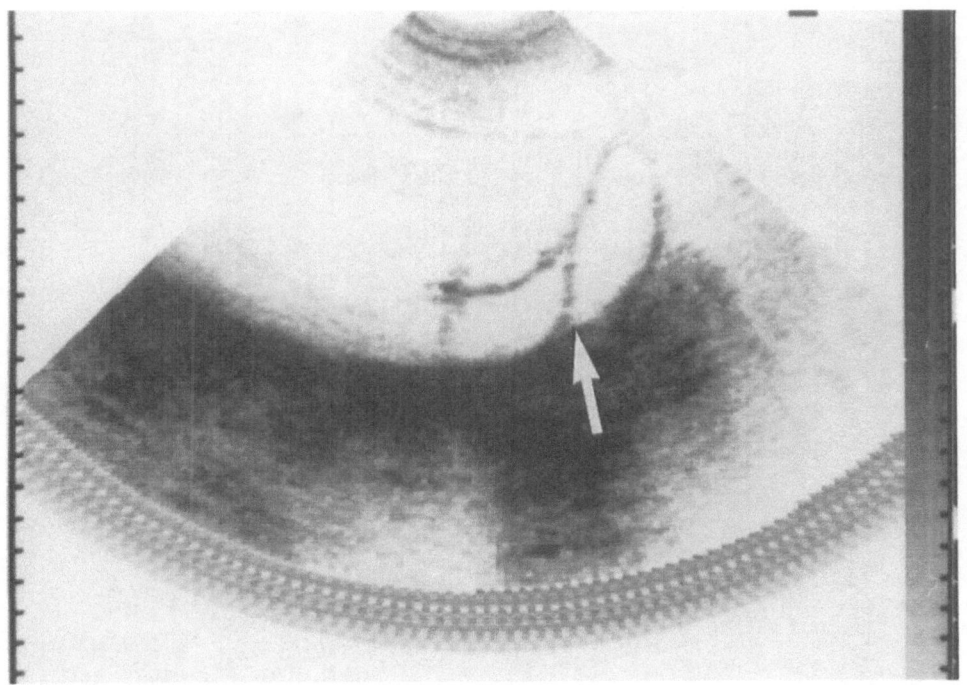

Figure 6-8. Septated cystic ovarian mass (arrow) representing mucinous cystadenoma.

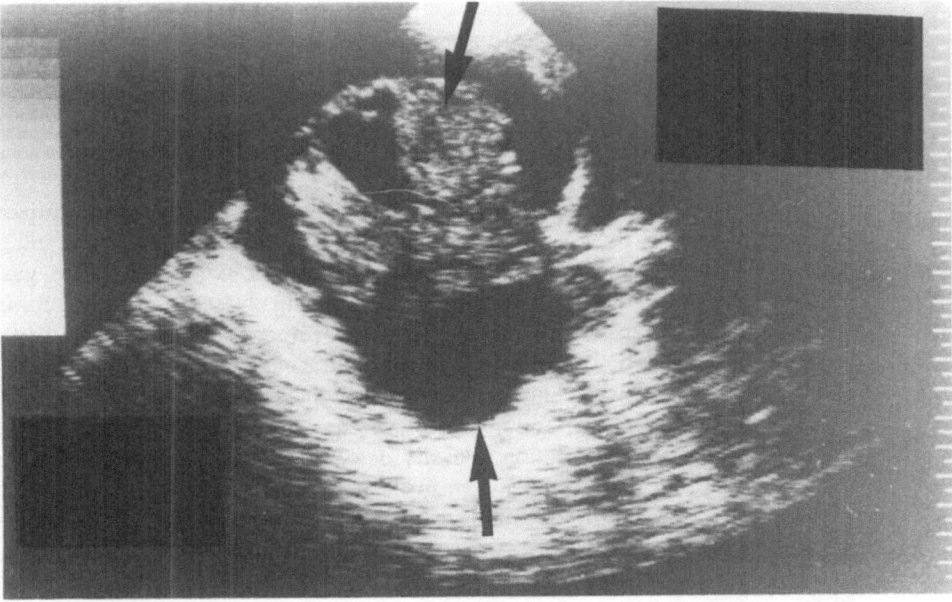

Figure 6-9. Mixed solid and cystic ovarian carcinoma (arrow) with ascites (lower arrow).

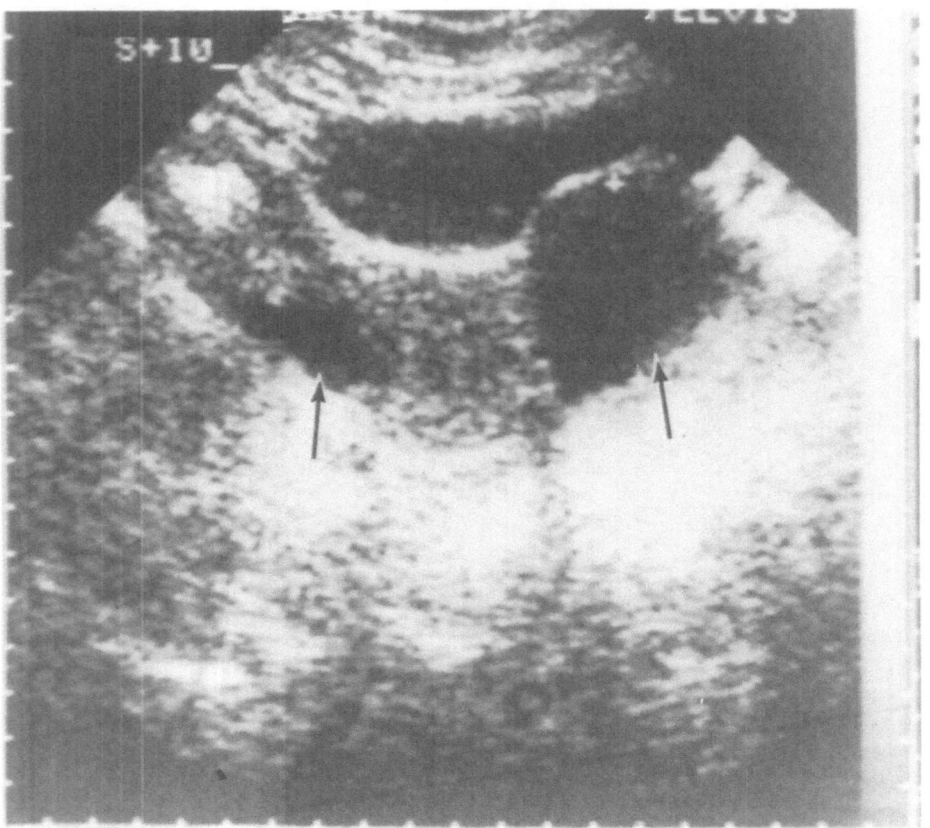

Figure 6-10. Bilateral mixed echogenic masses (arrows) representing endometriomas.

ing solid ovarian mass is strongly suggestive of malignancy until proven otherwise.

Computerized Tomography

Although ultrasound is the primary procedure utilized for imaging pelvic masses, CT can be helpful when ultrasound is unsuccessful because of either excessive gas, obesity, or postoperative scarring. It is also most helpful in patients who have had prior surgery such as cystectomy or bowel resection. As with ultrasound, the differentiation between uterine and ovarian masses can usually be made. Cystic and solid lesions can also be distinguished. Fat or calcification is easily detected. Air bubbles within lesions will usually signify the presence of abscess or infection. Utilizing oral or rectal contrast medium will help determine

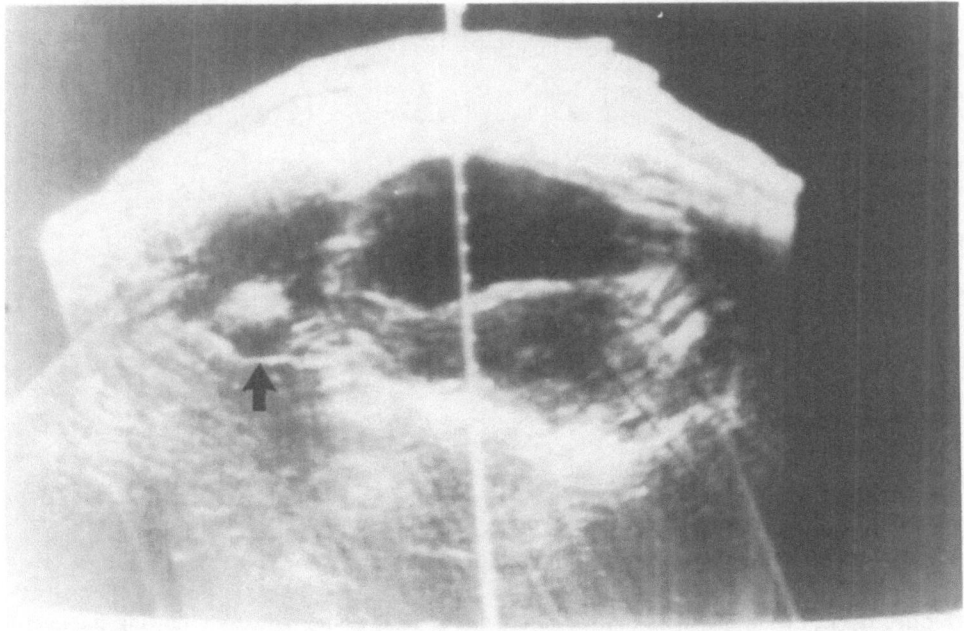

Figure 6-11. Cystic mass with echogenic collection of fat (arrow) consistent with ovarian dermoid.

the relationship between a mass and neighboring bowel or bladder. The local staging of neoplasm can be performed with accurate evaluation of parametrial infiltration, extension to the pelvic side wall, or the presence of pelvic and inguinal lymph nodes[5] and accompanying ascites. Omental implants may also be readily visualized.

Localization of Intrauterine Device

Ultrasound is frequently used in the detection of an intrauterine device when its location cannot be determined clinically. In cases of perforation of the uterus, hematoma or abscess can be visualized (Fig. 6-12).

Presacral Mass

Ultrasound is not as accurate as CT in the detection or determination of presacral masses owing to interference from bowel gas and shadowing related to the adjacent bone. CT can detect the presence of air, fat, or fluid within the mass, which would be helpful in arriving at a histologic diagnosis. Bony erosion or invasion can also be detected readily.

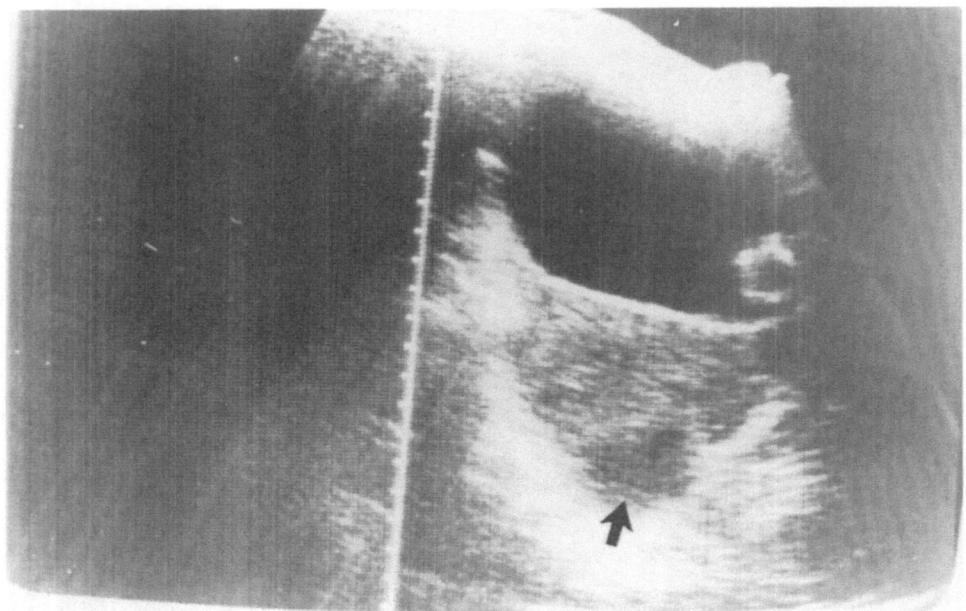

Figure 6-12. Echogenic mass (arrow) in cul-de-sac representing abscess following intrauterine device perforation.

Assessment of the Postoperative Pelvis

The detection of postoperative complications or local recurrence of benign or malignant disease has been difficult sonographically in patients with prior cystectomy or bowel resection, making CT the procedure of choice for these patients. CT is well suited for evaluation of the ileal bladder.[3] Recognition of alteration of symmetry of the remaining structures facilitates the diagnosis of pathologic conditions at an earlier stage. Local recurrence of bladder or rectal tumor (Fig. 6-13),[2] surgical complications, i.e., urinoma, lymphocele, hematoma, or abscess (Figs. 6-14 and 6-15), or metastasis can be recognized on postoperative scans. Occasionally when postoperative masses are seen, histologic diagnosis may be made based on the appearance of the lesion. In equivocal cases, CT-directed, percutaneous needle biopsy can be easily performed without complication. If a tumor is present, radiation therapy fields may be planned and the patient can be followed with serial studies.

Radionuclide Study

The gallium scan may be useful in patients with previous surgery in whom one is trying to detect the presence of a postoperative abscess. The study, however, is non-

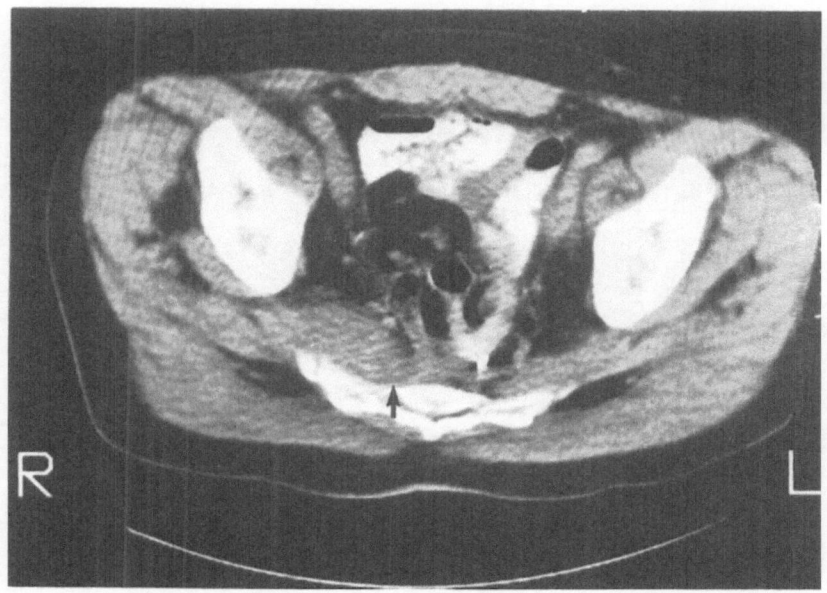

Figure 6-13. Solid mass (arrow) anterior to sacrum representing recurrent rectal tumor.

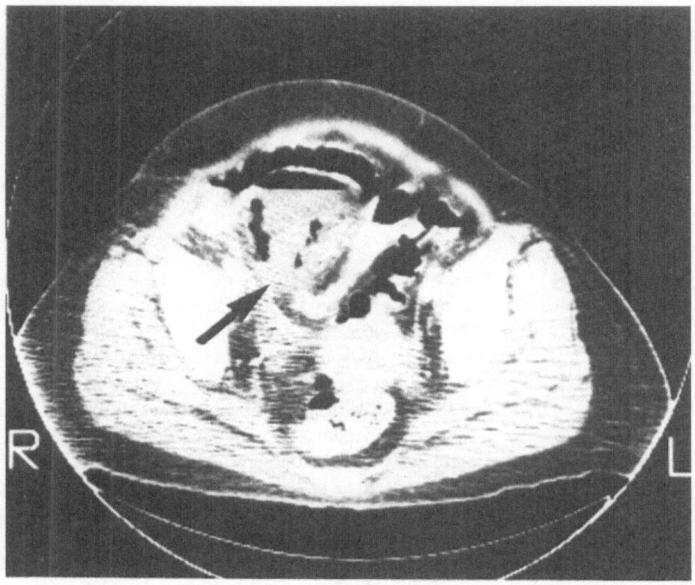

Figure 6-14. Fluid-filled right-lower-quadrant mass (arrow) with air bubbles representing appendiceal abscess.

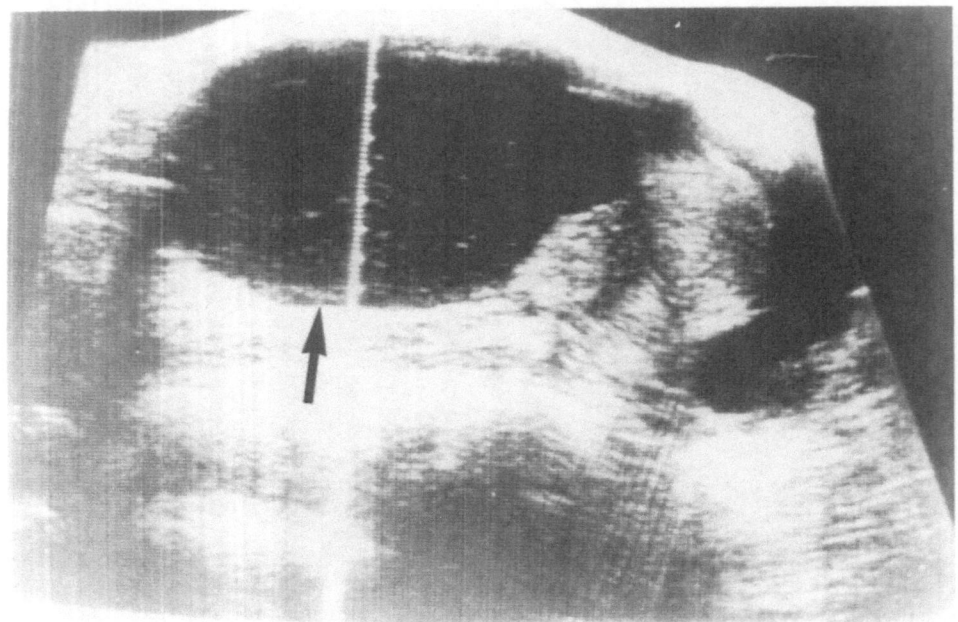

Figure 6-15. Fluid-filled mass with echogenic debris (arrow) representing tuboovarian abscess.

specific owing to abnormal gallium uptake in certain tumors, lymphadenopathy, or normal bowel loops. Many institutions now use Indium 111 oxine tagged to leukocytes, which does not localize in normal bowel and has been found to be useful in the localization of pelvic infections.

REFERENCES

1. Guttman PH: In search of the elusive benign cystic teratoma: Application of the ultrasound "tip of the iceberg sign." *J Clin Ultrasound* 1977;5:403–406.
2. Husband JE, Jodson NJ, Parsons CA: The use of computed tomography in recurrent rectal tumors. *Radiology* 1980;134:677–682.
3. Lee JKT, McClennan BL, Stanley RJ, et al: Use of CT in evaluation of postcystectomy patients. *Am J Radiol* 1981;136:483–487.
4. VonMicksky LI: Sonography study of uterine fibromyomata in the nonpregnant state and during gestation, in Sanders RC, James AE (eds): *Ultrasonography in Obstetrics and Gynecology.* New York, Appleton-Century-Crofts, 1977.
5. Walsh JW, Amendola MA, Konerding KF, et al: Computed tomographic detection of pelvic and inguinal lymph node metastases from primary and recurrent pelvic malignant disease. *Radiology* 1980;137:157–166.

7 Respiratory System

For many years, the only means of evaluating the respiratory tract had been plain film radiography, tomography, and radiopaque contrast examinations such as bronchography and laryngography. Gradually radionuclide studies were added to the diagnostic armamentarium of the radiologist, and in recent years ultrasound has been found useful as well. However, computerized tomography (CT) has become the primary examination for evaluation of thoracic disease following the initial chest radiograph.

INFLAMMATORY DISEASE

Uncomplicated pulmonary parenchymal disease is most effectively and economically diagnosed utilizing the plain posteroanterior and lateral chest radiograph. However, in the more complicated cases other modalities may be necessary to supplement information obtained on the chest film. The noninvasive imaging modalities have become utilized widely in these circumstances.

Nuclear Medicine

Pulmonary ventilation scanning utilizing xenon and perfusion scans with technetium macroaggregates are useful in helping to assess pulmonary function prior to proposed thoracotomy for chronic inflammatory disease such as tuberculosis or bronchiectasis. These studies can also be used to determine whether pulmonary function of the nonresect-

93

ed portions of the lungs is capable of sustaining the patient following thoracotomy for either carcinoma, tuberculosis, or emphysematous bullae.[2]

Ultrasound

Many inflammatory parenchymal processes are associated with pleural effusions, either free or loculated in nature. Ultrasound is a useful technique both to detect the loculated fluid (Fig. 7-1) as well as to localize the collection for thoracentesis.

Computerized Tomography

CT is not necessary in patients with parenchymal disease except in selected instances. CT can help detect endobronchial obstructing lesions in patients with chronic localized infections for whom other causes have been excluded. It is also quite useful in differentiating lung abscess from empyema and directing percutaneous drainage of pleural and mediastinal collections (Figs. 7-2 and 7-3).

PULMONARY EMBOLUS

Pulmonary embolus is a common clinical problem with frequent dire consequences and has remained a very difficult condition to diagnose clinically. The chest radiograph is usually of little assistance, either appearing normal or showing nonspecific findings such as atelectasis or lo-

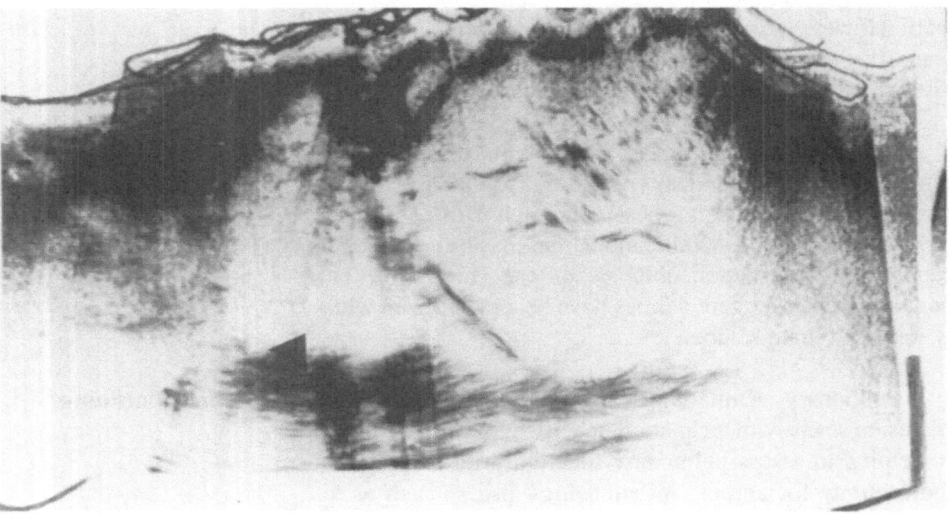

Figure 7-1. Large sonolucent collection representing right pleural effusion (arrow).

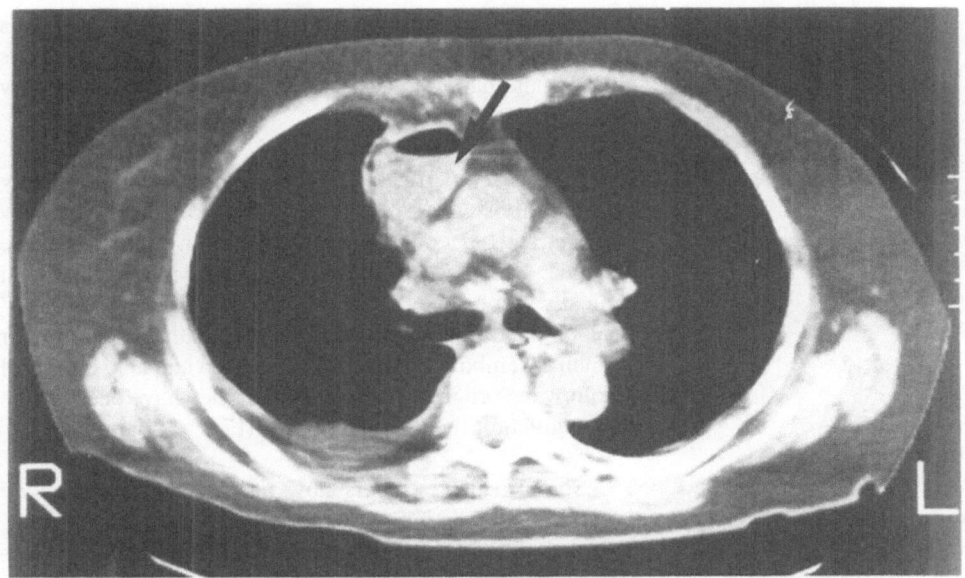

Figure 7-2. Anterior mediastinal mass with air–fluid level representing mediastinal abscess (arrow).

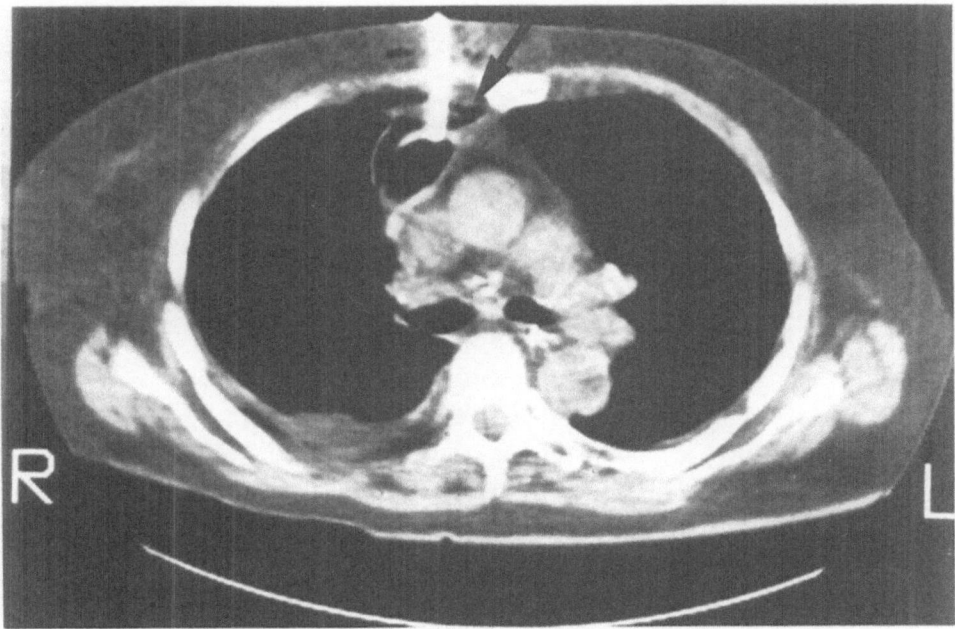

Figure 7-3. Von Sonnenberg drain inserted into abscess (arrow) with decreased pus accumulation.

calized infiltrate. Pulmonary contrast angiography remains the definitive diagnostic modality. However, this study is invasive and has a small, but real, morbidity and mortality rate associated with it.

Nuclear Medicine

Pulmonary perfusion and ventilation scans have very high sensitivity and specificity in diagnosis of pulmonary embolus and, in conjunction with a plain radiograph, are now the screening procedure of choice in patients with clinically suspected emboli.[1] A perfusion defect in the presence of a normal ventilation scan is pathognomonic for pulmonary embolus (Fig. 7-4). This scan can also be useful to follow the progress of patients after they have been put on anticoagulation therapy for emboli (Figs. 7-5 and 7-6).

Computerized Tomography

Some medical centers now utilize contrast-enhanced dynamic CT scanning to evaluate the presence of pulmonary emboli; however, this technique has not gained widespread acceptance owing to the increased cost, radiation, and necessity for utilization of iodinated contrast material.

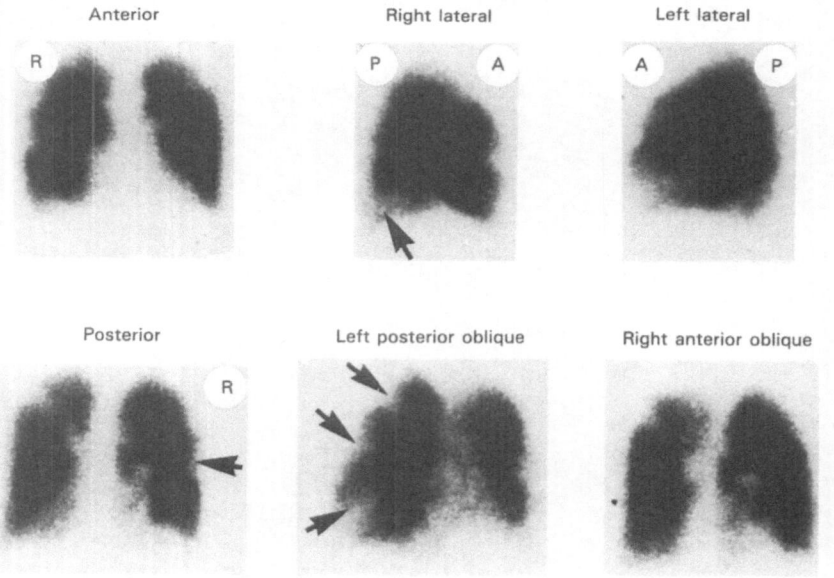

Figure 7-4. Focal wedge-shaped perfusion defects (arrows) in patient with pulmonary emboli.

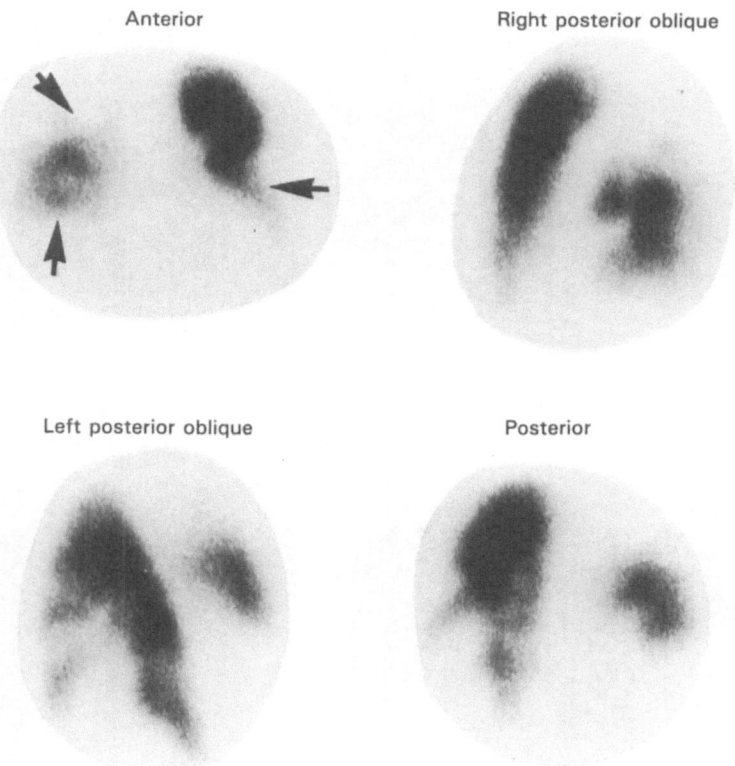

Anterior   Right posterior oblique

Left posterior oblique   Posterior

Figure 7-5. Multiple large perfusion defects (arrows) representing extensive emboli.

LUNG NEOPLASM (PRIMARY)

Primary neoplasms of the lung were originally detected utilizing chest radiographs and locally staged utilizing tomography or angiography. The radiograph remains the primary screening procedure for detection of lung masses; however, CT has taken over the role of staging the tumors both preoperatively and postoperatively to evaluate the possibility of recurrence.

Computerized Tomography

CT is the procedure of choice for evaluating pulmonary and parenchymal masses following their original detection on plain radiograph. The presence or absence of calcification can fairly easily be determined. Mediastinal or pleural infiltration by the tumor is easily detected, as is

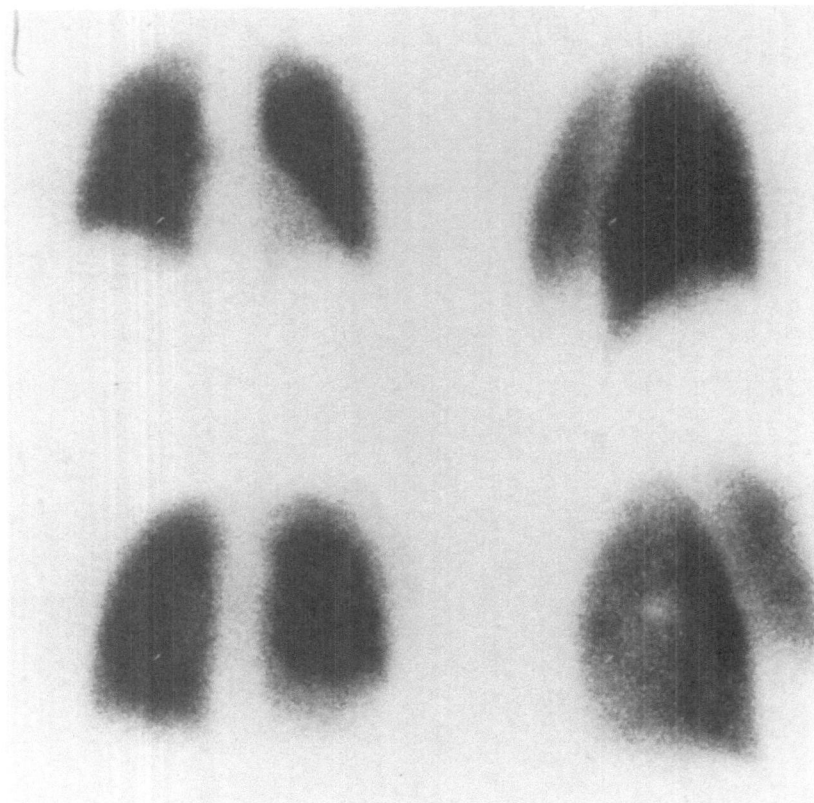

Figure 7-6. Relatively normal perfusion scan following anticoagulation therapy.

invasion of vital organs such as pulmonary arteries, aorta, esophagus, or superior vena cava (Fig. 7-7).[6] The presence of hilar or mediastinal lymphadenopathy is well documented. Pleural-based nodules associated with a primary lesion can be detected. In equivocal cases CT-directed biopsy allows cytologic aspiration of lesions. CT is also the method of choice for postoperative or other therapeutic follow-up in patients following treatment for known lung neoplasms.

Radionuclide Studies   In patients with known malignancy who are being considered for resection, perfusion and ventilation studies may be utilized to evaluate the functions of the lungs prior to thoracotomy.

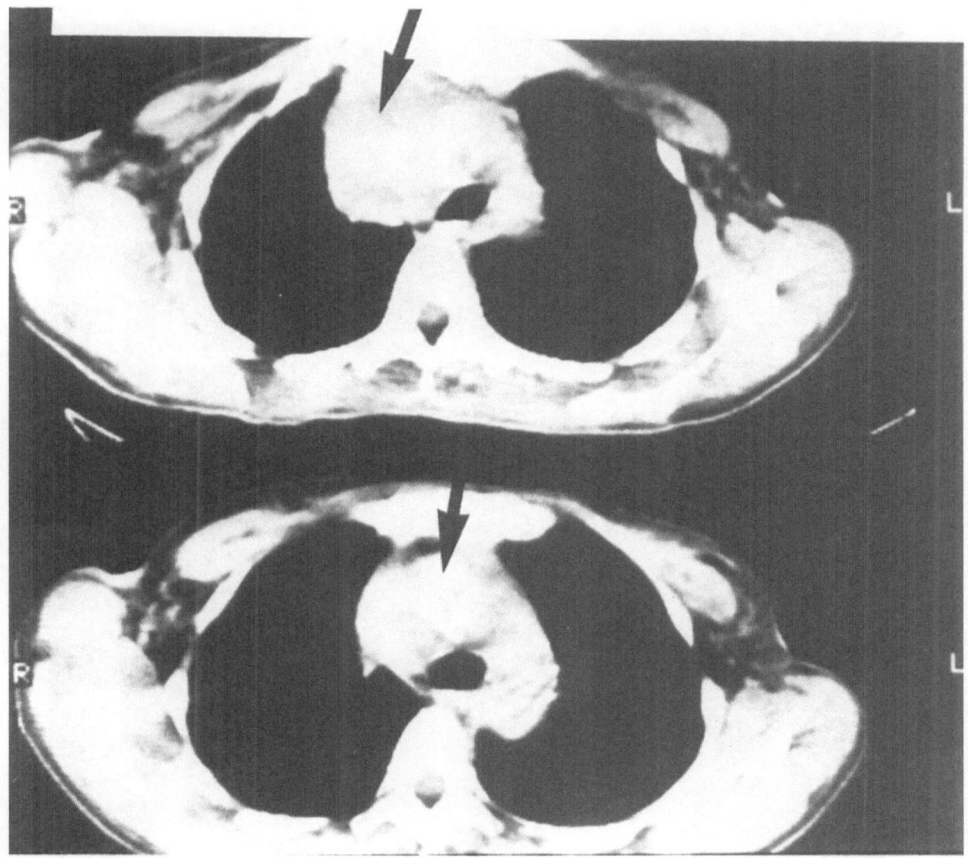

Figure 7-7. Large anterior mediastinal mass (arrow) compressing superior vena cava.

Occasionally gallium scanning may be useful in the detection of hilar or mediastinal nodes (Figs. 7-8 and 7-9). This study, however, is less sensitive than CT and is usually utilized in institutions without CT scanners.

CT has virtually replaced plain-film tomography in the evaluation of patients with extrapulmonary tumors that frequently metastasize to the lungs such as melanoma, breast tumors, and bone or soft tissue sarcomas. Computerized tomography is capable of detecting far more parenchymal and subpleural nodules than plain-film tomography (Fig. 7-10).[5]

PULMONARY METASTASES

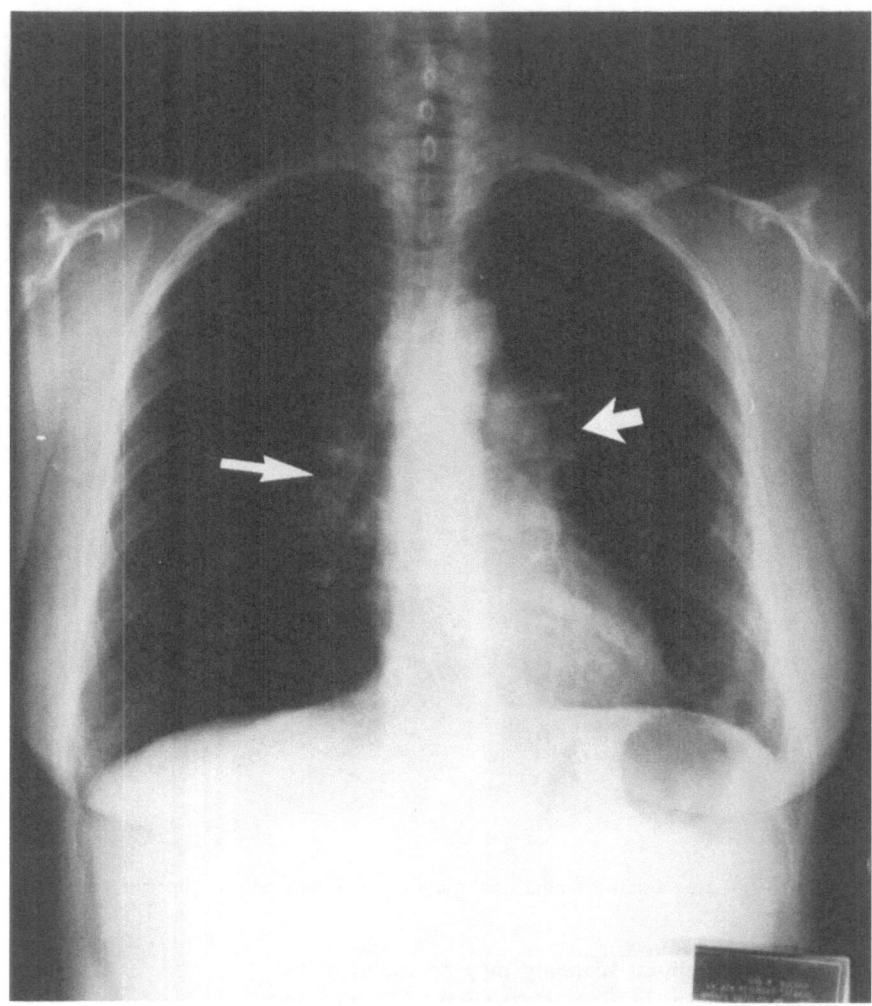

Figure 7-8. Enlarged paratracheal and hilar nodes (arrows) in patient with sarcoid.

THE WIDENED MEDIASTINUM AND MEDIASTINAL MASS

The widened mediastinum on plain chest radiography in the past had been evaluated utilizing plain-film tomography or other contrast examinations such as barium swallow or angiography. However, many patients underwent thoracotomies for mediastinal widening that ultimately proved to be based on increased fat deposition or tortuosity of the great vessels. CT has been most effective in alleviating these problems.[3]

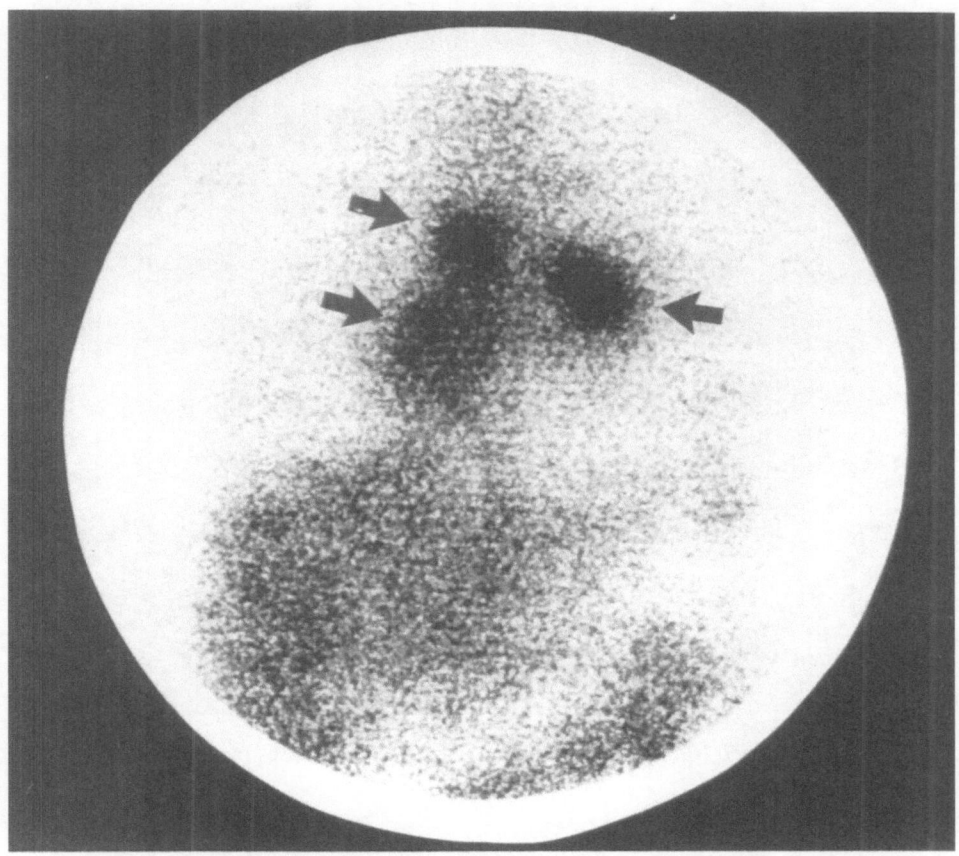

Figure 7-9. Gallium accumulation in lymph nodes (arrows) in same patient.

Computerized Tomography

Because of its excellent soft tissue contrast discrimination, CT has been an effective means of differentiating benign mediastinal widening, such as that produced by mediastinal lipomatosis or tortuous vessels, from actual mediastinal masses (Fig. 7-11). In the presence of an abnormal mediastinal mass, the presence or absence of calcification can be ascertained as well as the vascularity of the lesion. Involvement of adjacent organs and presence of multiple lesions can readily be detected. CT-directed percutaneous biopsy can be performed. CT is also useful in evaluating patients in whom the radiograph appears normal but a thymic tumor,[4] lymphadenopathy, or parathyroid adenoma is strongly suspected clinically. In patients being treated for

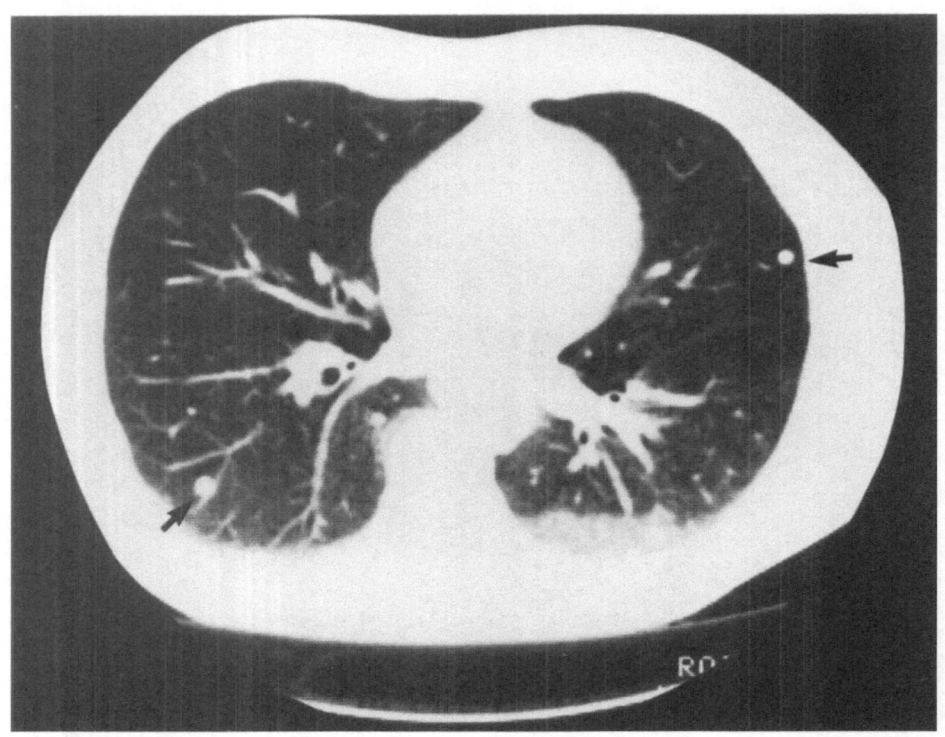

Figure 7-10. Multiple peripheral pulmonary metastases (arrows).

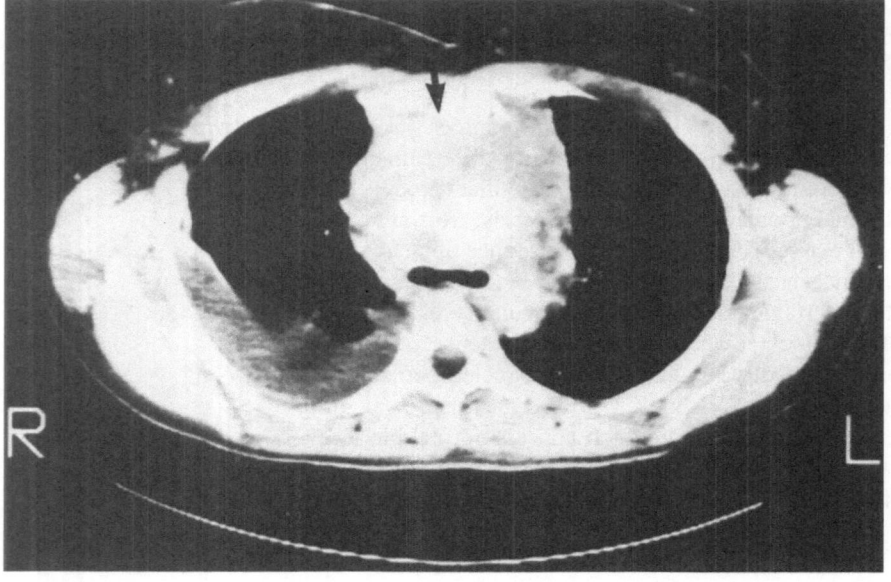

Figure 7-11. Extensive anterior mediastinal mass in patient with lymphoma (arrow).

mediastinal malignancy, serial scans following therapy are easily obtained to evaluate progression or regression of disease.

1. Biello DR, Mattar AG, McKnight RC: Ventilation perfusion studies in suspected pulmonary embolism. *Am J Roentgenol* 1979;133:1033–1039.
2. Boysen PG, et al. Prospective evaluation for pneumonectomy using the 99m Tc quantitative perfusion lung scan. *Chest* 1977;72:422.
3. Larde D, Bellar C, Vasile N, et al: Computed tomography of aortic dissection. *Radiology* 1980;136:147–151.
4. Moore AV, Korobkin M, Powers B, et al: Thymoma detection by mediastinal CT: Patients with myasthenia gravis. *Am J Radiol* 1982;138:217–222.
5. Muhm JR, Brown LR, Crowe JR: Comparison of whole lung tomography and computed tomography for detecting pulmonary nodules. *Am J Radiol* 1978;131:981–984.
6. Rea HH, Sherland JE, House AJS: Accuracy of computed tomographic scanning in assessment of the mediastinum in bronchial carcinoma. *J Thorac Cardiovasc Surg* 1981;81:823–829.

8   Cardiovascular System

Prior to the institution of newer imaging modalities, the diagnosis and evaluation of congenital heart disease was restricted to plain radiographic techniques and contrast angiographic studies. The introduction of nuclear imaging for physiologic information and cross-sectional anatomic studies utilizing ultrasound, computerized tomography (CT), and nuclear medicine has enabled the radiologist to make earlier diagnoses in often critically ill patients with utilization of less invasive procedures.

CARDIAC DISEASE

Congenital Heart Disease

The radionuclide angiogram is often useful as an ancillary procedure in evaluation of congenital heart disease and may be useful following surgical repair. This is a simple method for evaluating patients with intracardiac shunts (Fig. 8-1) and other anatomic anomalies. Postoperative evaluation following closure of shunts and corrections of transposition can also be easily evaluated. It is a relatively inexpensive, quick, and safe procedure. In patients with known congenital valvular disease, the gated heart study can determine the approximate regurgitant fraction as well as provide evaluation of size and wall motion of the ventricles as well as the atria.

Radionuclide Study

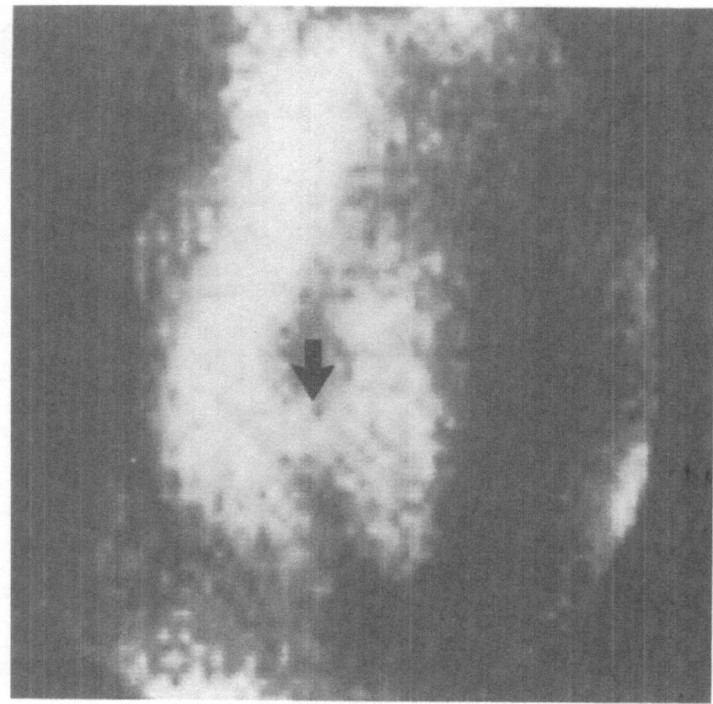

Figure 8-1. Large posttraumatic ventriculoseptal defect (arrow) on gated cardiac study.

Echocardiography

Owing to the excellent cross-sectional anatomic display of structures and lack of ionizing radiation, two-dimensional echocardiography has provided a significant contribution to the noninvasive evaluation of congenital heart defects (Fig. 8-2), often providing the definitive anatomic diagnosis. It is of particular value in defining septal defects, positional anomalies of the great vessels, and atrial ventricular valves. Structures such as coronary arteries, interatrial septum, aortic arch, pulmonary artery bifurcation, vena cava (Figs. 8-3 and 8-4) and pulmonary veins can often be recognized.[2]

Radionuclide Scan

The original procedure devised for this purpose was the myocardial pyrophosphate scan, which was useful in patients with atypical chest pain, nondiagnostic electrocardiogram, and nondiagnostic enzyme changes. It has a high sensitivity for acute transmural infarct within 72 hr of the event and a lesser degree for subendocardial infarct.[5]

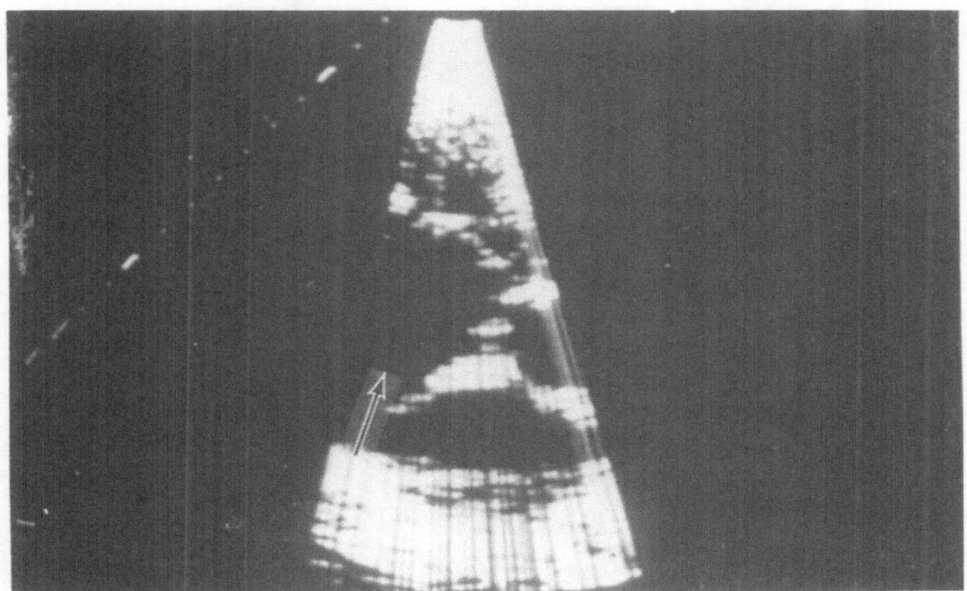

Figure 8-2. Apical view demonstrating huge right atrium (arrow) in patient with Ebstein's malformation.

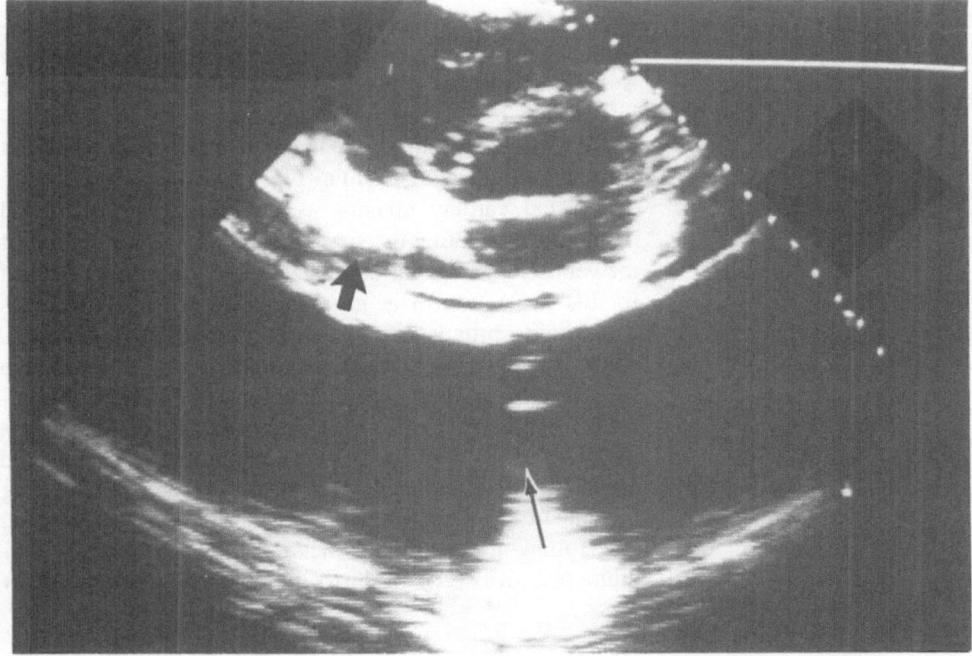

Figure 8-3. Left superior vena cava (arrow) entering right atrium. Incidental finding of large pericardial effusion (longer arrow).

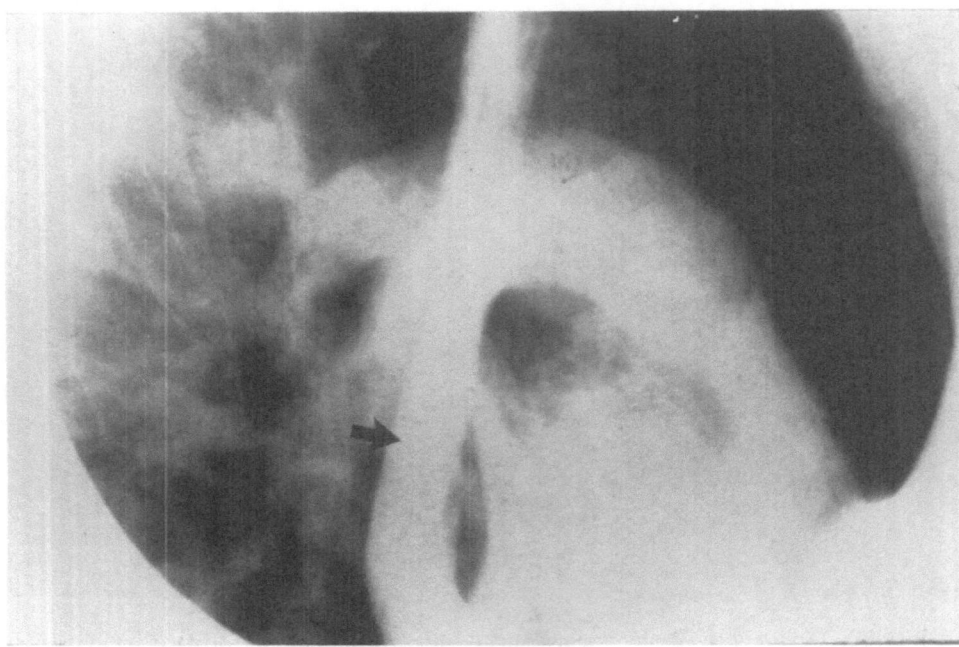

Figure 8-4. Left lateral view of angiogram confirming presence of persistent left superior vena cava (arrow).

Thallium scans performed at rest were useful for detecting and sizing myocardial infarcts (Fig. 8-5). The study is limited because it does not distinguish between acute infarct and old scarring. The thallium stress test and redistribution study will enable the distinction of actual infarct from stress-induced ischemia (Figs. 8-6 and 8-7).

Gated cardiac imaging is an accurate, fairly rapid method of evaluating the size, wall motion, and function of the ventricles as well as atrial size.[8] The procedure is useful for the evaluation of acute myocardial infarcts insofar as determining prognosis and extension to the inferior wall. Right ventricular infarct and valvular regurgitation can also be evaluated. Patients in intractable heart failure in the intensive care and cardiac care units can be evaluated with portable cameras. Ventricular aneurysms may be detected and followed after medical or surgical therapy. Coupling the gated heart study with exercise will aid in the detection and follow-up of organic heart disease, especially cardiomyopathies, valvular heart disease, and coronary artery

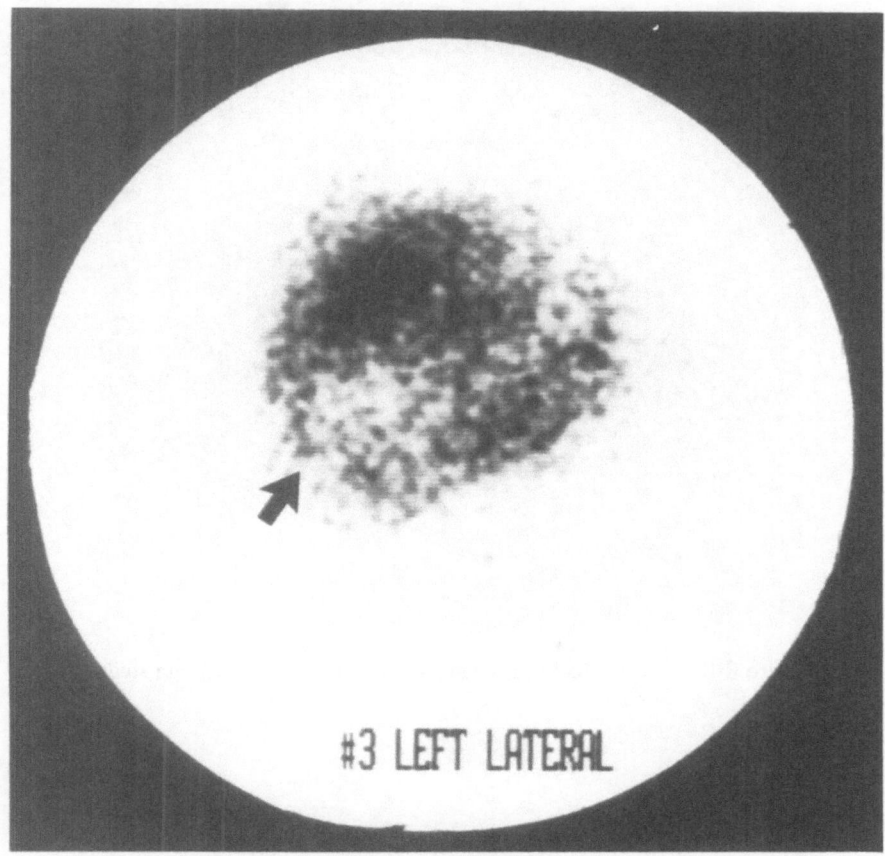

Figure 8-5. Myocardial infarct involving anteroinferior wall (arrow) demonstrated on resting thallium study.

disease.[1] The test measures physiologic response of the ventricular chambers to stress as well as changes in ejection fraction with increasing exercise loads or following utilization of chemotherapeutic agents such as Adriamycin.

Ultrasound

Two-dimensional echocardiography has found increasing utilization in the study of regional cardiac function such as the qualitative and quantitative evaluation of ventricular wall motion. Wall thickening can be detected. Infarct sizes can be estimated. Coronary arteries can be directly visualized. Complications of ischemic heart disease and acute myocardial infarcts can be detected such as papillary muscle

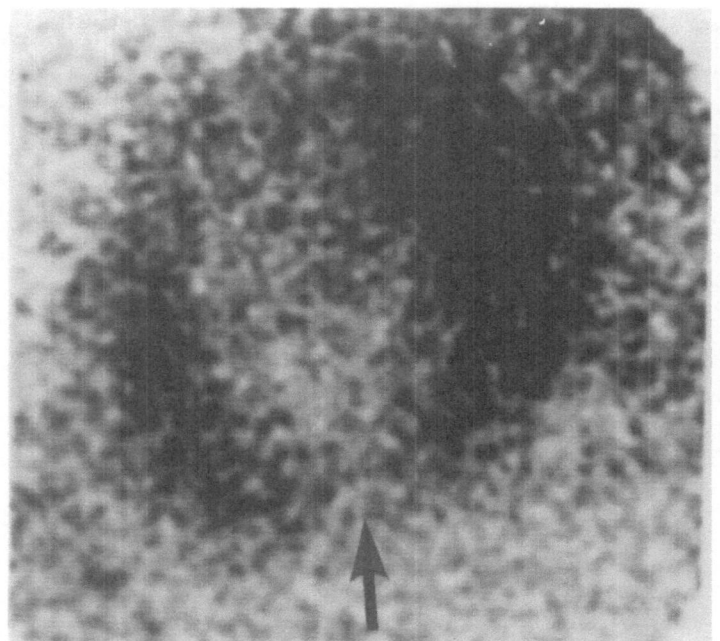

Figure 8-6. Apical defect (arrow) demonstrated on stress thallium study.

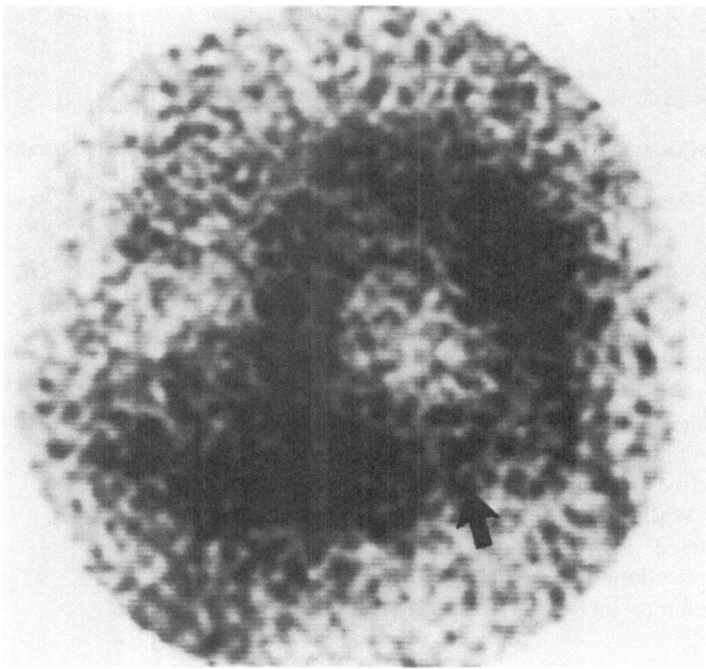

Figure 8-7. Apical defect of Fig. 6 reperfuses on resting image (arrow) compatible with stress-induced ischemia.

dysfunction, ventricular septal rupture (Fig. 8-8), ventricular aneurysms (Fig. 8-9), or left ventricular thrombus.[10]

Coronary artery disease, a common disabling disease, has often been difficult to detect radiographically owing to the often normal-appearing chest radiograph; this necessitates use of coronary angiography, which carries a fairly significant morbidity and mortality rate. Although coronary angiography and cardiac ventriculography remains the procedure of choice, radionuclide procedures supplemented by echocardiography have developed as inexpensive, noninvasive, fairly sensitive screening modalities.

Ischemic Heart Disease

The evaluation of patients with valvular disease, either congenital or postinflammatory (rheumatic heart disease, subacute bacterial endocarditis), had previously been largely based on clinical parameters, radiographic findings,

Valvular Disease

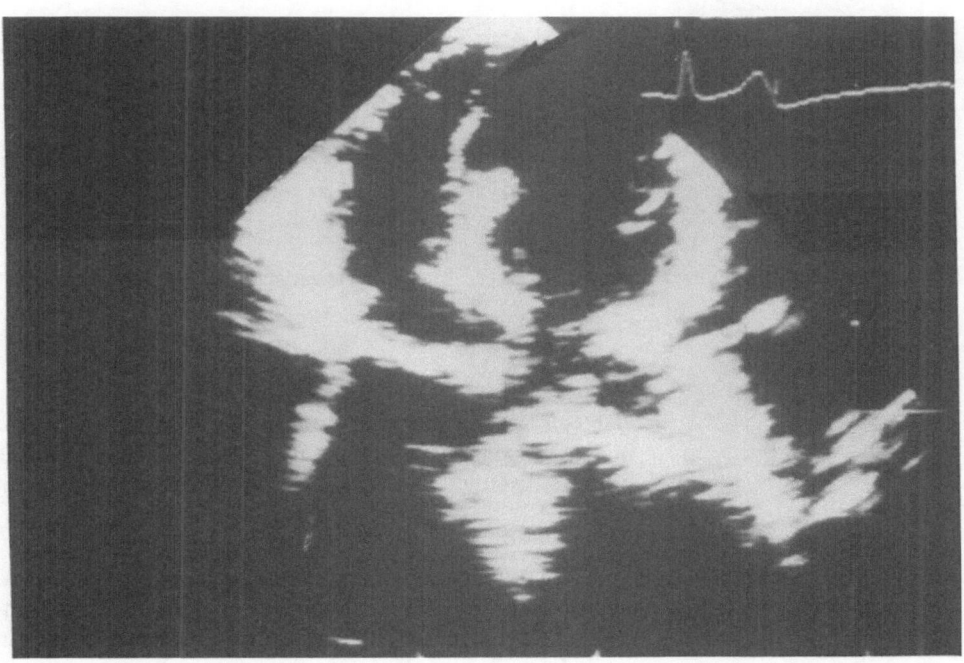

Figure 8-8. Modified four-chamber view demonstrating posttraumatic ventriculoseptal defect (arrow) (same case as in Fig. 2).

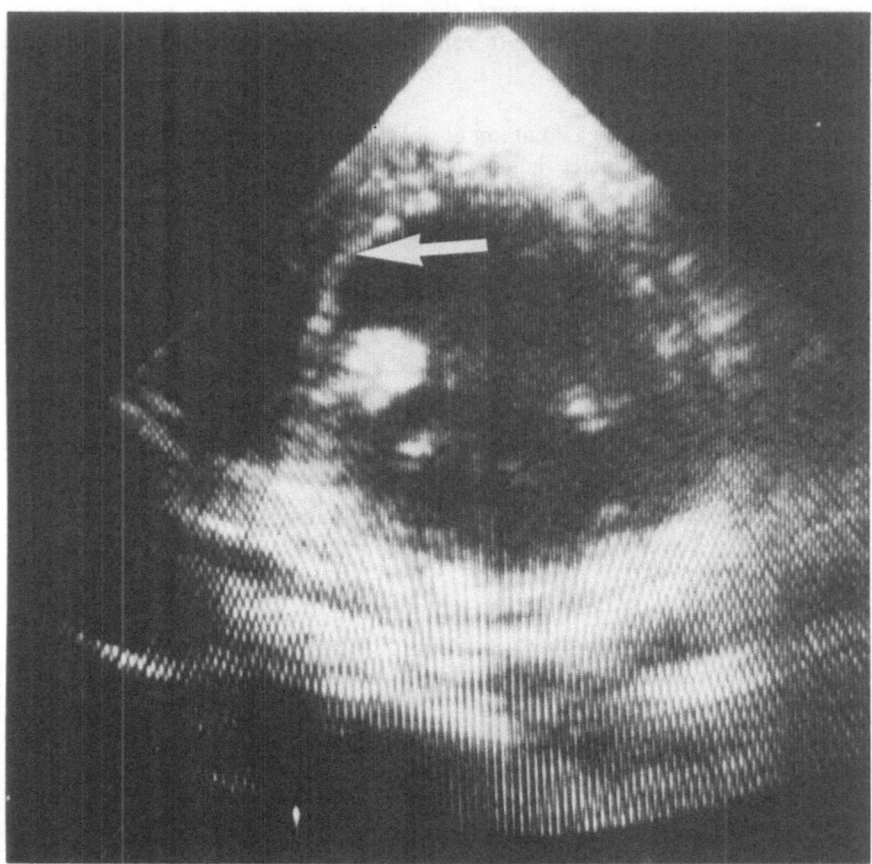

Figure 8-9. Short-axis view demonstrating large, thin-walled aneurysm involving interventricular septum (arrow).

and contrast angiographic procedures. Use of the newer imaging modalities has markedly facilitated early diagnosis of these disorders and earlier and more effective treatment (Fig. 8-10).

Ultrasound The primary noninvasive imaging modality for evaluation of valvular disease is two-dimensional echocardiography. The diagnosis of valvular stenosis or insufficiency can easily be made as well as detection of the subsequent effects of these lesions on the cardiac chambers. Vegetations on the valves are easily detected and distinguished from thrombus

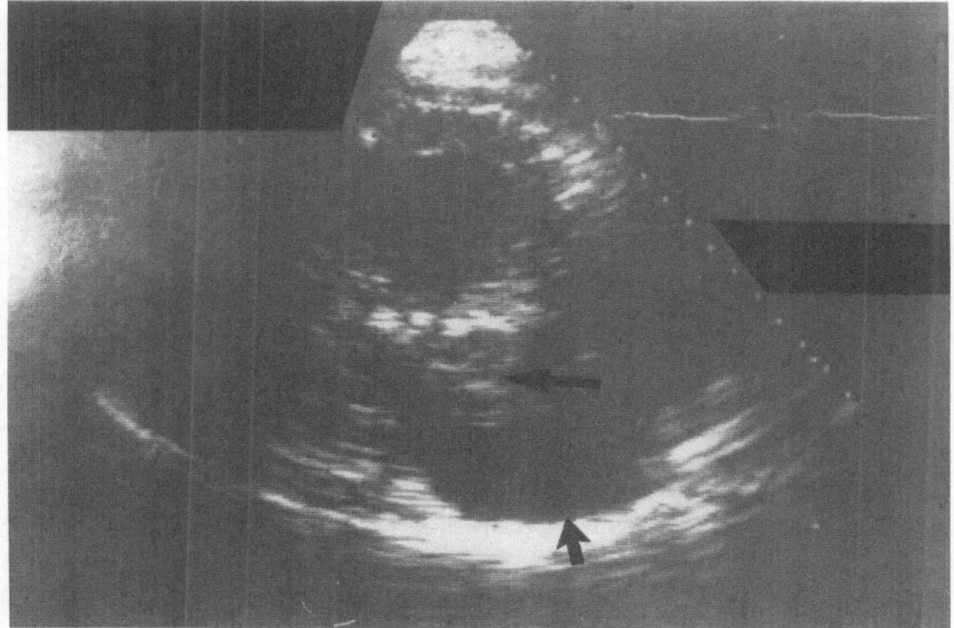

Figure 8-10. Short-axis view showing *Escherichia coli* abscess (arrow) following atrioventricular valve replacement with accompanying effusion (arrowhead).

or tumor such as atrial myxoma (Figs. 8-11 and 8-12). Postoperatively, patients with valve prosthesis can be evaluated.[6]

Primary and Secondary Cardiomyopathy

In many instances, the clinical differentiation between diffuse ischemic heart disease and cardiomyopathy has been a difficult task. The use of radionuclide scans and echocardiography has significantly facilitated making the clinical diagnoses.

Radionuclide Scan

The gated cardiac study has been useful in detecting ischemic cardiac disease and localizing the disease to a specific vessel as determined by the focal areas of decreased wall motion. The patient afflicted with a cardiomyopathy will usually demonstrate an enlarged heart with a more diffuse hypokinesis of the ventricular chamber walls as well as exhibiting coexistent atrial enlargement.

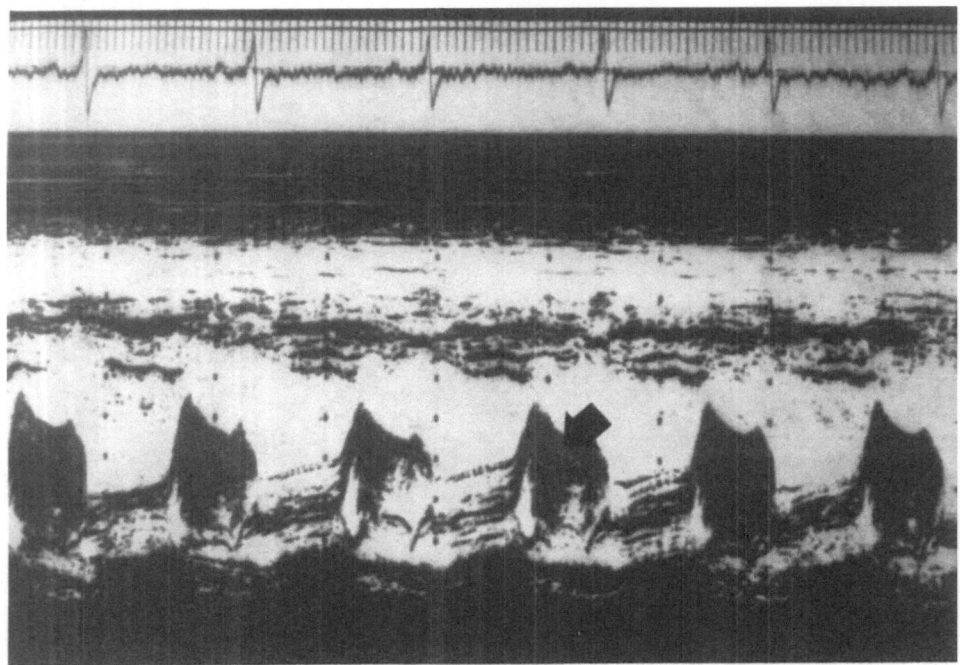

Figure 8-11. M-mode echocardiogram demonstrating large atrial myxoma (arrow) attached to mitral valve.

Ultrasound

Over the past several years echocardiography has shown increasing utilization in recognizing various cardiomyopathies and assessing them anatomically as well as functionally. The basic subgroups of cardiomyopathies (dilated, hypertrophic, restrictive) may be differentiated, and the degree of global or regional myocardial function can be assessed. In the proper clinical settings, occasionally secondary cardiomyopathies such as amyloidosis,[9] glycogen storage disease, and Fabry's disease can be recognized and characterized without resorting to the invasive myocardial biopsy.

Pericardial Disease

The diagnosis of pericardial disease has previously been limited to plain radiographs, contrast angiography, and iatrogenic pneumopericardium prior to introduction of the newer, less invasive procedures.

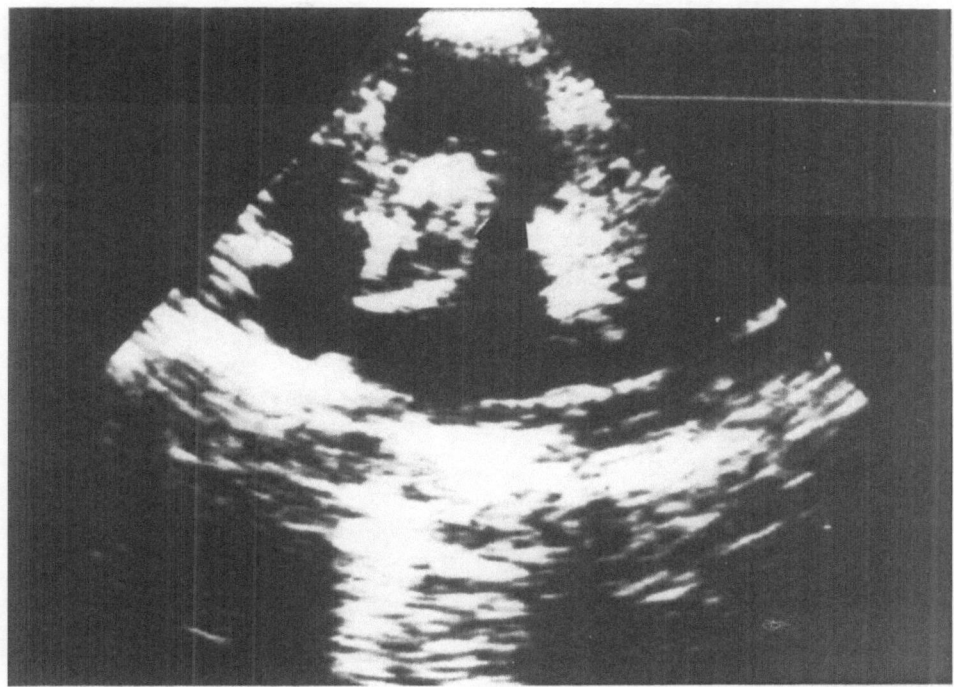

Figure 8-12. Modified four-chamber view demonstrating large myxoma (arrow) prolapsing through mitral valve.

Radionuclide Study

Static blood pool imaging utilizing dynamic radionuclide angiography has proven useful in the diagnosis of pericardial effusion although this study is limited to relatively larger collections than those detected by ultrasound or CT.[11]

Ultrasound

Echocardiography is the cheapest, least invasive means of detecting and quantitating pericardial effusions (Figs. 8-13 to 8-15). Cardiac tamponade, pericardial thickening, and constriction can also be detected without the utilization of intravenous contrast or ionizing radiation.[3]

Computerized Tomography

CT can be used to supplement or complement sonography when diagnostic problems arise. It may prove beneficial in patients requiring evaluation following thoracic surgery, when pleural effusions are present, and in the diag-

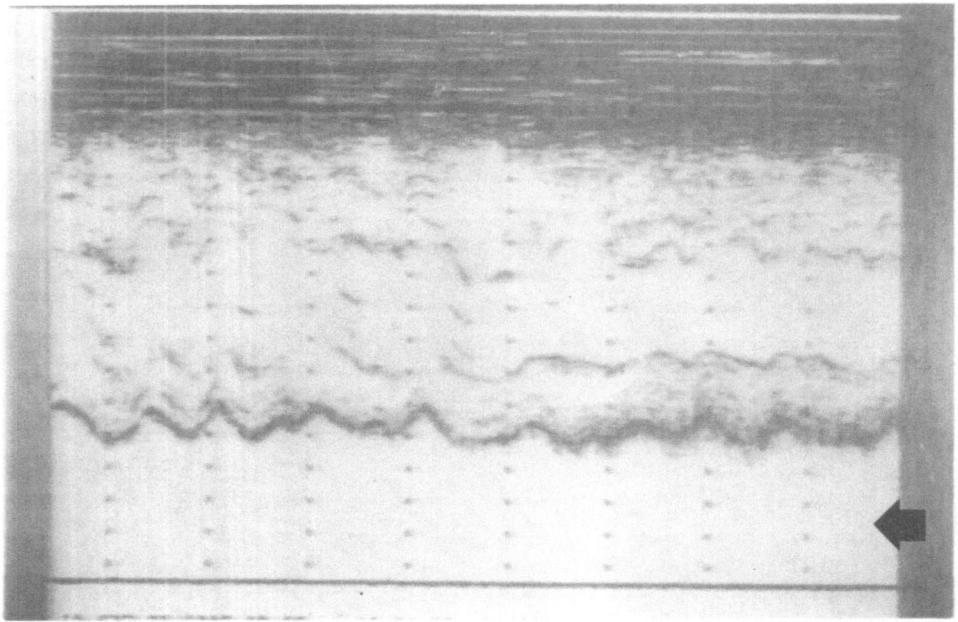

Figure 8-13. M-mode echocardiogram demonstrating large, posterior pericardial fluid collection (arrow).

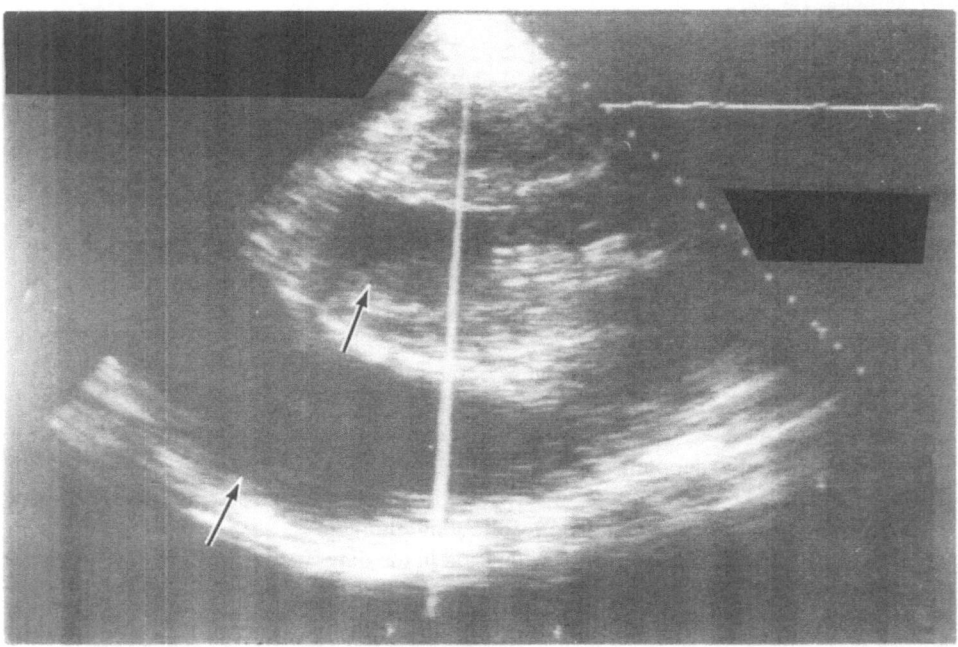

Figure 8-14. Long-axis view demonstrating left ventricular hypertrophy (arrow) in renal patient with large pericardial effusion (arrowhead).

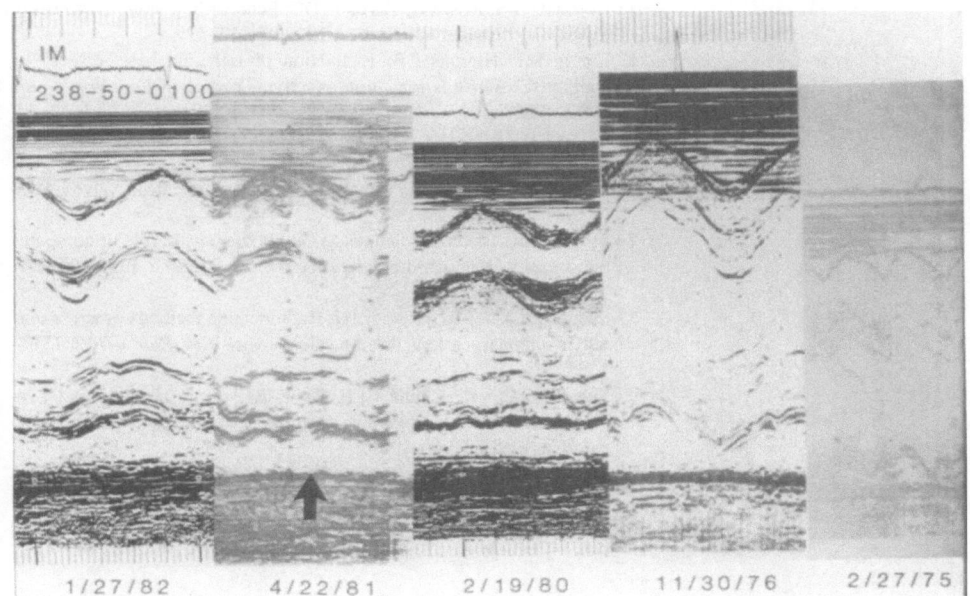

Figure 8-15. Serial M-mode echocardiograms demonstrating patient with idiopathic asymptomatic pericardial effusion (arrow). Figs. 1–4 and 8–15 are courtesy of Dr. Michael Goldman, Cardiology Department, Jewish Hospital, Louisville, Kentucky.

nosis of loculated pericardial effusions. The presence of a thickened pericardium can help distinguish a restrictive from infiltrative cardiomyopathy such as that produced by amyloidosis. CT is also an excellent tool for diagnosis of neoplastic pericardial disease, which usually manifests as an exudative effusion with plaquelike thickening or nodular masses localized to the pericardium.[7]

In some centers, CT has proven useful in quantitating the size of myocardial infarcts and detecting regional myocardial ischemia by alteration in wall thickening or wall dynamics utilizing cardiac gating.[4] Left ventricular aneurysms can be detected. One can also evaluate the patency of a coronary bypass graft utilizing CT.

Ischemic Heart Disease

Computerized Tomography

REFERENCES

1. Berger HJ, Zaret BL: Nuclear cardiology. *N. Engl J Med* 1981;305:799–807.
2. Feigenbaum H: *Congenital Heart Disease in Echocardiography*, ed. 3. Philadelphia, Lea & Febiger, 1981, p 352.

3. Horowitz MS, Rosen R, Harrison DC: Echocardiographic diagnosis of pericardial disease. *Am Heart J* 1979;97:420–427.
4. Lipton MJ, Higgins CB: Evaluation of ischemic heart disease by computed transmission tomography. *Radiol Clin North Am* 1980;18:557–576.
5. Lyons KP, Olson HG, Aronow WS: Pyrophosphate myocardial imaging. *Semin Nucl Med* 1980;10:168–177.
6. Mehlman DJ: Ultrasonic visualization of prosthetic heart valves. *Semin Ultrasound* 1981;2:134–142.
7. Moncada R, Baker M, Salinas M, et al: Diagnostic role of computed tomography in pericardial heart disease. *Am Heart J* 1982;100:263–282.
8. Sands MJ, Zaret BL, Berger HJ: Radionuclide methods of stress testing in coronary artery disease. *Cardiovasc Rev Rep* 1976;3:1317–1338.
9. Siqueira-Filho A, Cunha CLP, Tajik AJ, et al: M-mode and two-dimensional echocardiographic features in cardiac amyloidosis. *Circulation* 1981;63:188–196.
10. Talano JV, Gardin JM: *Textbook of Two Dimensional Echocardiography.* New York, Grune & Stratton Inc, 1983, pp 187–202.
11. Wagner HN, McAffee JG, Mozley JM: Diagnosis of pericardial effusion by radioisotope scanning. *Arch Intern Med* 1961;108:79.

VASCULAR DISEASE

Aortic Aneurysm

Aortic aneurysms are frequently palpable clinically and visualized on plain radiographs owing to their calcification when present. The preferred study for evaluation of aneurysms is the aortogram utilizing contrast medium. However, the study is somewhat invasive and carries a significant risk of morbidity. The newer imaging procedures[1] are now replacing the aortogram as a screening study to detect and evaluate the presence of aortic aneurysms, with angiography being reserved for more precise anatomic localization and preoperative assessment.

Nuclear Medicine

Radionuclide aortography is a technically simple and reliable procedure for detection of aortic aneurysms utilizing dynamic flow studies. It is useful as a screening procedure. However, there is limited spatial resolution, and other findings such as dissection, plaque, or thrombus cannot be detected thus necessitating the need for further investigation with either ultrasound or CT.[2]

Ultrasound

Ultrasound is the procedure of choice in screening of patients for detection of abdominal aortic aneurysms (Fig. 8-16). An accurate measurement of the aortic lumen can be obtained, and the presence of clot or thrombus can be deter-

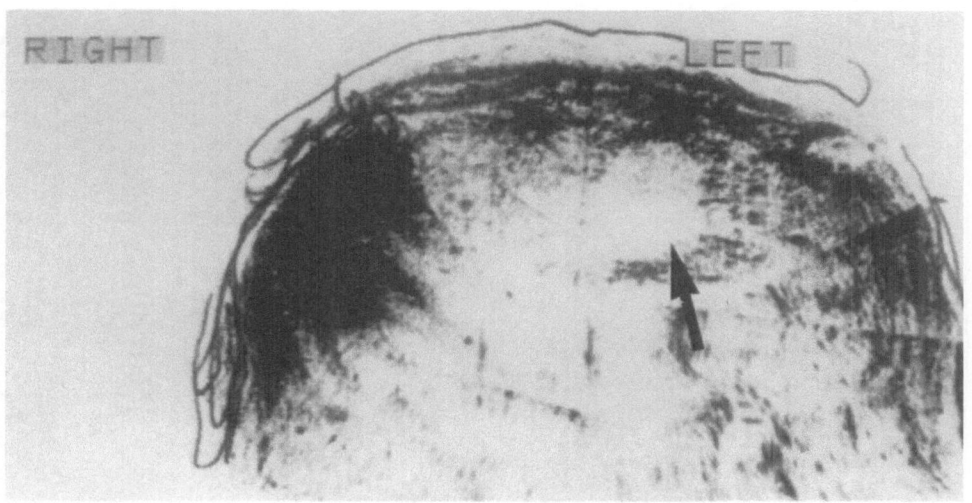

Figure 8-16. Large sonolucent mass representing abdominal aortic aneurysm (arrow).

mined.[9] Complications of aneurysms such as dissection or blood withing the abdomen can be ascertained. Localization of the aneurysm can be performed as well as detection of extension into the pelvic vessels.

CT is the screening procedure of choice for evaluation of possible thoracic aneurysms. By use of contrast enhancement, presence of dissection can be detected as demonstrated by the presence of an intimal flap (Fig. 8-17). CT is also useful in evaluation of complications resulting from aneurysmal grafts such as evaluating graft patency and the possibility of infection or leakage.[8] Although CT is a very useful means of detecting aneurysmal dissection, angiography is necessary preoperatively. Aortoiliac fistulae can also be detected utilizing CT (Figs. 8-18 and 8-19).

Computerized Tomography

Anatomic abnormalities involving the peripheral vessels such as aneurysms or pseudoaneurysms and occlusions of small vessels are best studied utilizing angiography or digital subtraction angiography. Some of the larger vessels can be studied with CT or ultrasound. Radionuclide procedures are useful in evaluating the physiologic perfusion of the extremities in patients with peripheral vascular disease.

Peripheral Vessels

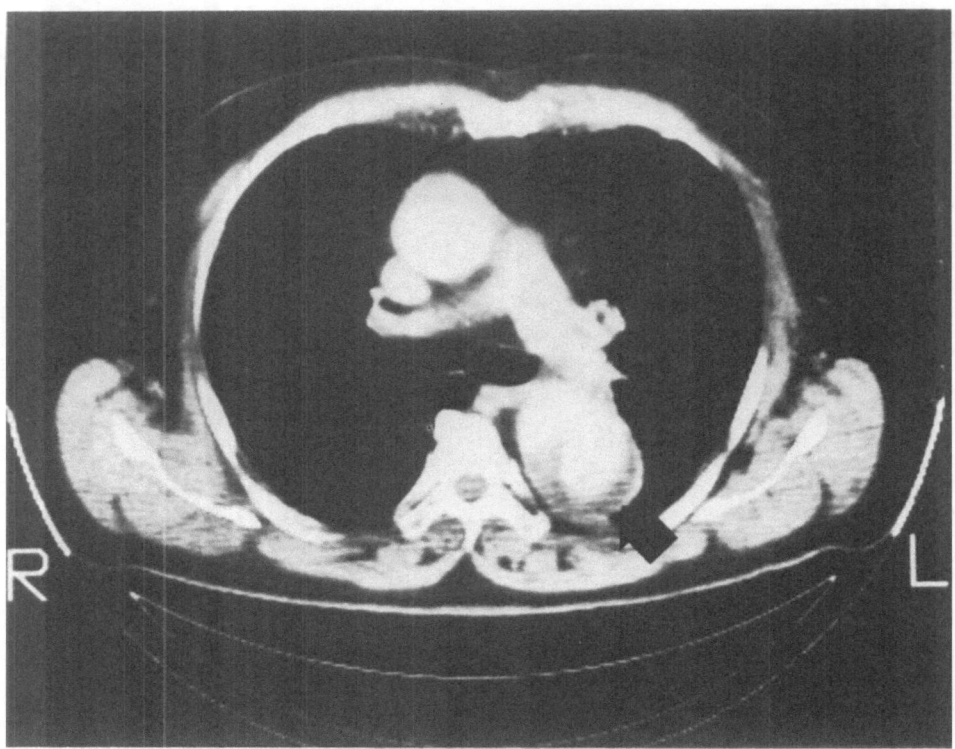

Figure 8-17. Posttraumatic dissection of thoracic aorta with false lumen (arrow).

Nuclear Medicine

Dynamic flow studies can produce useful information related to the degree of reduction of arterial flow, the presence of collateral circulation, and the efficiency of surgical intervention in peripheral arterial disease. The large vessels, such as the iliac, femoral, and subclavian arteries, are readily visualized on static images. In most cases of occlusive disease, flow images reveal the qualitative nature of abnormalities and sites of occlusion. Asymmetry of the flow between the left and right extremities can be detected. Semiquantitative measurements of flow rates can be obtained with analysis of time activity curves generated by computers utilizing tagged red blood cells. Raynaud's phenomenon can be evaluated successfully[6] as can soft tissue perfusion in patients with peripheral vascular injuries both pre- and postoperatively.[5]

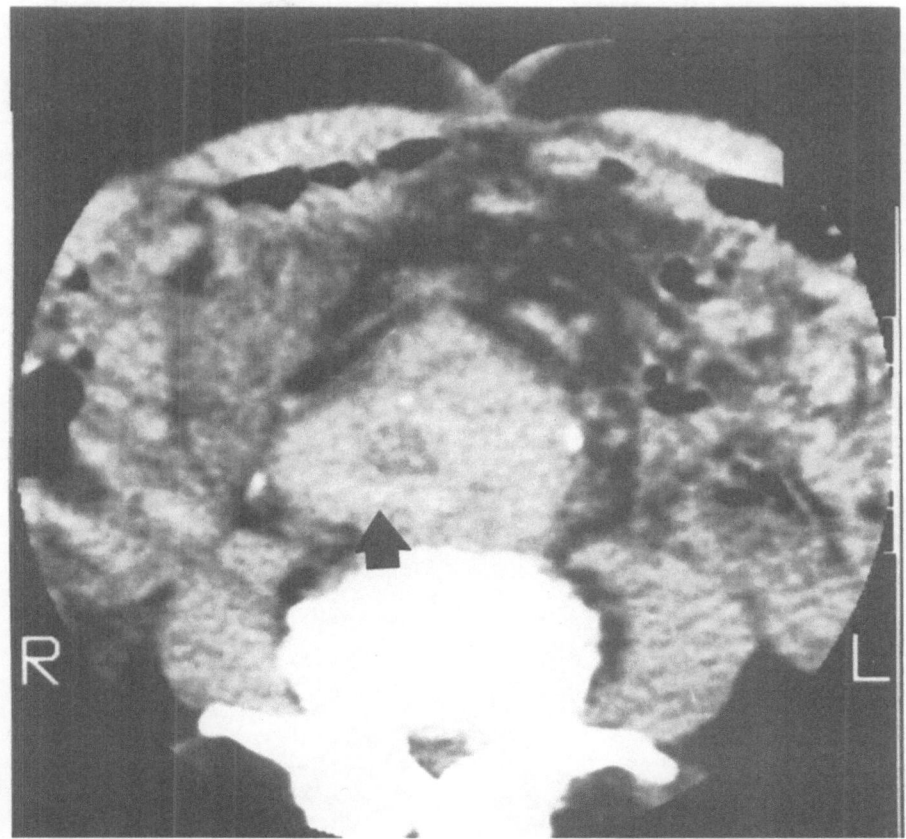

Figure 8-18. "Fused" aorta and inferior vena cava representing aortocaval fistula (arrow).

During the past 5–10 years, methods for detection of venous thrombosis have been devised utilizing the radi-oiodinated fibrinogen studies[4] and intravenous injection of technetium albumin particles. Sites of clot formation can be detected as well as the presence of collateral venous circulation. Superior vena caval obstruction can be determined in patients with suspected superior vena cava syndrome, and inferior vena caval abnormalities can be evaluated utilizing tagged albumin particles.[7]

Venous System

Nuclear Medicine

Ultrasound is a useful means of detecting the presence of a clot in the inferior vena cava in patients with pulmonary emboli. Tumor invasion of the inferior vena cava or portal

Ultrasound

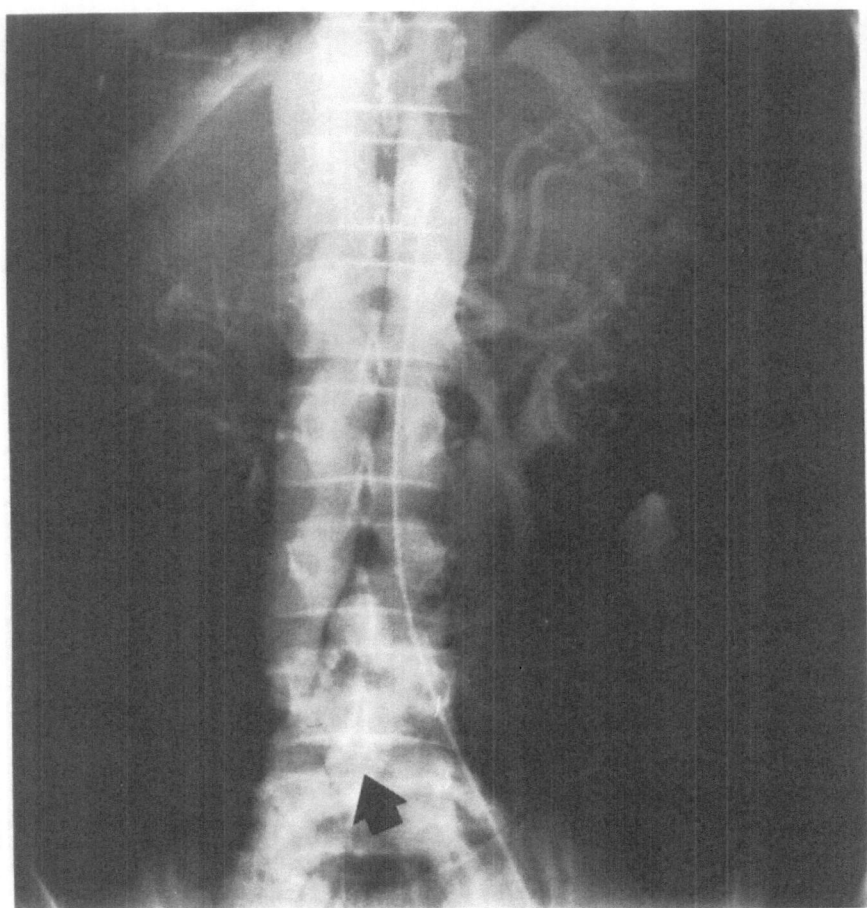

Figure 8-19. Angiogram confirming fistula.

veins can be detected in patients with hepatoma or renal cell carcinoma (Fig 8-20).[3] Congenital anomalies involving the inferior vena cava and other retroperitoneal venous structures can also be assessed. There have been reports of detection of esophageal varices in patients with portal hypertension. Splenic vein occlusion secondary to pancreatitis or pancreatic carcinoma can also be determined.

Computerized Tomography

Owing to the excellent cross-sectional anatomy provided by CT, the presence of a clot or tumor within the major retroperitoneal venous structures (Fig. 8-21) can be

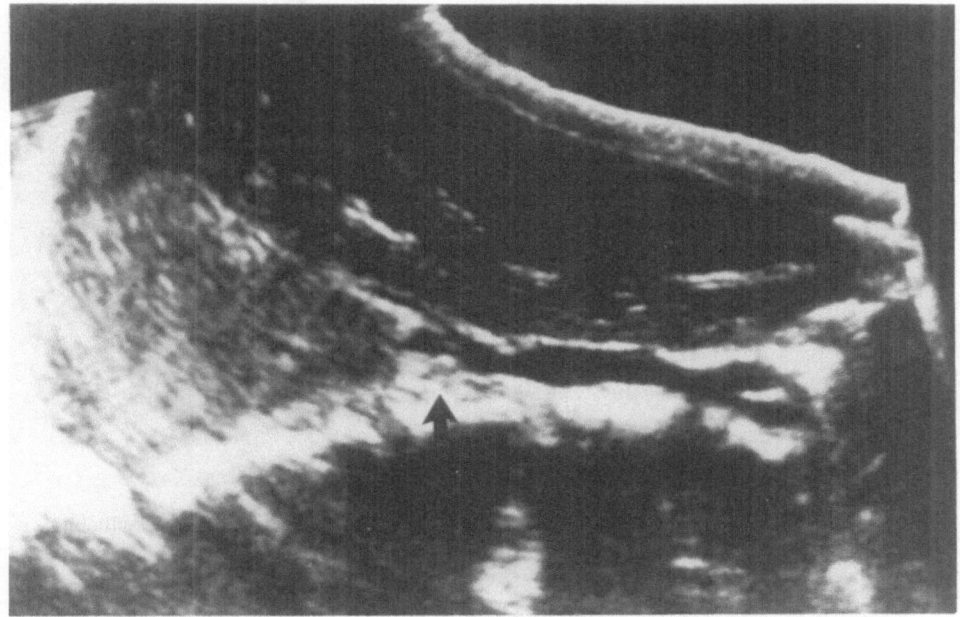

Figure 8-20. Renal cell tumor thrombus (arrow) in inferior vena cava.

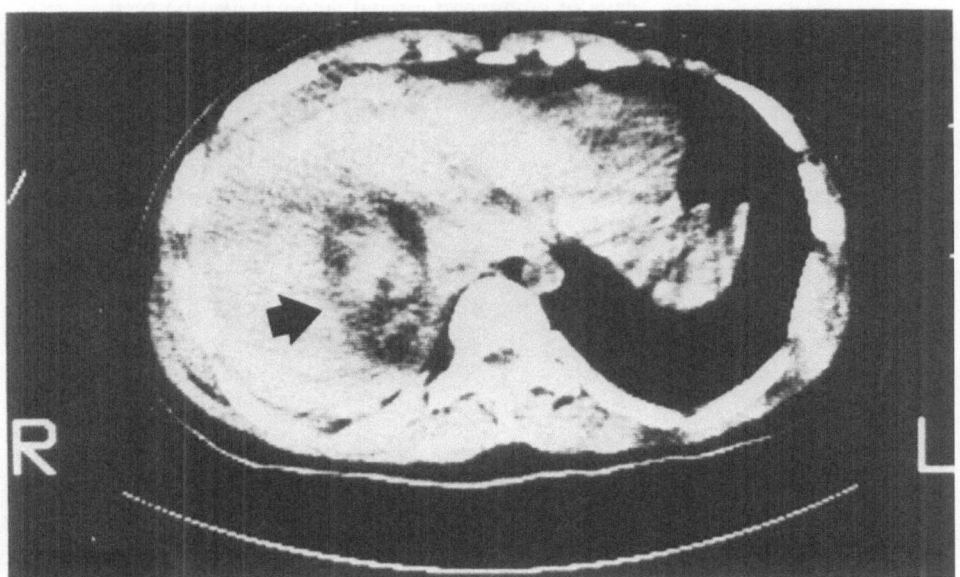

Figure 8-21. Hepatoma thrombus (arrow) in inferior vena cava.

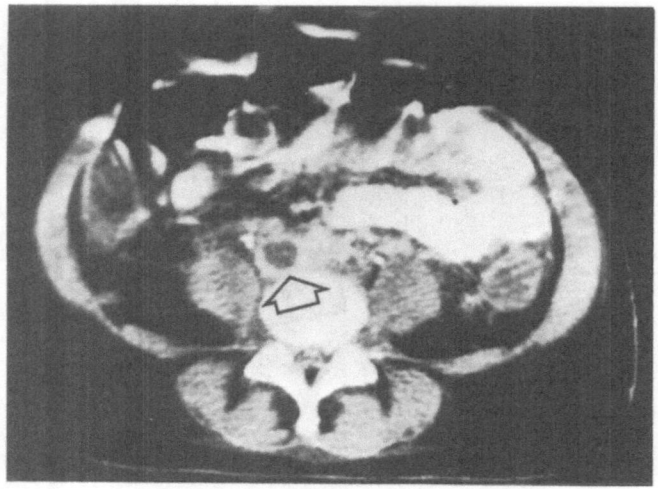

Figure 8-22. Large clot (arrow) in inferior vena cava in patient with pelvic thrombophlebitis.

evaluated.[10] Pelvic thrombophlebitis can be diagnosed utilizing intravenous contrast (Fig. 8-22). Retroperitoneal and gastroesophageal varices can also be detected (Fig. 8-23). Venous anomalies such as interruption of the inferior vena cava or circumaortic renal vein can also be seen.

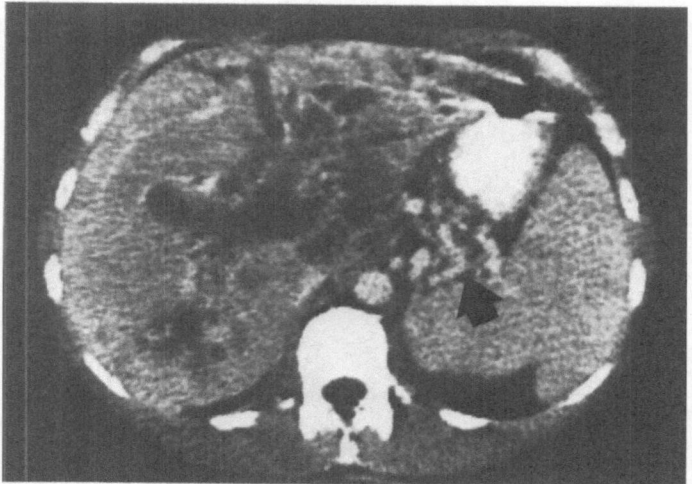

Figure 8-23. Multiple gastric varices (arrow) in patient with splenic vein obstructed by pancreatic tumor.

REFERENCES

1. Axelbaum SP, Schellinger D, Gomes MN: Computed tomographic evaluation of aortic aneurysms. *Am J Radiol* 1976;127:75–78.
2. Bergan JJ, Yao RST, Henkins RE, et al: Radionuclide aortography in the detection of arterial aneurysms. *Arch Surg* 1974;109:80–83.
3. Goldstein HM, Green B, Weaver MN: Ultrasonic detection of renal tumor extension into the inferior vena cava. *Am J Radiol* 1978;130:1083–1085.
4. Pollack EN, Webber MM, Victery W, et al: Radioisotope detection of venous thrombosis. *Arch Surg* 1975;110:613–616.
5. Rudavsky AZ, Moss CM: Radionuclide angiography for the evaluation of peripheral vascular injuries, in Freeman LM, Weissman HS (eds): *Nuclear Medicine Annual*. New York, Raven Press, 1981, pp 315–335.
6. Ryo UY, Siddiqui A, Ellman MH, et al: A study on usefulness of Tc99m RBC for an evaluation of hand blood flow in patients with Raynaud phenomenon. *J Nucl Med* 1976;17:564.
7. Ryo UY, Lee JI, Pinsky SM: Radionuclide venography in the upper extremity. *Clin Nucl Med* 1976;1:242–244.
8. Suchato C, Diedrich L: Indications of dissecting aneurysm on non-contrast CT. *J Comput Assist Tomogr* 1980;4:115–116.
9. Wheeler WE, Beachley MC, Ranniger K: Angiography and ultrasonography: A comparative study of abdominal aortic aneurysms. *Am J Radiol* 1976;126:95.
10. Zerhouni EA, Bourth KH, Siegelman SS: Demonstration of venous thrombosis by computed tomography. *Am J Radiol* 1980;134:753–758.

9   Central Nervous System

Evaluation of the central nervous system (brain and spine) was previously limited to plain skull films, tomography, and more invasive procedures such as pneumoencephalography, angiography, and venography. The advent of newer noninvasive imaging procedures has eliminated the pneumoencephalogram and restricted the utilization of contrast studies in many instances.

BRAIN

The first radiographic procedure performed in patients with suspected skull fractures or trauma to the brain is usually the plain skull series. Utilization of these films, however, has been the subject of much debate in recent times, and in many institutions they are considered unnecessary. It is now generally believed that computerized tomography (CT) is the procedure of choice in patients with recent head trauma, especially those exhibiting neurologic symptoms.

Trauma

CT is a very sensitive and specific examination for detecting the presence of extracerebral hemorrhage[12] and enabling the differentiation between subdural and epidural hemorrhage (Fig. 9-1). Intracerebral and subarachnoid hemorrhage is also easily detectable owing to the characteristic

Computerized Tomography

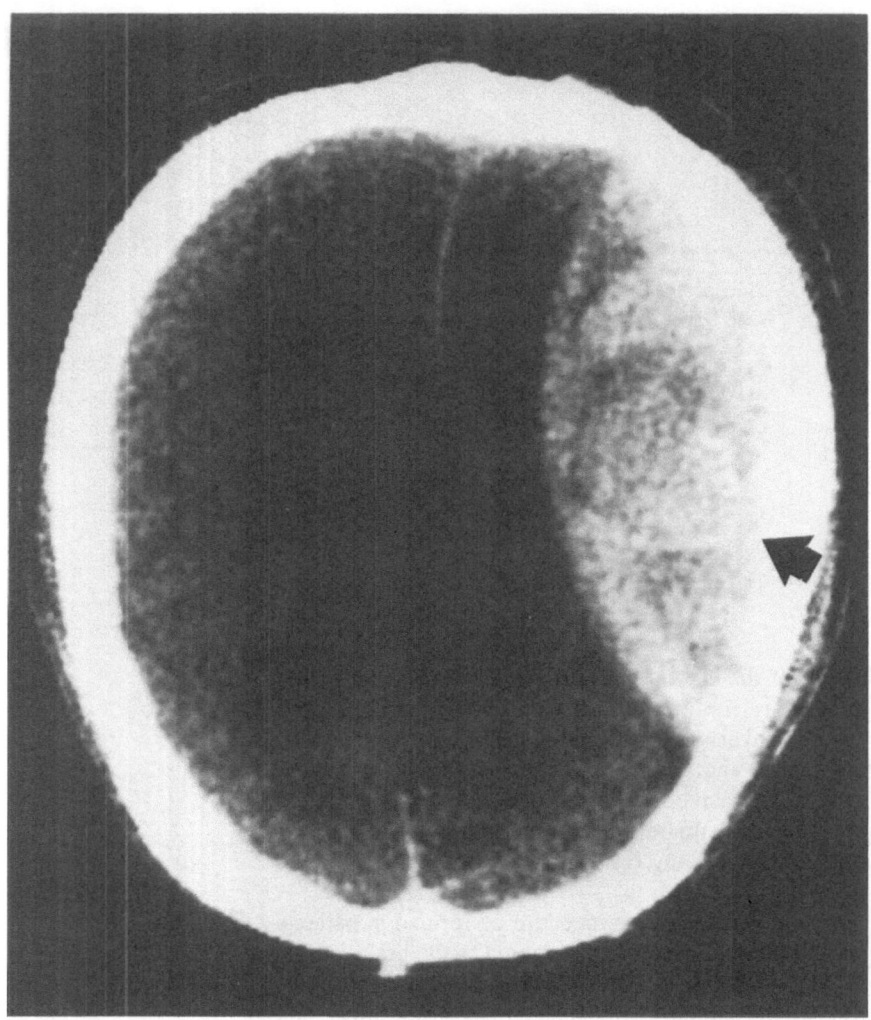

Figure 9-1. Large left epidural hematoma (arrow) in patient with recent trauma.

appearance of blood in the varying locations (Fig. 9-2). However, in addition to detection of the presence of hemorrhage, the deleterious side effects produced by the blood on the remainder of the brain, such as ventricular shift and subfalcine, transtentorial, or uncal herniation, are easily depicted without resorting to angiography or pneumoencephalography. Depressed skull fractures can be evaluated, and early detection of basilar skull fractures is possible.

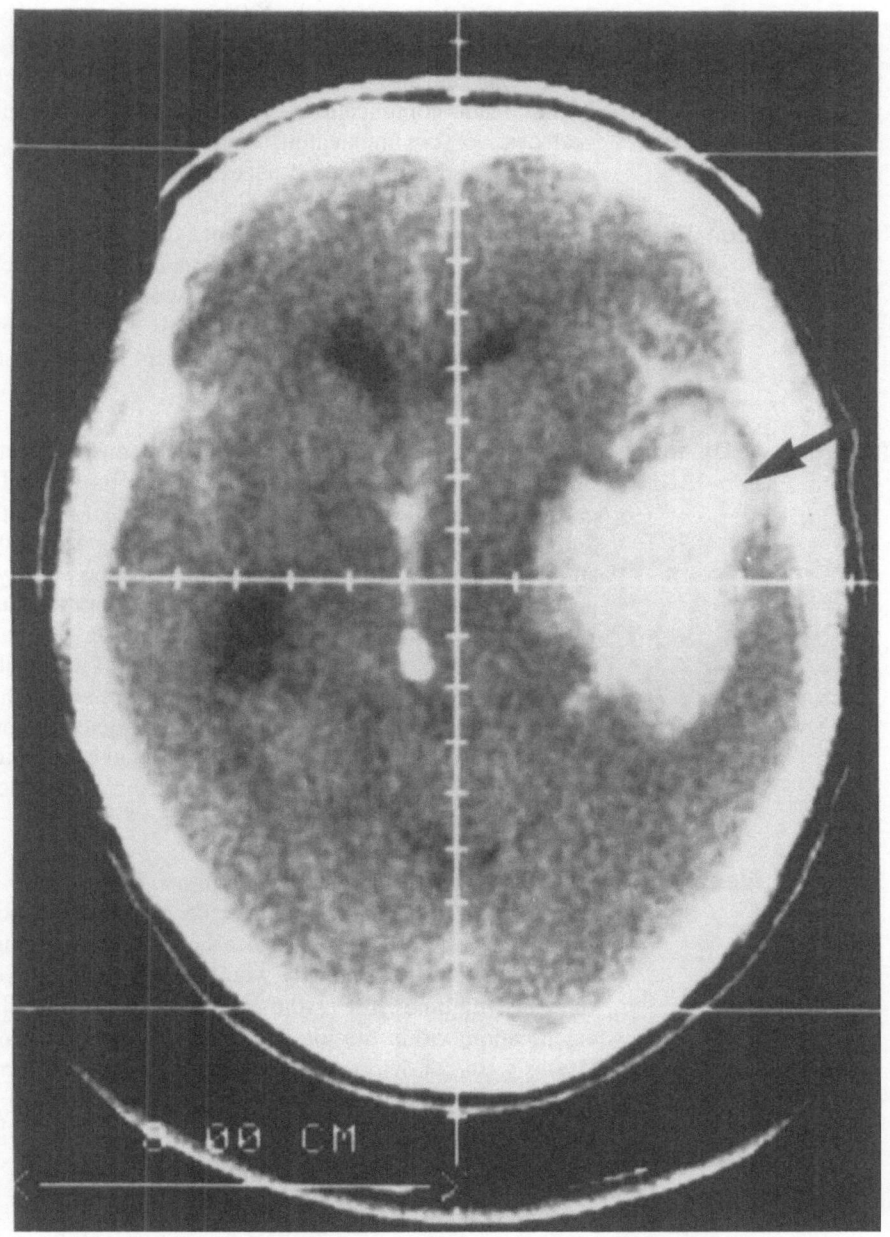

Figure 9-2. Subarachnoid and intraventricular bleeding (arrow).

Pneumocephalus secondary to fractures communicating with the paranasal sinuses is also easily detected. Trauma to the brain stem can also be evaluated utilizing this modality. Posttraumatic complications such as atrophy, leptomeningeal cyst, or communicating hydrocephalus can also be easily assessed and treated if necessary.

Radionuclide Scan

The radionuclide brain scan and flow study is a very sensitive means of detecting the presence of extracerebral hemorrhage,[4] although it is not nearly as sensitive in the detection of intracerebral bleeding. This study, however, has been universally replaced by CT except in small institutions where CT is not readily available.

Inflammatory Disease

CT with and without contrast is a very sensitive method of detecting diffuse meningitis, focal cerebritis, and localized abscess (Fig. 9-3) in varying stages of formation. Serial scans can evaluate patients following surgical or antibiotic therapy as well as detecting the possibility of postinflammatory complications such as communicating hydrocepalus or focal areas of encephalomalacia. The radionuclide scan has been largely replaced by CT in most instances for detection of inflammatory disease, although occasionally meningitis or encephalitis can be detected earlier utilizing this examination on the basis of focal hyperemia or increased flow to the affected areas prior to the actual changes becoming present on the CT scan.[9]

Neoplasm

In the past, most intracranial neoplasms went undetected until attaining a large size because few diagnostic modalities were available to detect them at the early stages. Plain skull films occasionally would reveal signs of hydrocephalus, midline shift of the calcified pineal, or perhaps calcification within the intracranial mass. However, most lesions were not detected until angiography was performed on symptomatic patients. The radionuclide brain scan and now the CT scan have facilitated earlier detection of these lesions.

Computerized Tomography

CT is the best and most sensitive screening procedure in evaluation of patients with neurologic symptoms suspected of harboring intracranial neoplasm.[1] The location and relative vascularity of the lesions in some instances will

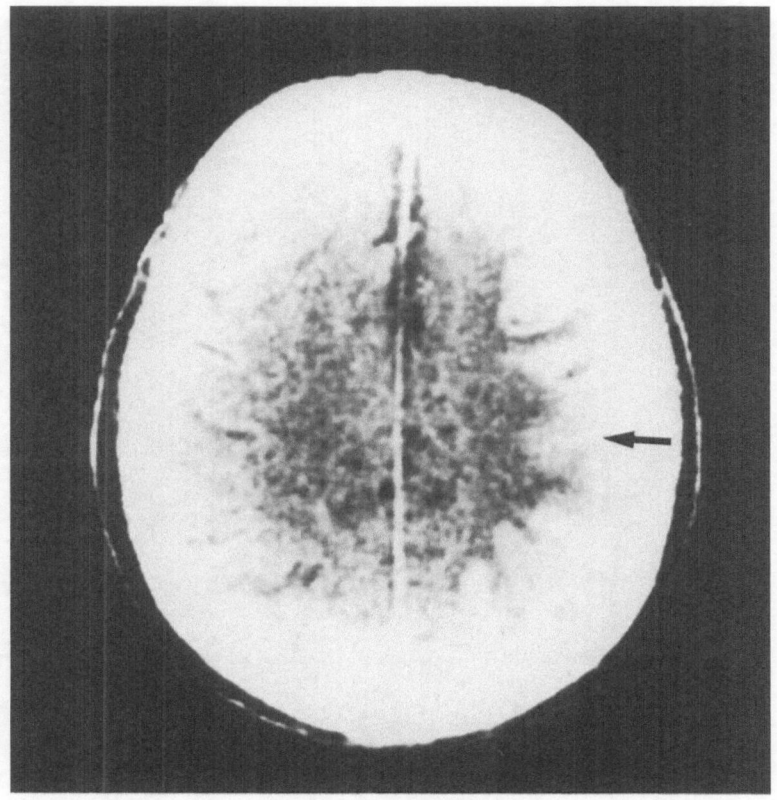

Figure 9-3. Enhancing area of focal cerebritis (arrow) prior to development of abscess.

enable the radiologist to make a definitive tissue diagnosis such as in the calcified or hypervascular meningioma (Fig. 9-4), or in fat-containing midline lesions such as the dermoid or epidermoid (Fig. 9-5). In many instances, the patient will be spared angiography prior to therapy, either surgical ablation or radiotherapy. The full anatomic extent of the lesion can be evaluated as well as the pressure effects exerted on the ventricular system or other centers of the brain. The presence of multiple lesions usually signifies the presence of metastases from either known or unknown primary tumors. CT is also the best way to evaluate the lesion following therapy, and at some institutions CT directed biopsies are performed to obtain tissue diagnosis.

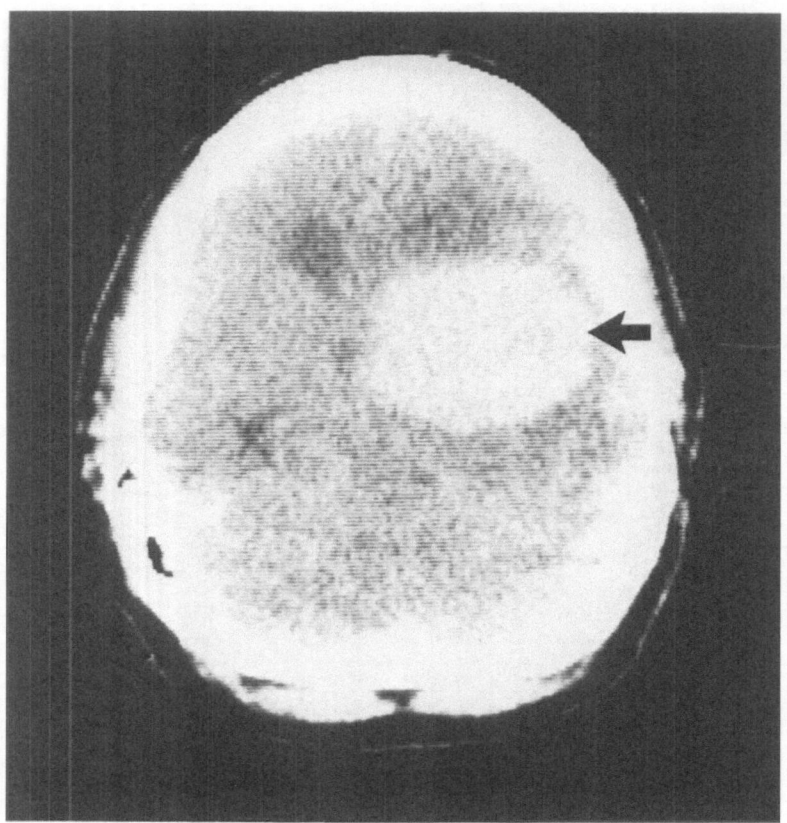

Figure 9-4. Enhancing temporal lobe meningioma (arrow) arising from petrous ridge.

Radionuclide Scan   The radionuclide brain scan, which had been utilized prior to the invention of CT for detecting intracranial lesions, has been largely replaced by CT scanning in most institutions. However, the brain scan is still useful in institutions where CT is not available or for patients who are allergic to iodine.

Vascular Lesions   The diagnosis of intracerebral vascular lesions has been difficult to make because of the occult nature of the disease prior to rupture of the vessels with resultant subarachnoid hemorrhage. In the past, angiography was necessary for detection of all such lesions. The radionuclide brain scan and CT now can detect the hemorrhage secondary to these lesions and can occasionally detect the lesions them-

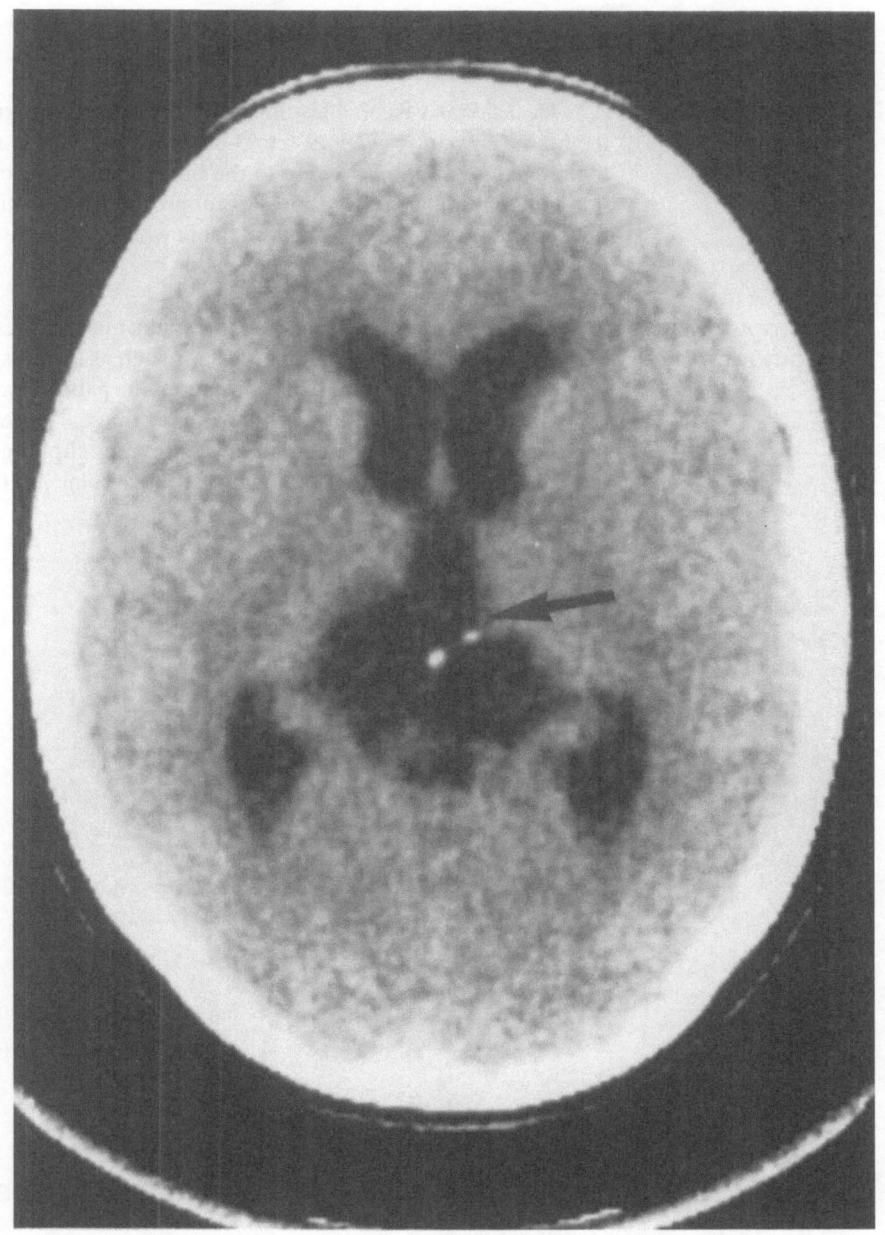

Figure 9-5. Midline epidermoid tumor (arrow) with calcifications and obstructive hydrocephalus.

selves. However, angiography will still be necessary prior to corrective surgery.

Radionuclide Scan

Occasional vascular lesions will be detected utilizing the brain flow study (Figs. 9-6 to 9-8). However, this is not the procedure of choice owing to the limited spatial resolution inherent in the study. It is a useful procedure in institutions that do not have CT or for patients who are allergic to iodinated contrast material.

Computerized Tomography

CT with and without contrast is the most useful means of detecting unsuspected vascular lesions such as aneurysms (Fig. 9-9) or arteriovenous malformations in patients with or without spontaneous subarachnoid hemorrhage.[8] Patients can then be followed postoperatively following clipping of the aneurysms or surgical removal of the vascular malformation.

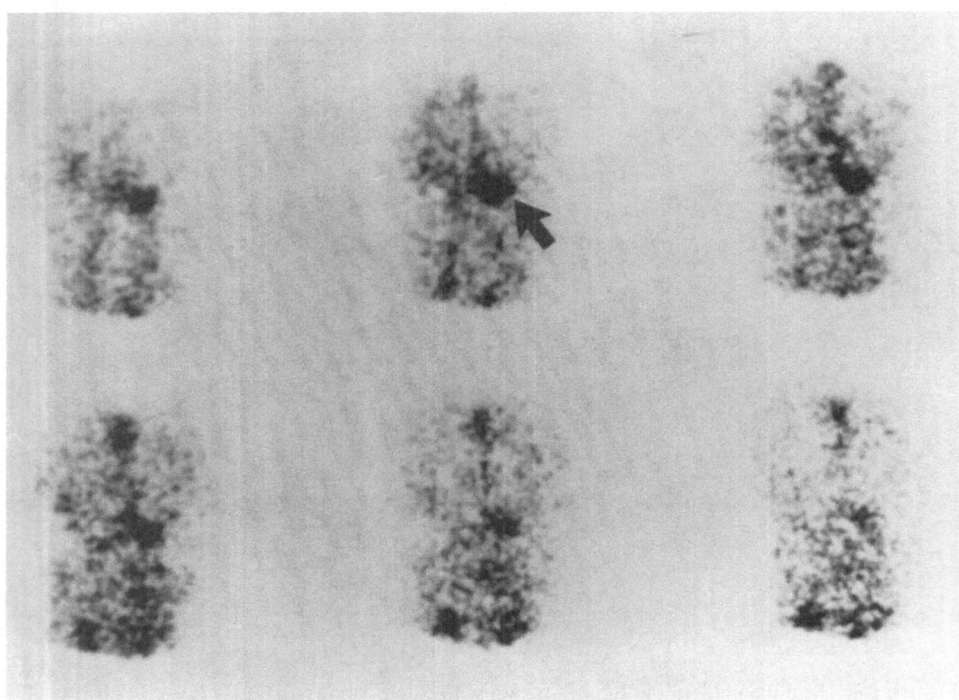

Figure 9-6. Focal area of increased early persisting vascularity (arrow) on radionuclide brain scan.

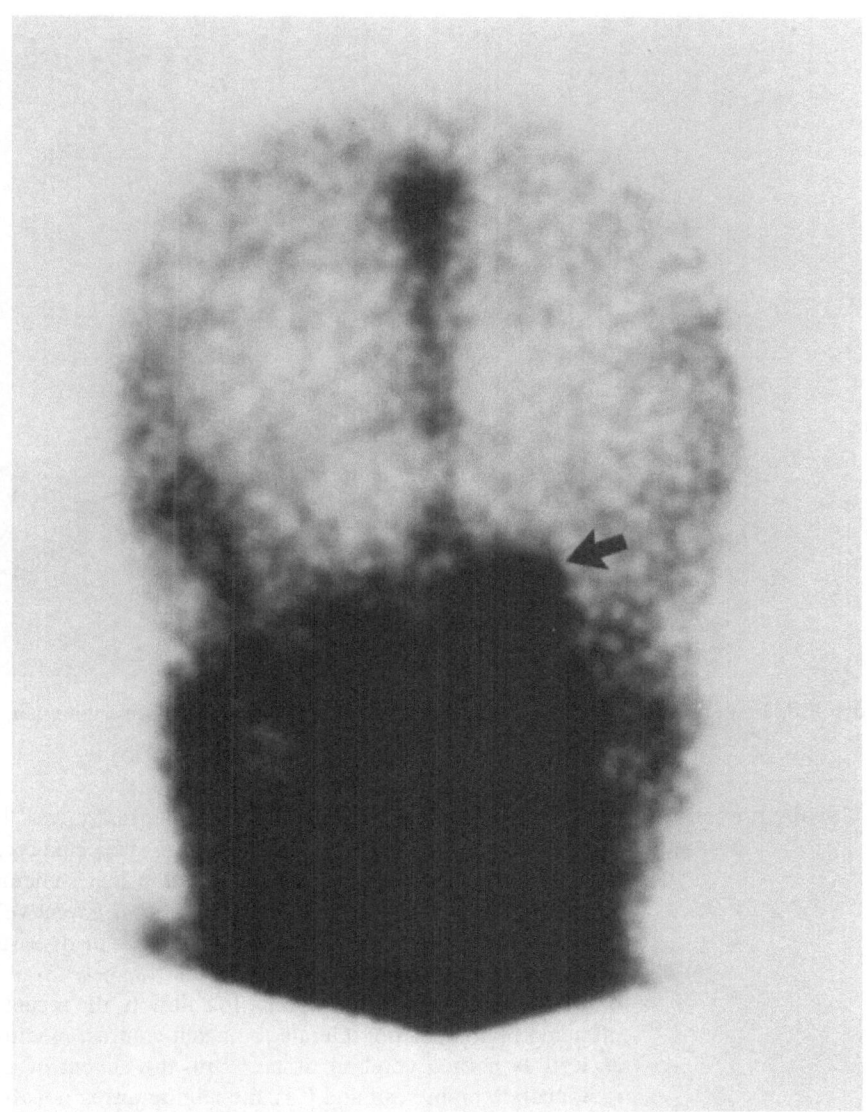

Figure 9-7. Area of increased radionuclide accumulation (arrow) on early image of brain scan compatible with aneurysm.

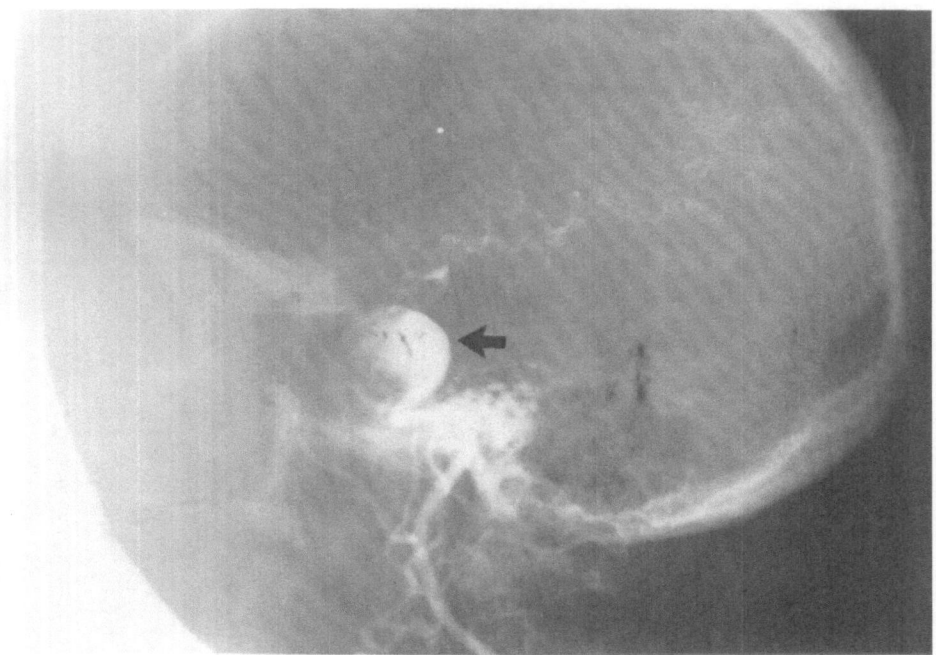

Figure 9-8. Large, partly thrombosed aneurysm of internal carotid (arrow) on angiogram.

Cerebrovascular Disease

Prior to the introduction of CT, angiography was the primary diagnostic modality in patients with suspected cerebral vascular disease such as infarcts or transient ischemic attacks. Unfortunately, although angiography is a relatively safe procedure, the manipulation of catheters in diseased vessels in some instances was responsible for new infarcts or progression of previous infarcts. In addition, the recently infarcted brain does not tolerate iodinated contrast medium as well as normal cerebral tissue. With the advent of the radionuclide brain scan and CT, the angiogram is not routinely utilized as a screening procedure in these patients although angiograms are performed in many instances following documentation of infarct on the CT scan.

Radionuclide Scan

The brain flow and static scan is occasionally able to detect early infarcts in patients prior to visualized changes on the CT examination. One can assess both intracranial and extracranial carotid flow and gross carotid stenosis (Figs. 9-10 to 9-12).[3]

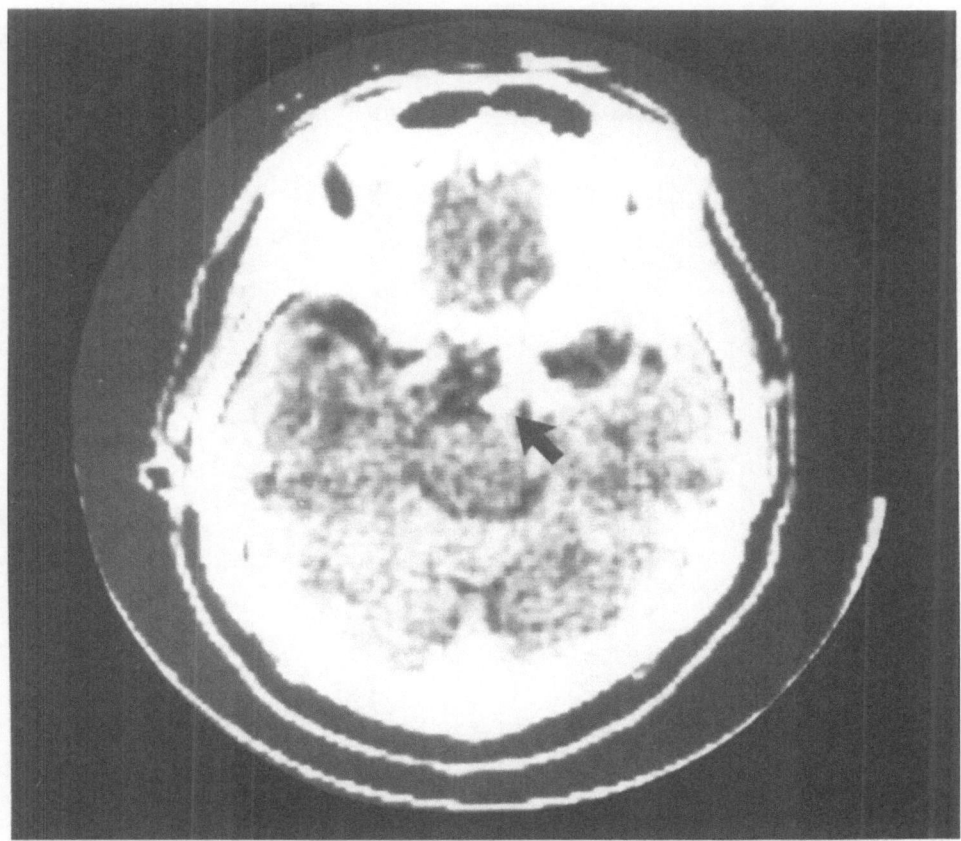

Figure 9-9. Enhanced axial computerized tomography scan demonstrating basilar artery aneurysm (arrow).

Computerized Tomography

CT is the most sensitive noninvasive means of detecting cerebral infarction and differentiating ischemic from hemorrhagic infarcts (Fig. 9-13).[5] The localization of lesions on the scan makes it possible to determine the diseased vessels prior to cerebral angiography. Patients can then be followed with serial scans to evaluate the possible resolution or progression of infarcts following therapy.

Ultrasound

In many institutions, duplex Doppler B mode carotid scanning has been used effectively in patients with symptoms of transient ischemic attack or asymptomatic patients with detectable cervical bruits prior to the more conven-

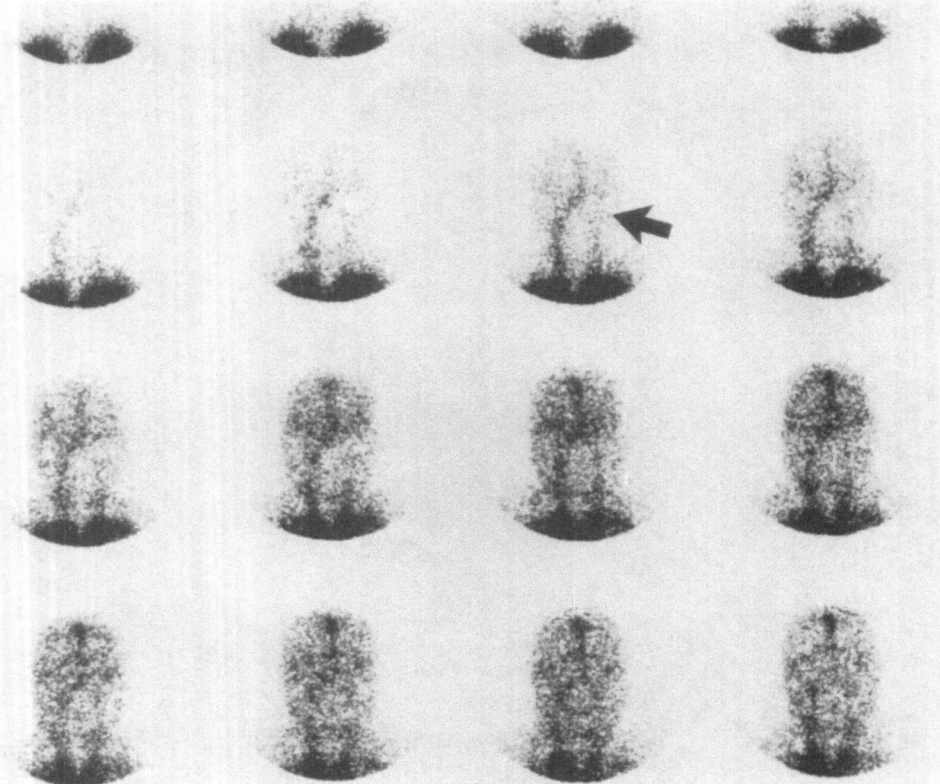

Figure 9-10. Delayed and decreased flow of left common carotid with decreased perfusion left cerebral hemisphere (arrow).

tional contrast arteriogram. The sonographic examinations can accurately and easily demonstrate major areas of stenosis, aneurysms, or ulcerative plaque formation (Figs. 9-14 and 9-15).[6]

Brain Death

Radionuclide Scan

The radionuclide flow study is utilized in many institutions for medicolegal purposes to detect the presence of brain death in patients who are on cardiac or respiratory assistance devices. The absence of intracranial cerebral perfusion and the lack of activity within the sagittal sinus has been termed diagnostic for presence of brain death.[2]

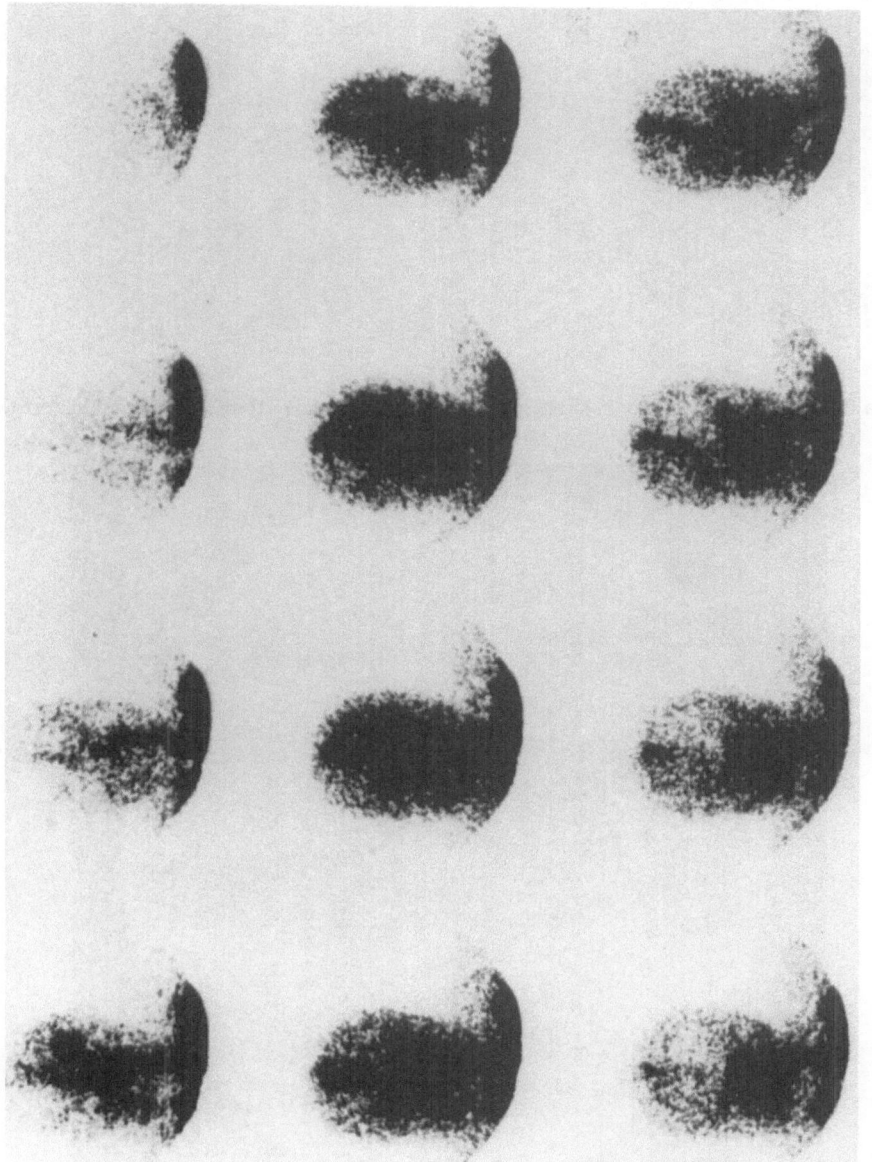

Figure 9-11. Increased and delayed perfusion in left cerebral hemisphere secondary to luxury perfusion of infarct.

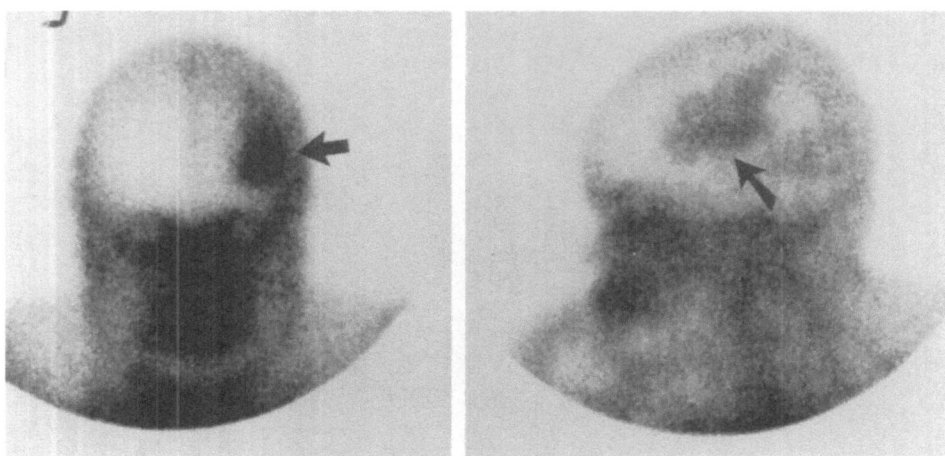

Figure 9-12. Increased activity in left cerebral hemisphere on delayed image from infarct (arrow).

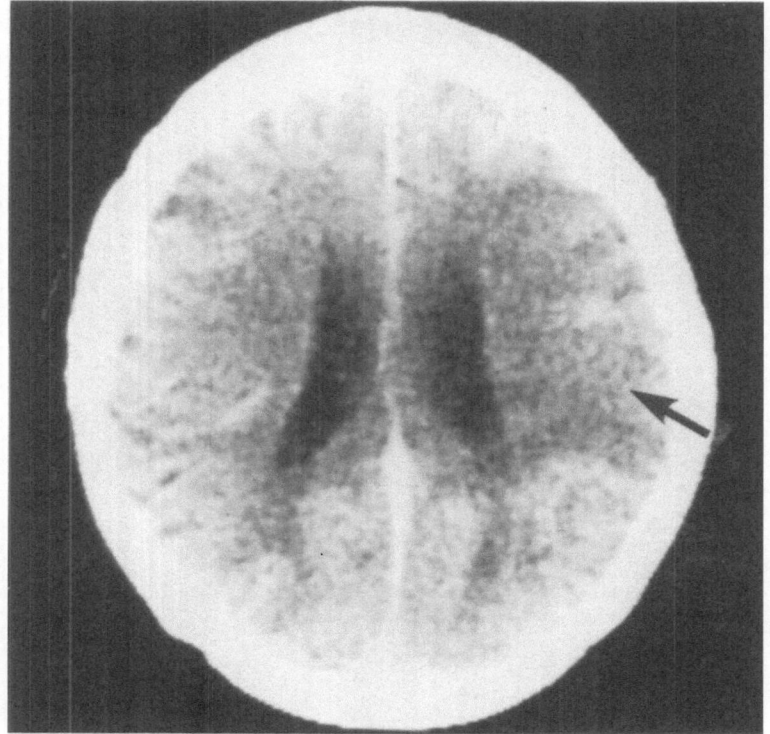

Figure 9-13. Diffusely decreased attenuation in left cerebral hemisphere (arrow) representing early ischemic infarct.

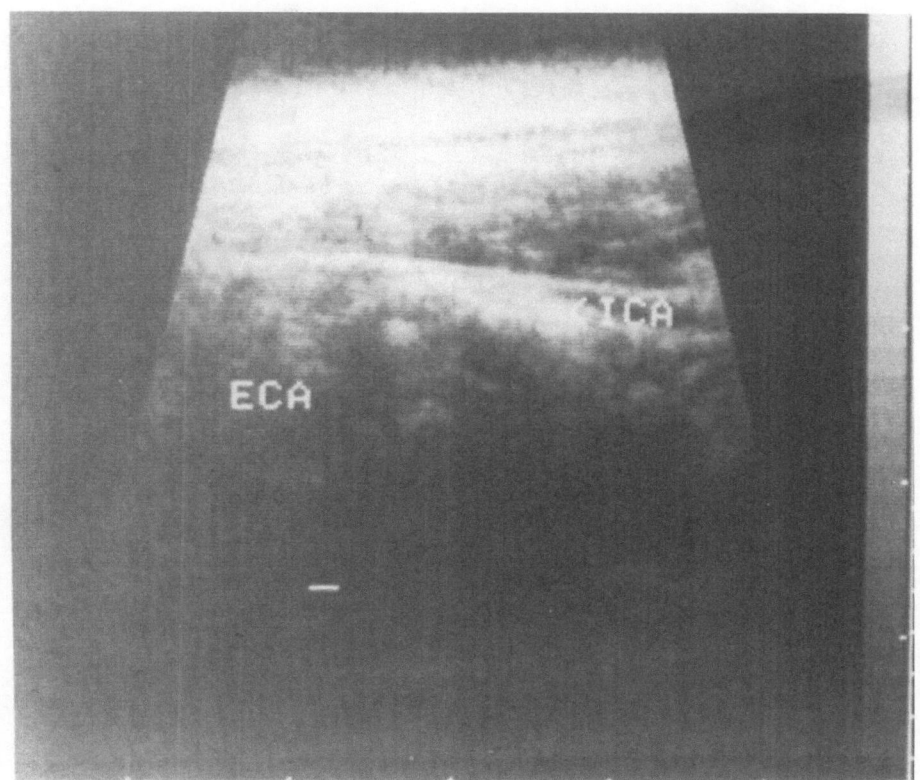

Figure 9-14. sonogram showing obstructed left internal carotid.

White-Matter Disease

Computerized Tomography

The ability of CT to distinguish between gray and white matter has enabled the detection of many white-matter diseases such as multiple sclerosis or other diseases resulting in demyelinization or dysmyelinization at an earlier stage.[10] Research studies with magnetic resonance imaging (MRI) have revealed an even better discrimination between gray and white matter enabling earlier detection of white-matter disease than with CT scanning. MRI will ultimately replace CT as the examination of choice in these patients when the equipment becomes routinely accessible.

Hydrocephalus

In former years, the detection of hydrocephalus had been determined utilizing indirect findings present on skull radiographs such as pressure erosion on the bony sella or by the more invasive procedures of pneumoencephalography

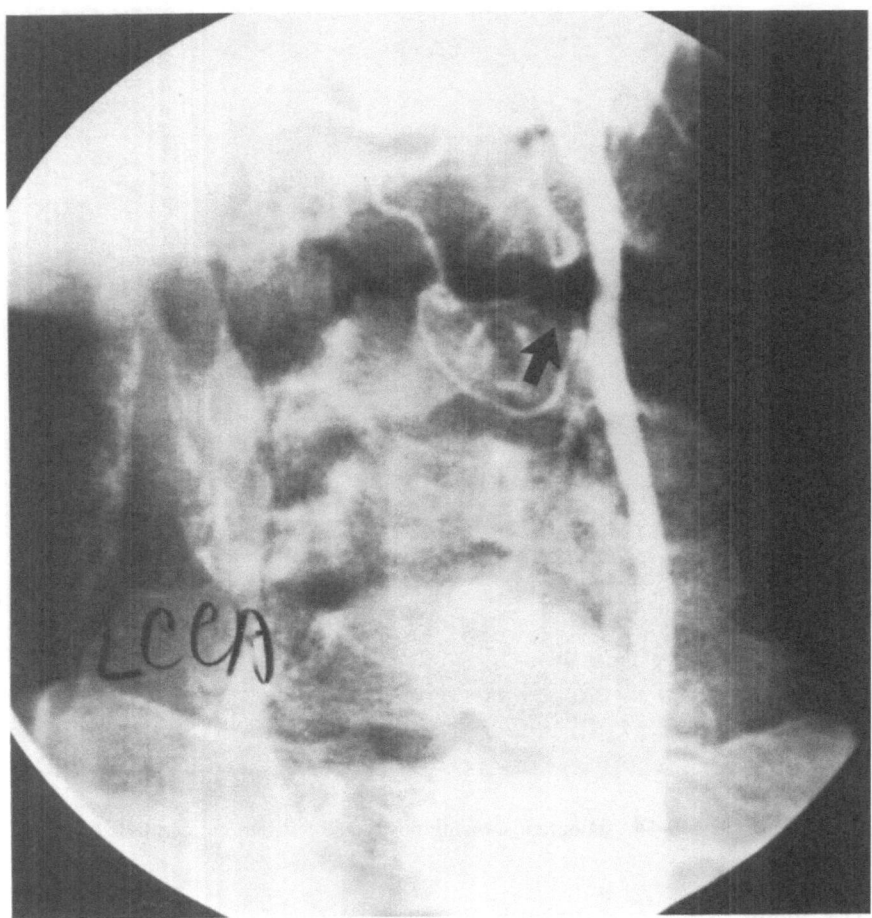

Figure 9-15. Confirmation of obstructed left internal carotid (arrow) on digital subtraction angiogram.

and cerebral angiography. The introduction of CT has made the detection of hydrocephalus easier, less traumatic, and cheaper for the patient.

Computerized Tomography

CT is a sensitive means of detecting the presence of hydrocephalus and differentiating between communicating and noncommunicating or obstructive hydrocephalus (Figs. 9-16 and 9-17). In cases of obstructive hydrocephalus, the level of obstruction and the offending lesion can often be detected. The patients can then be evaluated following in-

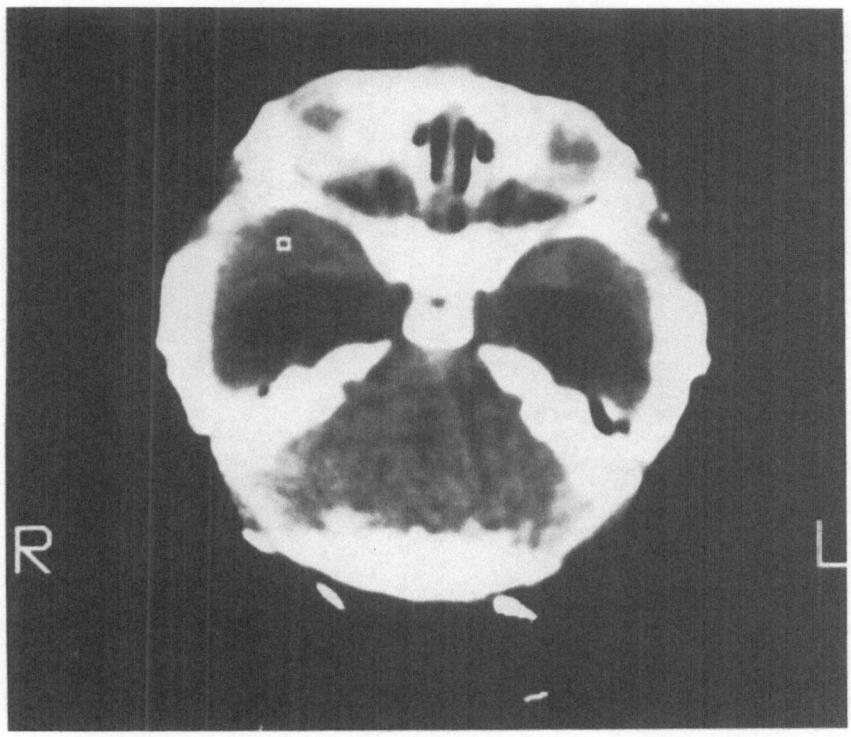

Figure 9-16. Hydrocephalus in newborn due to aqueduct stenosis.

traventricular shunting or postoperatively to evaluate the progression or regression of ventricular dilatation.

Radionuclide Scan

While CT will demonstrate the morphologic abnormalities of the ventricular system, the radionuclide cisternogram is a better means of evaluating physiology of the subarachnoid spaces and ventricular system. It is useful in cases of suspected block in the cerebrospinal fluid pathways such as those caused by subarachnoid adhesions, which may be due to either previous surgery or inflammatory disease (Fig. 9-18). It will document and localize a cerebrospinal fluid leak such as that which occurs in otorrhea or rhinorrhea. It may be useful in differentiating between etiologies of communicating hydrocephalus due to cerebral atrophy or that caused by normal-pressure hydrocephalus.[7] It may also be useful in determining which patients are most

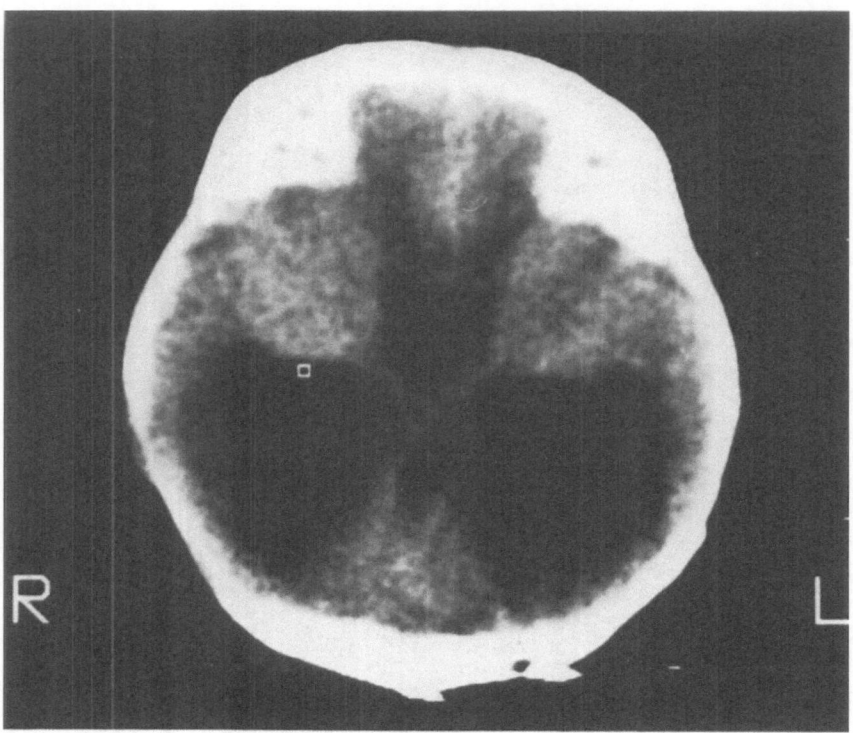

Figure 9-17. Hydrocephalus in newborn due to aqueduct stenosis.

likely to be aided by intraventricular shunting. Shunt patency and complications secondary to shunting can also be evaluated utilizing injection of radioactive tracer into the shunt reservoir.

Sellar Lesions

Sellar lesions may be discovered incidentally on routine skull radiographs or may be discovered in patients presenting with such diverse findings as acromegaly, galactorrhea, disturbed vision, or other neurologic signs and symptoms. Previous modalities of diagnosis included plain tomograms of the sella turcica followed by angiography or pneumoencephalography.

Computerized Tomography

CT is the screening procedure of choice for detecting the parasellar lesions and evaluating local extension into neighboring structures. Highly vascular lesions such as aneurysms, meningiomas, or occasionally pituitary ade-

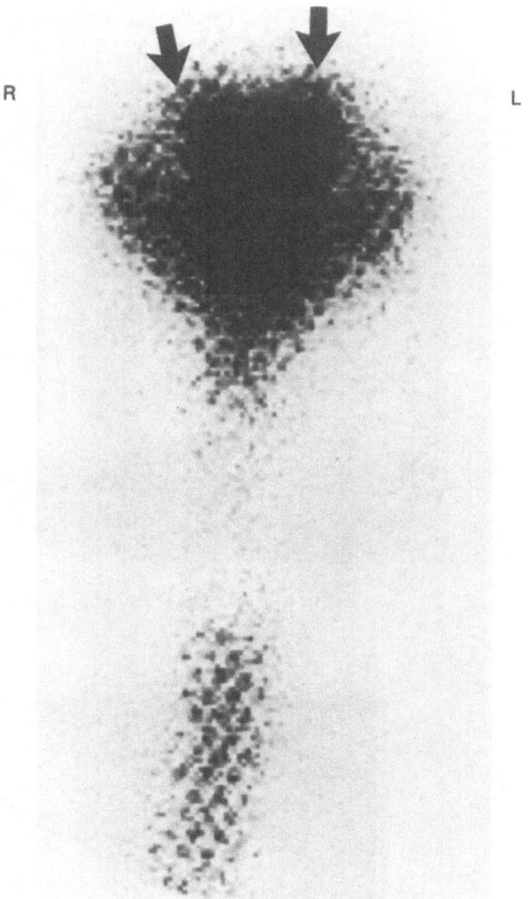

R   L

Figure 9-18. Radionuclide cisternogram revealing marked dilatation of ventricles containing radionuclide (arrows) in patient with communicating hydrocephalus.

nomas (Figs. 9-19 and 9-20) may be distinguished from other parasellar masses such as craniopharyngioma, which in many cases may exhibit calcification. In certain instances, metrizamide cisternography may be useful in cases that are equivocal on the routine CT examination.

A large number of premature neonates may develop intracerebral hemorrhage several days following birth. Ultrasound is an inexpensive, easy way of detecting the presence and extent of intracerebral hemorrhage and possible

Neonatal Echoencephalography

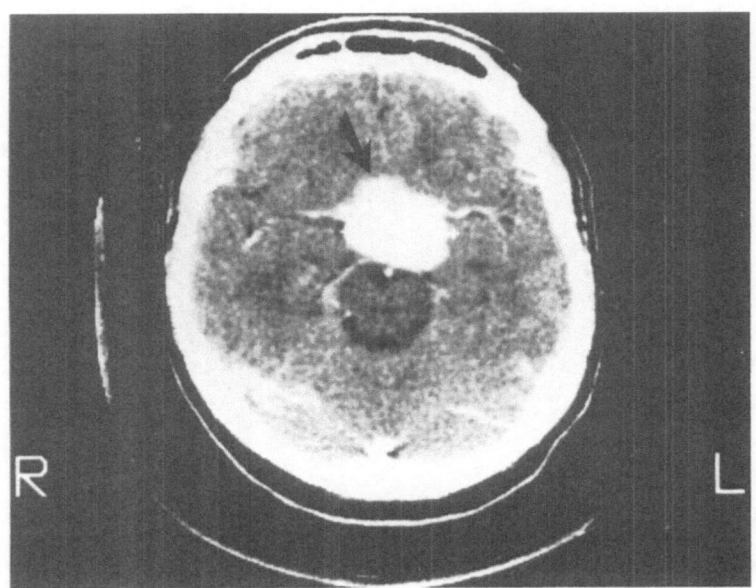

Figure 9-19. Large enhancing parasellar mass (arrow).

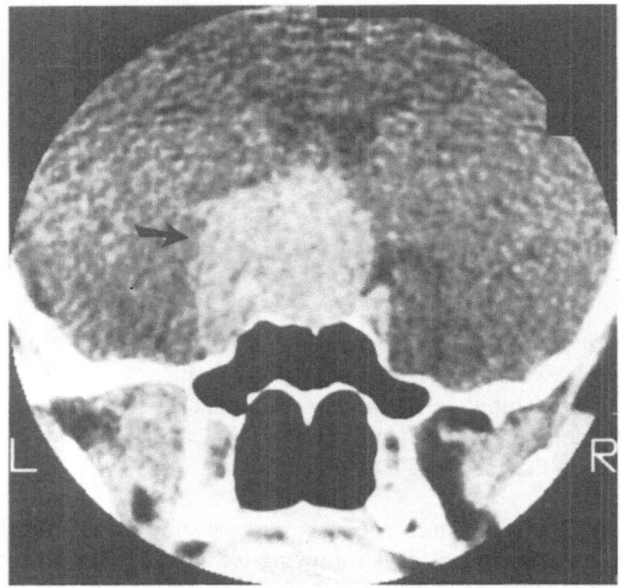

Figure 9-20. Coronal image revealing large enhancing pituitary adenoma (arrow).

concurrent hydrocephalus (Fig. 9-21).[11] Patients may then be followed with serial examinations for several days to evaluate the progression or regression of clot and/or hydrocephalus.

MRI has proven to be quite valuable in the detection of intracranial disease. As noted previously, MRI is much more sensitive in the detection of demyelinating plaques in multiple sclerosis than high-resolution CT. MRI is also a valuable tool in the evaluation of posterior fossa lesions and disease within the temporal lobes (Figs. 9-22 and 9-23) because of the lack of artifact production from the surrounding bone that is created on routine CT examinations. The early results indicate that MRI, because of its greater sensitivity in detecting intracranial disease, may eventually replace CT as the screening procedure of choice in patients with neurologic symptoms. However, because of the lesser

Magnetic Resonance Imaging

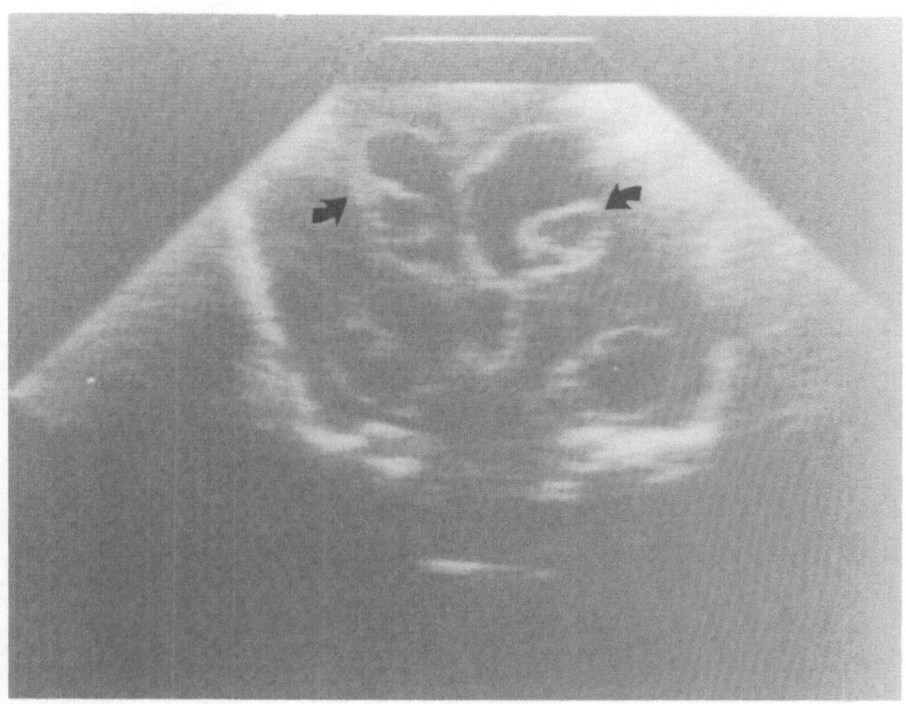

Figure 9-21. Hydrocephalus with bilateral intraventricular blood clots (arrow) in echoencephalogram of premature neonate.

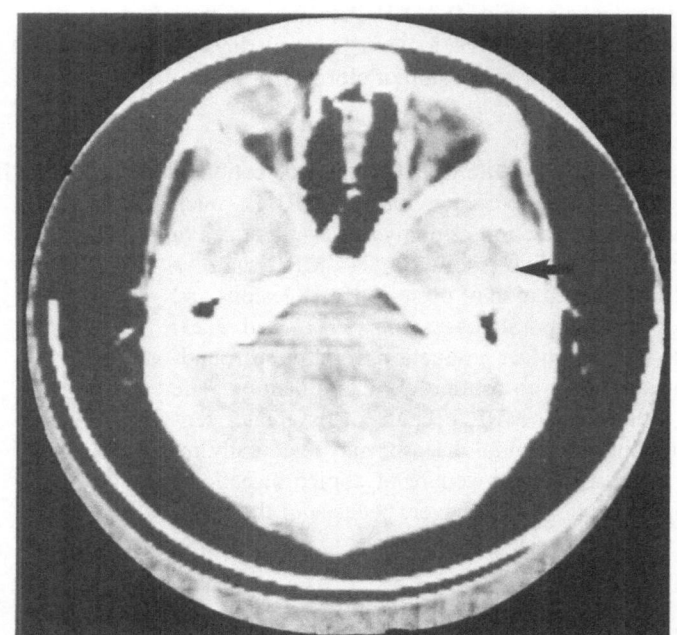

Figure 9-22. Artifact (arrow) obscuring visualization of temporal lobe.

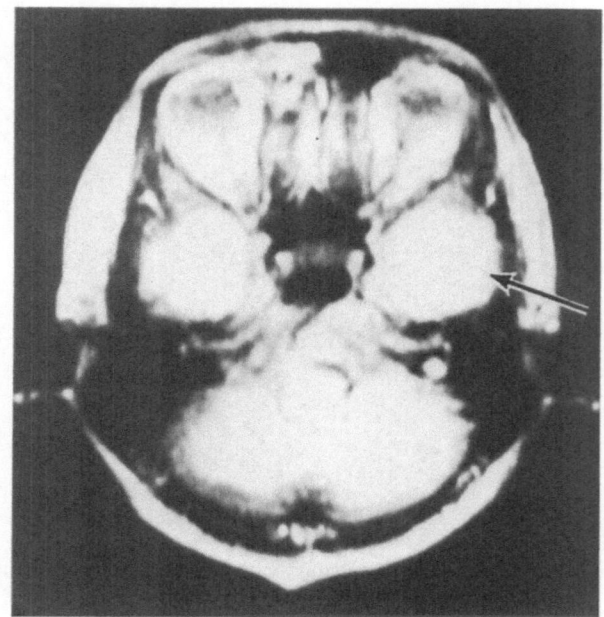

Figure 9-23. Same patient as in Fig. 22 with excellent visualization of normal temporal lobe (arrow) on magnetic resonance imaging.

expense and greater specificity afforded at this time, CT still remains the imaging modality of choice in most patients with suspected intracranial disease.

REFERENCES

1. Baker HL, Houser OW, Campbell JK: National Cancer Institute Study—Evaluation of CT in the diagnosis of intracranial neoplasms: Overall results. *Radiology* 1980;136:91–96.
2. Braunstein P, et al: Cerebral death: A rapid reliable diagnostic adjunct using radioisotopes. *J Nucl Med* 1973;14:122.
3. Campbell JK, Houser OW, Stevens JC, et al: Computed tomography and radionuclide imaging in the evaluation of ischemic stroke. *Radiology* 1978;126:695–702.
4. Cowan RJ, Maynard CD: Trauma to brain and extracranial structures. *Semin Nucl Med* 1974;4:319.
5. Davis KR, Ackerman RH, Kistler JP, et al: Computed tomography of cerebral infarction: Hemorrhagic, contrast enhancement and time of appearance. *Comput Tomogr* 1977;1:71–86.
6. Dreisbach JN: Duplex ultrasound evaluation of carotid disease. *Clin Diag US* 1984;13:69–105.
7. Harbert JC: Radionuclide cisternography. *Semin Nucl Med* 1971;1:90.
8. Kendall BE, Lee BOP, Claveria E: Computerized tomography and angiography in subarachnoid hemorrhage. *Br J. Radiol* 1976;49:483–501.
9. Kim EE, DeLand FH, Mantebella J: Sensitivity of radionuclide brain scan and computed tomography in early detection of viral meningoencephalitis. *Radiology* 1979;132:425–429.
10. Lane B, Carroll BA, Pedley TA: Computerized cranial tomography in cerebral diseases of white matter. *Neurology* 1978;28:534–544.
11. Shankaran S, Slovis TL, Bedard MP, et al: Sonographic classification of intracranial hemorrhage. A prognostic indication of mortality, morbidity and short term neurologic outcome. *J Pediatr* 1982;100:469.
12. Zimmerman RD, Danziger A: Extracerebral trauma. *Radiol Clin North Am* 1982;20:105–121.

SPINE

Radiographic evaluation of the spine in the past had been limited to plain films, tomography, and contrast myelography utilizing either iodinated contrast medium or air. Occasionally, spinal arteriography or epidural venography was necessary. At this time, however, CT has effectively replaced myelography and, in many cases, angiography for most clinical situations.

Trauma

CT is a useful adjunctive means of evaluating spinal fractures after their initial documentation on plain radiographs.[2] Extension of fractures into the posterior neural arch elements or displacement of bony fragments into the spinal canal can be demonstrated (Figs. 9-24 and 9-25), allowing assessment of stability of the injury. This is aided by sagittal and coronal reconstructions. Serial examinations can be performed postoperatively; however, in many instances, metallic artifact may degrade the images. The utilization of intrathecal metrizamide will demonstrate the presence of spinal cord compression.

Neoplasm   CT with or without metrizamide has effectively replaced myelography in the evaluation of spinal cord lesions presenting as either diffuse enlargement or focal tumor.[1] The presence of contrast filling a central canal effectively demonstrates syringomyelia. The presence of fatty lesions

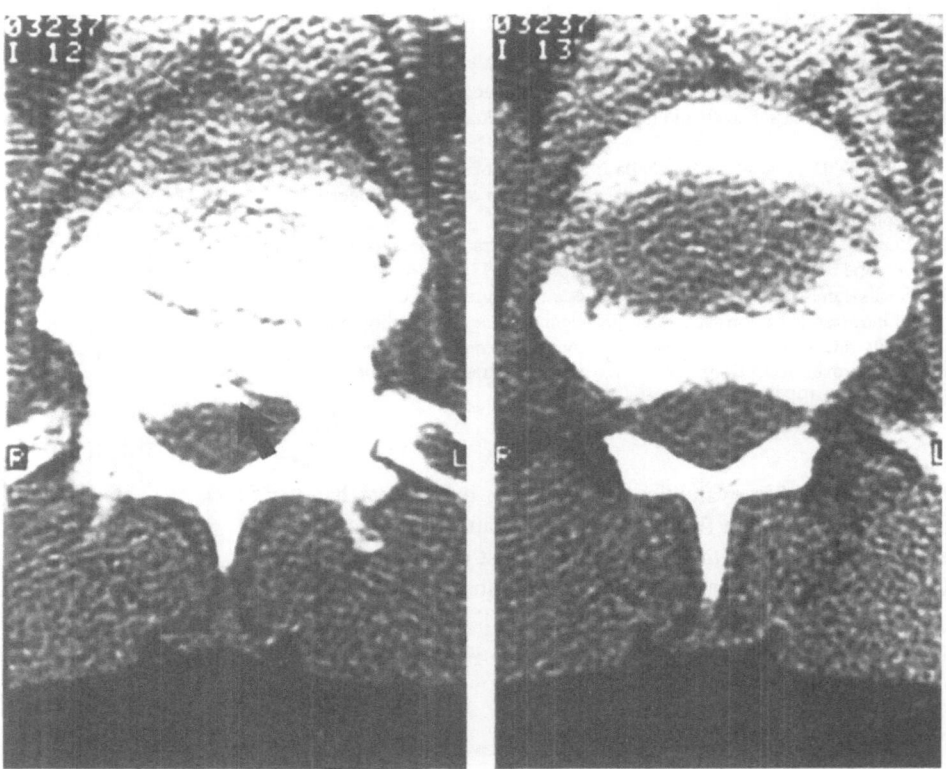

Figure 9-24. Axial image of patient with vertebral body compression fracture with displacement of bone fragment into spinal canal (arrow).

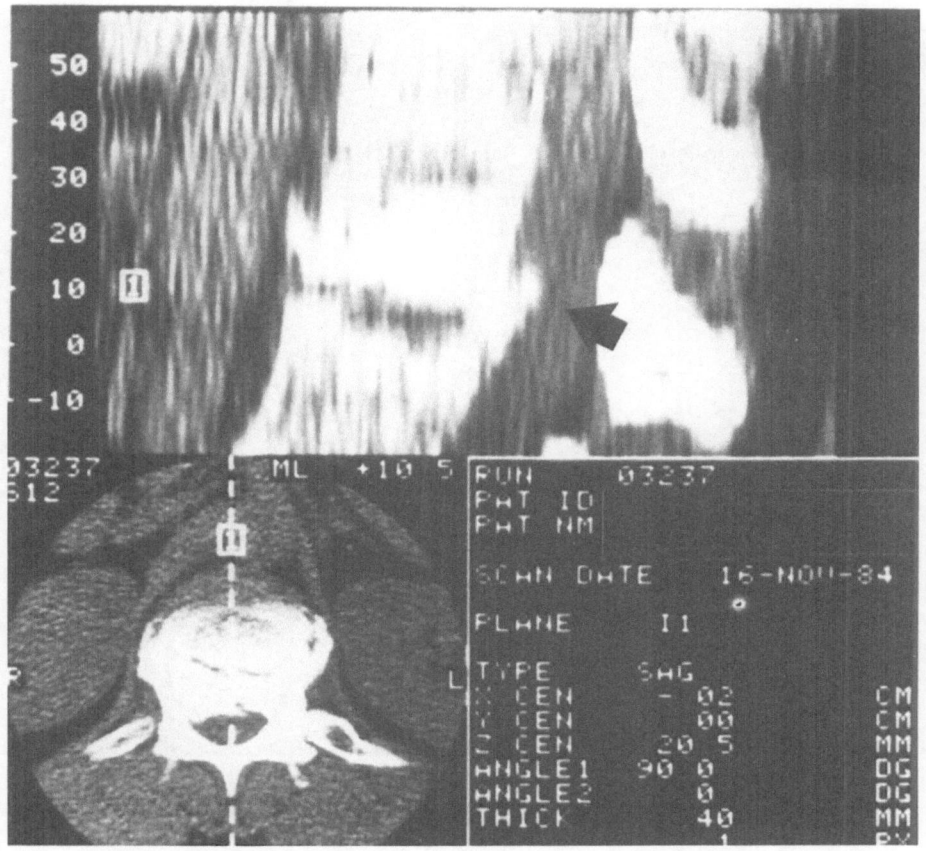

Figure 9-25. Sagittal image of same patient as in Fig. 24 showing displaced bone fragment (arrow).

in patients with spinal dysraphism is useful in the diagnosis of tethered cord secondary to lipoma or lipomeningocele. Meningoceles (Fig. 9-26) and myelomeningoceles can be readily detected and often differentiated. CT can also be used to evaluate bone metastases to the spinal column with resultant soft tissue spread into the spinal canal (Fig. 9-27).

Ultrasound

Ultrasound has recently been utilized in several institutions intraoperatively to enable the neurosurgeon to better localize spinal cord lesions in the operating room, resulting in less disruption of the normal spinal tissues.

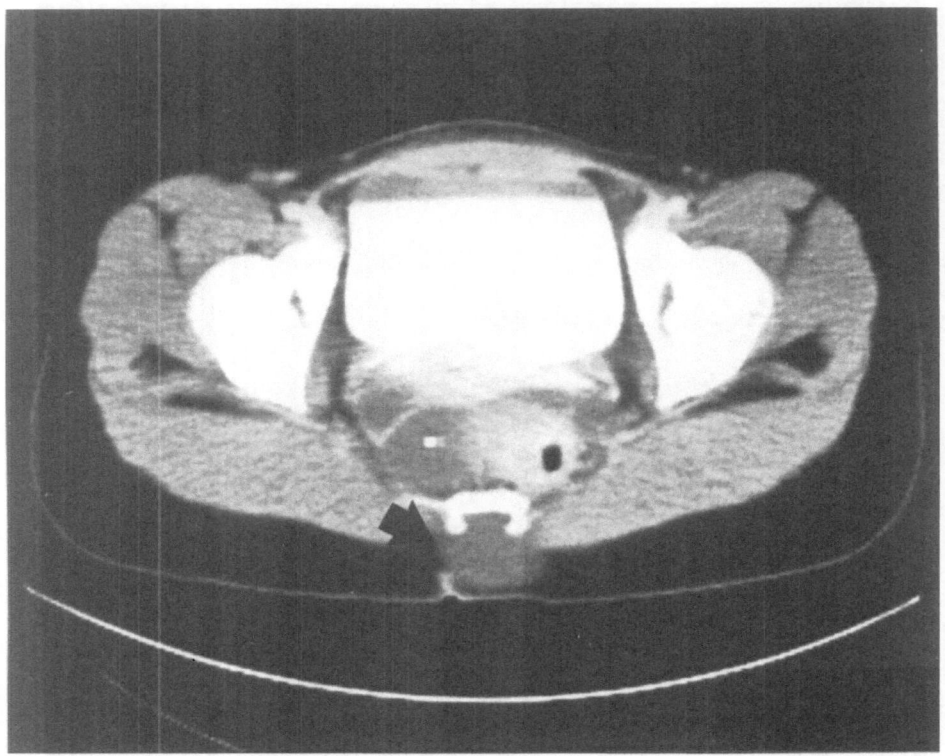

Figure 9-26. Fourteen-year-old girl with sacral spinal dysraphism and meningocele (arrow).

Inflammatory Disease

Radionuclide Studies

Utilized in conjunction with plain films, the radionuclide bone scan and gallium scans are fairly sensitive although not specific methods of detecting discitis and osteomyelitis involving adjacent vertebral bodies (Fig. 9-28).

Computerized Tomography

CT is an excellent means of evaluating the extraosseous extent of osteomyelitis, which may result in prevertebral or adjacent psoas abscesses. Extent of spread of infection into the spinal canal can also be assessed both prior to and following therapy.[4]

Low-Back Pain

Low-back pain is the most common disability afflicting the ranks of the employed in this nation today. Formerly, radiographic evaluation of low-back pain included

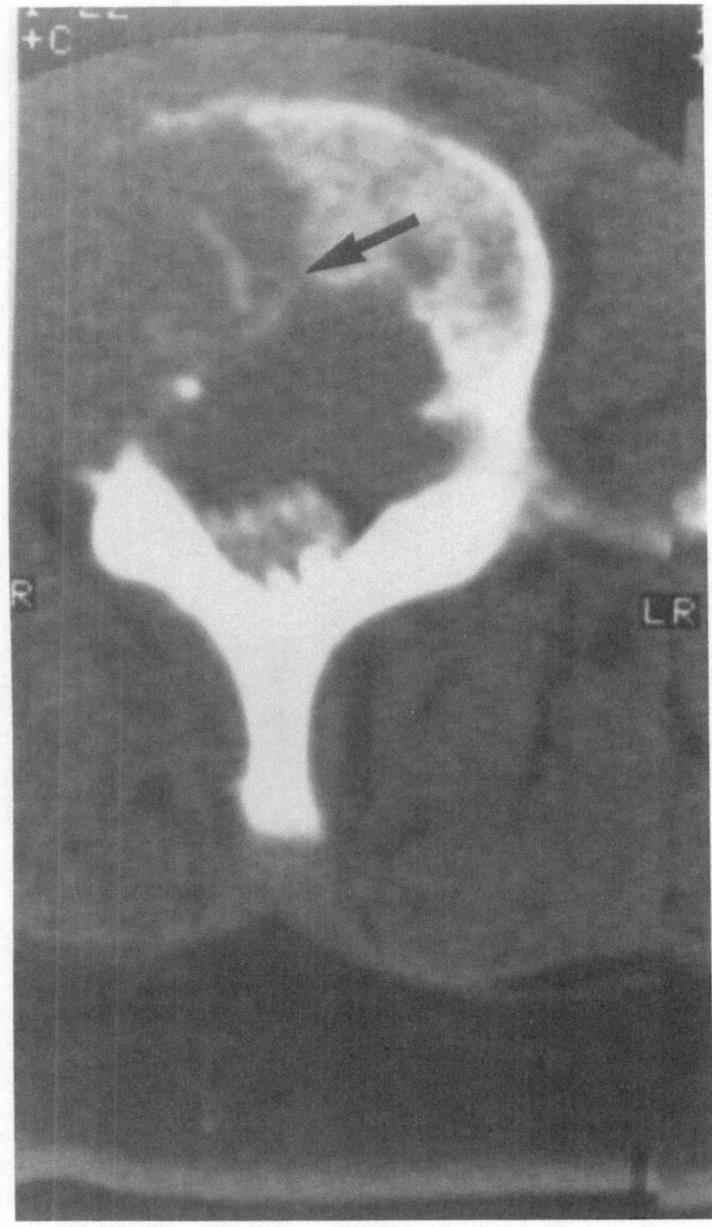

Figure 9-27. Spinal cord compression secondary to vertebral body metastasis that has invaded spinal canal (arrow).

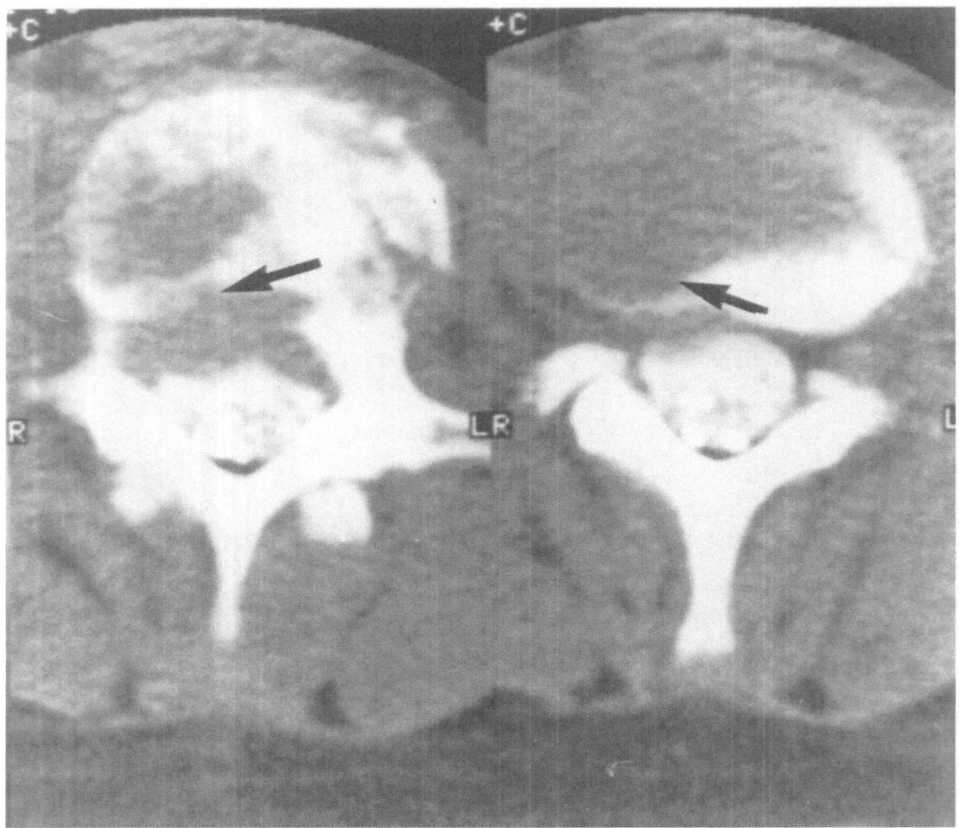

Figure 9-28. Osteomyelitis resulting in bony destruction and epidural abscess (arrow).

lumbar spine films, occasionally tomograms, or myelography in certain circumstances. High-resolution CT has virtually replaced the myelogram as the screening procedure of choice for patients with sciatica or disc syndrome symptomatology.

Computerized Tomography

CT with or without intrathecal contrast medium is an effective means of detecting herniated disc fragments and differentiating this entity from the bulging anulus fibrosus, which is usually treated more conservatively (Fig. 9-29).[3] Other etiologies of low-back pain, such as spondylolysis or degenerative arthritis involving the facets, are readily demonstrated. Early changes of sacroiliitis can also be easily detected.

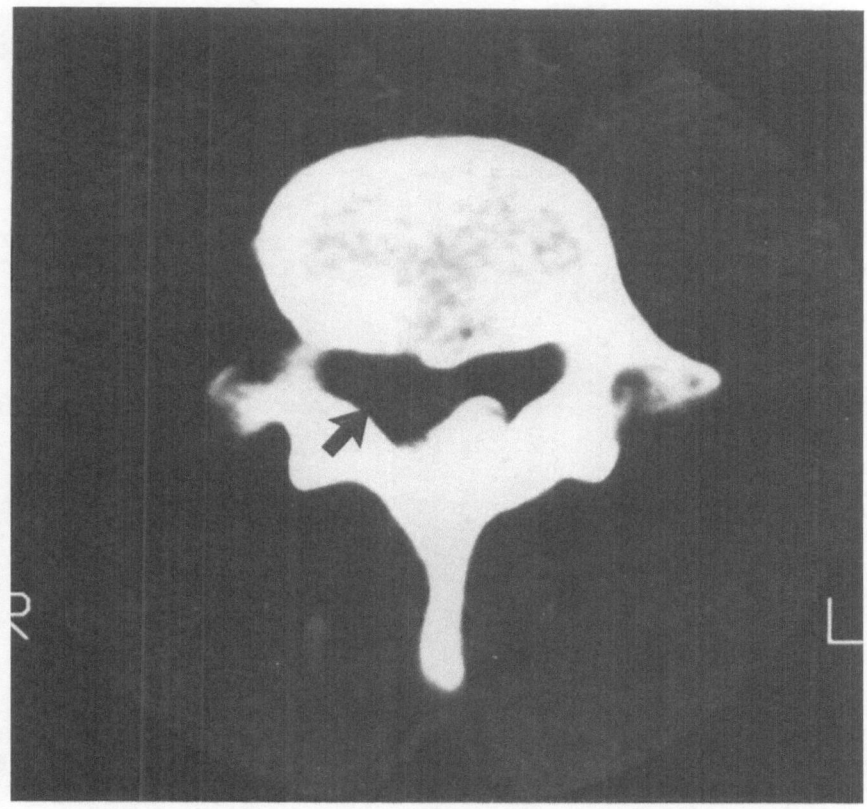

Figure 9-29. Large, herniated disc fragment (arrow) displacing metrizamide-filled thecal sac.

MRI, although still in the experimental stages, has thus far shown to have great promise in the early detection of spinal cord lesions. Owing to the markedly improved contrast resolution and lack of necessity for ionizing radiation and iodinated contrast medium, this study will become the initial screening procedure of choice in patients suspected of harboring these lesions. Owing to excellent characterization of soft tissue enabling differentiation between a normal and degenerating intervertebral disc, patients with degenerative disc disease will also be detected at an earlier stage, which will subsequently facilitate and improve treatment (Fig. 9-30).

Magnetic Resonance Imaging

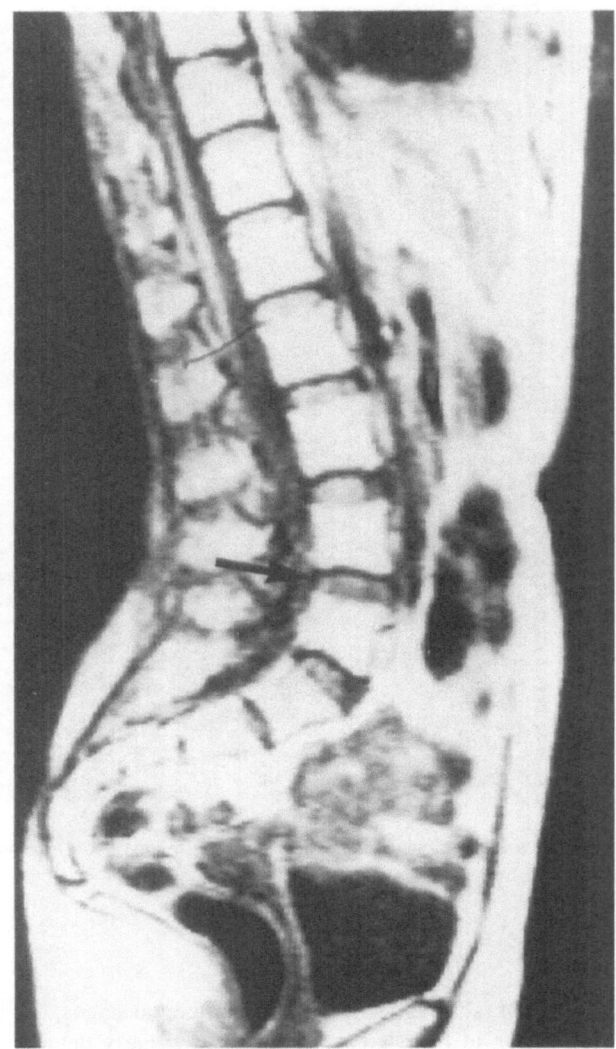

Figure 9-30. Sagittal magnetic resonance imaging scan demonstrating appearance of normal lumbar disc (arrow).

REFERENCES

1. Aubin ML, Jardin C, Bar D, et al: Computerized tomography in 32 cases of intraspinal tumor. *J Neuroradiol* 1979;6:81–92.
2. Brant-Zawadzki M, Miller EM, Federle MP: CT in the evaluation of spine trauma. *Am J Radiol* 1981;136:369–375.
3. Haughton VM, Williams AL: *Computed Tomography of the Spine.* St. Louis, CV Mosby Co, 1982.
4. Kuhn JP, Berger PE: Computed tomographic diagnosis of osteomyelitis. *Radiology* 1979;130:502–506.
5. Williams AL, Haughton VM: Computed tomography in the diagnosis of herniated nucleus pulposus. *Radiology* 1980;135:95–99.

10 Neck and Facial Structures

This chapter deals with disease processes, both benign and malignant, involving the facial bones, paranasal sinuses, orbits, mouth, salivary glands, and respiratory system proximal to the trachea (pharynx and larynx). Prior to the advent of newer noninvasive imaging modalities the radiographic evaluation of these structures had been largely limited to plain-film tomography or more invasive contrast studies such as sialography, laryngography, and, occasionally, angiography or venography in limited circumstances.

ORBITS

Trauma

The initial study in the evaluation of trauma to the orbit is plain-radiographic examination of the facial bones and orbits. Once significant trauma is detected on the radiograph or if the patient is experiencing visual difficulties, computerized tomography, is the procedure of choice.

Computerized Tomography

CT of the orbits is an excellent means of evaluating and delineating orbital fractures with reliable identification of medial (Figs. 10-1 and 10-2) or inferior orbital blowout fractures as well as identifying the presence of retrobulbar hemorrhage.[10] Intraorbital foreign bodies can be localized and the possibility of optic nerve entrapment secondary to bony injury can be easily detected. Anterior or posterior chamber hemorrhage can also be seen.

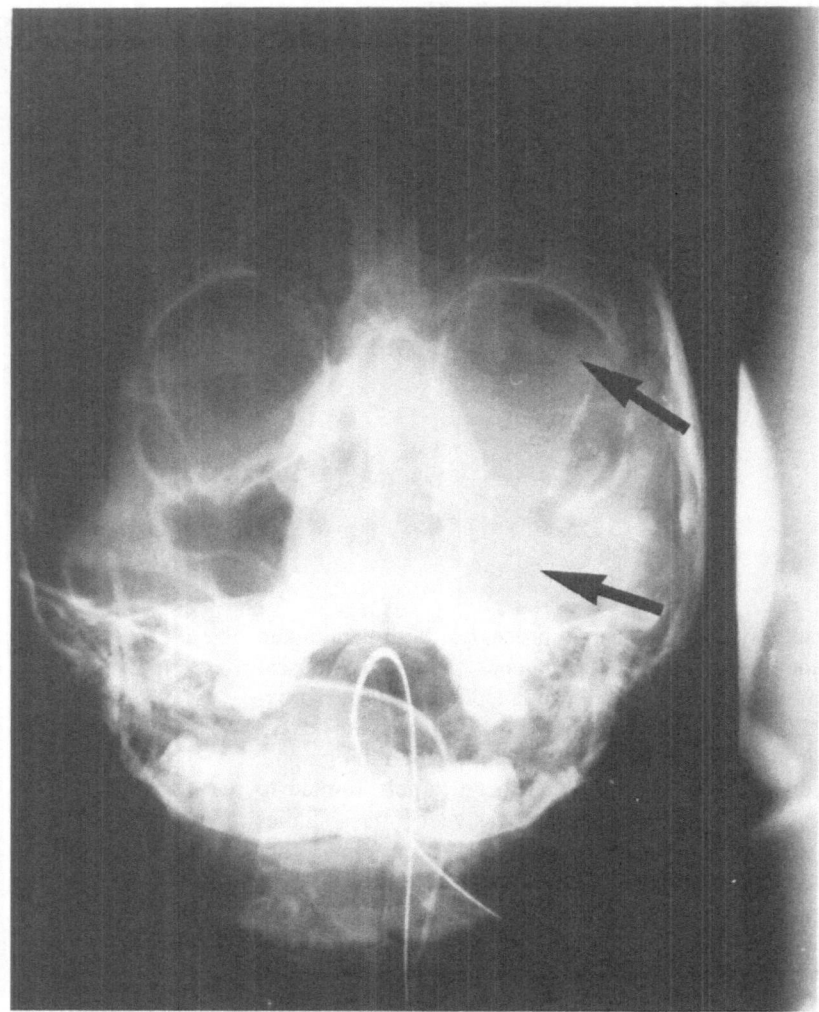

Figure 10-1. Waters view of facial bones demonstrating facial bone fractures with air in left orbit (arrow).

Ultrasound   Sonography is also utilized in identifying post-traumatic hemorrhage into the anterior and posterior chambers of the eye. Intraorbital foreign bodies can be identified as well as the presence of optic nerve swelling. Retinal detachment with coexistent vitreous hemorrhage can be easily detected.

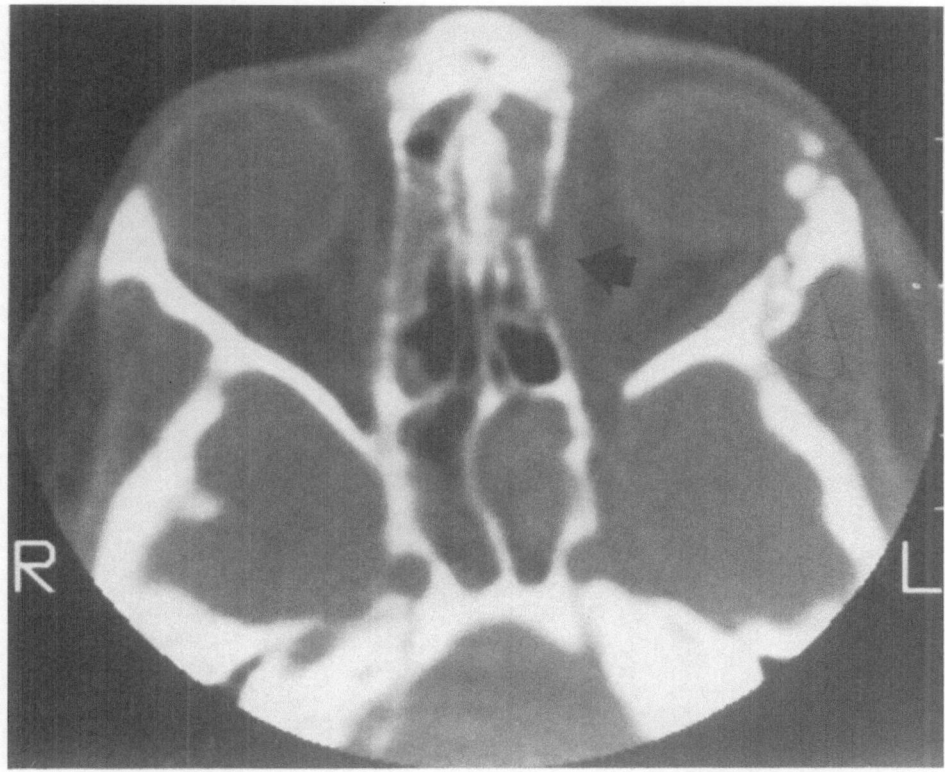

Figure 10-2. Computerized tomography confirming fracture of lamina papyracea (arrow) resulting in intraorbital air.

Proptosis

Following plain radiography, CT is the examination of choice in evaluating patients with proptosis. A variety of inflammatory conditions can cause swelling of the extra-ocular muscles such as that seen in orbital myositis and granulomatous diseases as well as in Graves' disease.[9] Retrobulbar masses resulting in anterior displacement of the optic globe, such as that produced by hemorrhage, lymphoma, or carcinoma invading from the paranasal sinuses (Fig. 10-3), can be identified as the probable etiology of proptosis.

Loss of Vision

CT of the orbits is the examination of choice following inadequate fundoscopic examination and plain radiography of the orbits or optic canals. The etiology of visual loss such

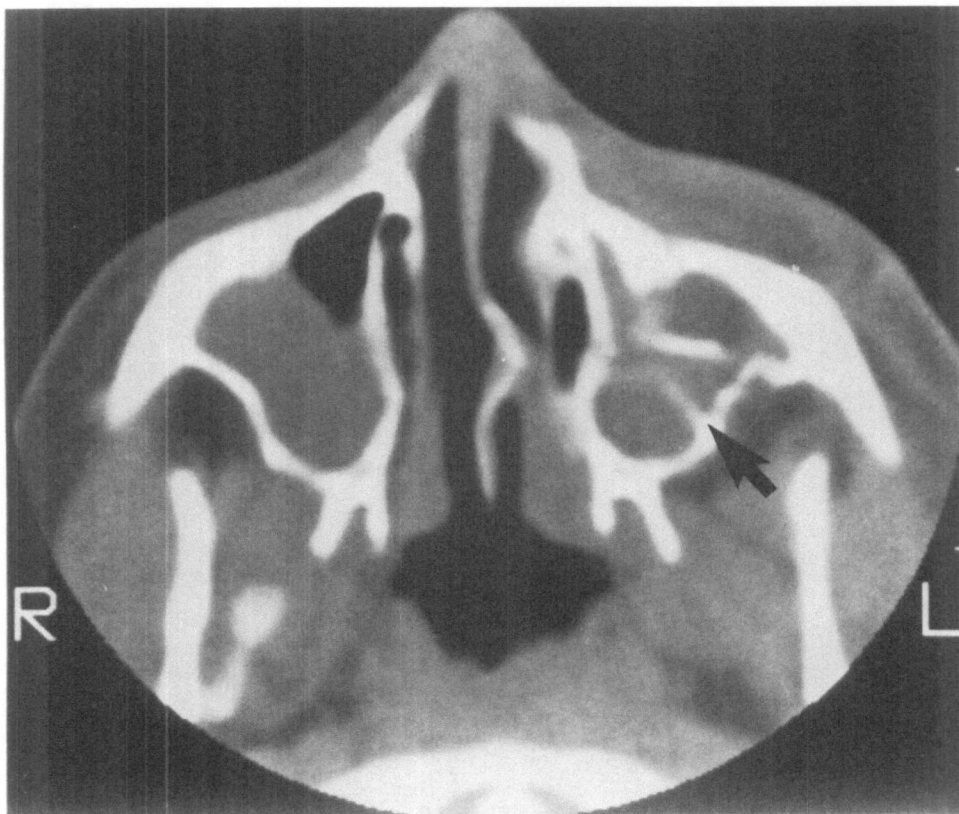

Figure 10-3. Computerized tomography demonstrating carcinoma in left maxillary antrum (arrow) with sinusitis on right.

as optic nerve tumors, lesions involving the choroid such as metastasis, or posttraumatic entrapment of the optic nerve can be easily visualized. Postinflammatory changes of the orbit such as phthisis bulbi or congenital lesions such as retinoblastoma can also be detected as the cause of visual loss. In addition, however, CT can also afford visualization of intracerebral causes of visual disturbance such as lesions affecting the optic chiasm, diseases involving the intracerebral optic pathways, or disturbances afflicting the visual center within the occipital lobes (Fig. 10-4).[1]

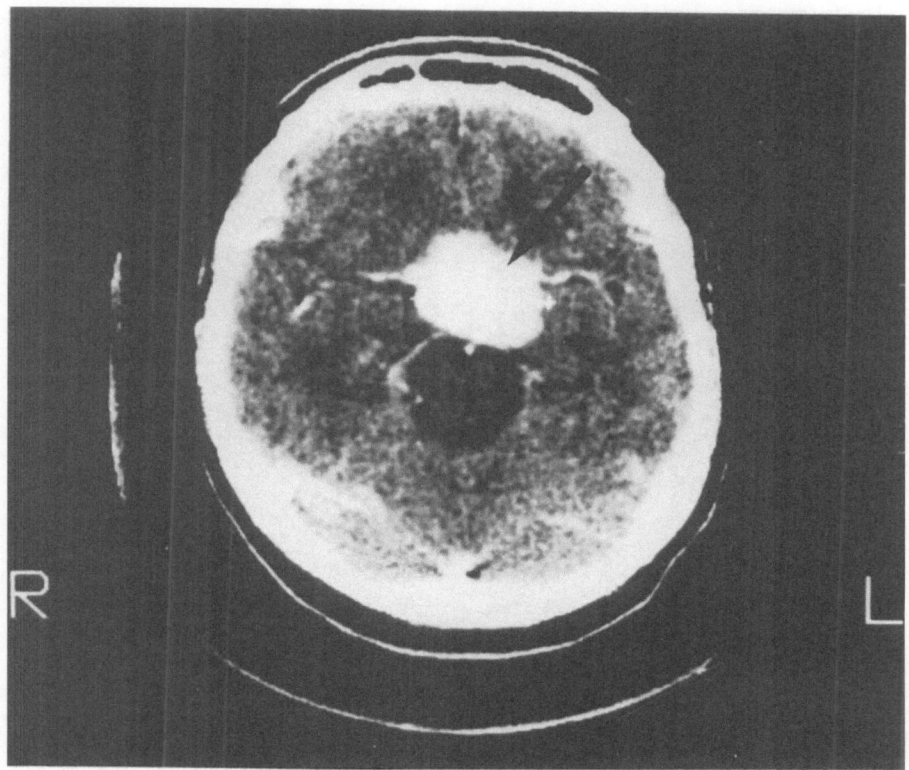

Figure 10-4. Large parasellar mass (arrow) compressing optic chiasm.

CT is a very effective noninvasive means of visualizing lacrimal gland tumors (Fig. 10-5) or lesions adjacent to the lacrimal glands that may affect the function of the gland itself or could result in decreased emptying of the ductal system.[3]

Dacryocystography utilizing radiopharmaceuticals is very useful in the evaluation of patients with epiphora in whom routine clinical tests cannot determine either etiology or site of lacrimal duct obstruction. The presence of lacrimal ductal abnormalities can be detected, as can the relationship of orbital masses adjacent to the ductal system.

LACRIMAL GLAND DYSFUNCTION

Computerized Tomography

Radionuclide Studies

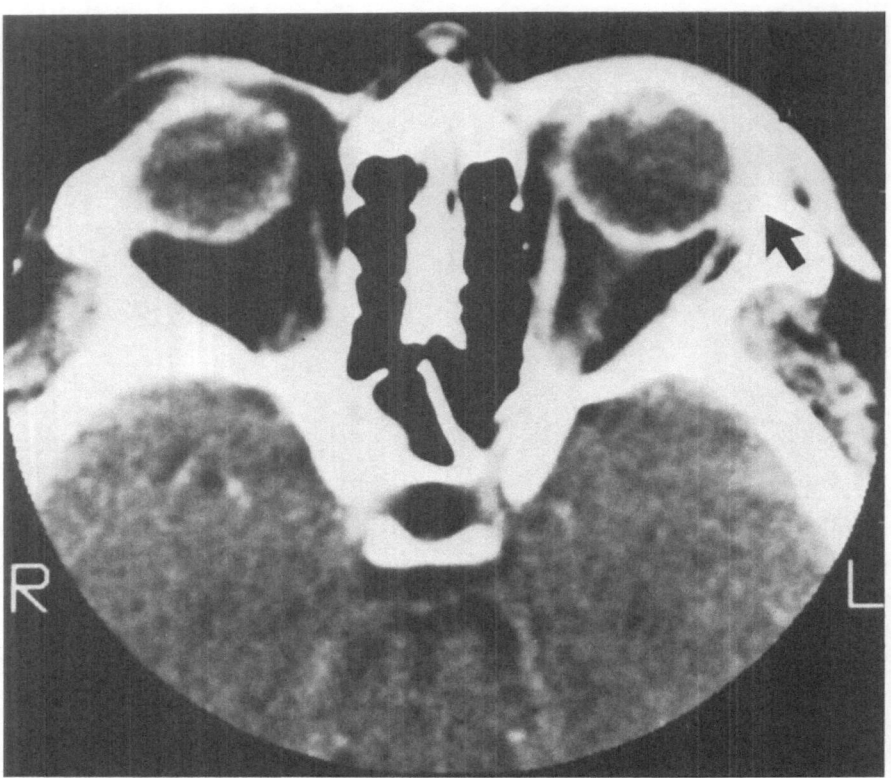

Figure 10-5. Enhancing enlarged left lacrimal gland (arrow) with conjunctival enhancement secondary to sarcoid.

PARANASAL SINUSES

Inflammatory disease of the paranasal sinuses is quite common resulting from either bacterial or allergic sinusitis, which may be acute or chronic in duration. Chronic inflammatory disease may result in space-occupying lesions subsequent to blockage of the ducts that normally empty the sinuses into the nasal cavity. Postinflammatory lesions such as retention cysts, polyps, or mucoceles can be detected radiographically. However, in patients with extensive mucosal thickening, these lesions may not be adequately visualized on plain-radiographic examinations.

Sinusitis

Computerized Tomography

Sinusitis is a fairly easily clinically diagnosed disease, which can be documented utilizing plain radiographs. CT of the sinuses should be reserved for patients in whom paranasal sinus masses are suspected. CT is an excellent means of identifying postinflammatory conditions involving the sinuses such as polyps, retention cysts, mucoceles, or pyocele (Fig. 10-6). In addition to detection of the presence of a lesion, the extent of disease can be evaluated, such as possible bone erosion or destruction. Serial examinations can also detect the response to therapy.

Trauma involving the facial bones frequently involves injury to the paranasal sinuses with resultant mucosal thickening or hemorrhage. Extent of the fractures and displacement of bony fragments is easily identified utilizing CT. The excellent cross-sectional anatomic display will enable the plastic surgeon to identify and classify Le Fort fracture and aid in the determination of reconstruction procedures.[4]

Trauma

Computerized
Tomography

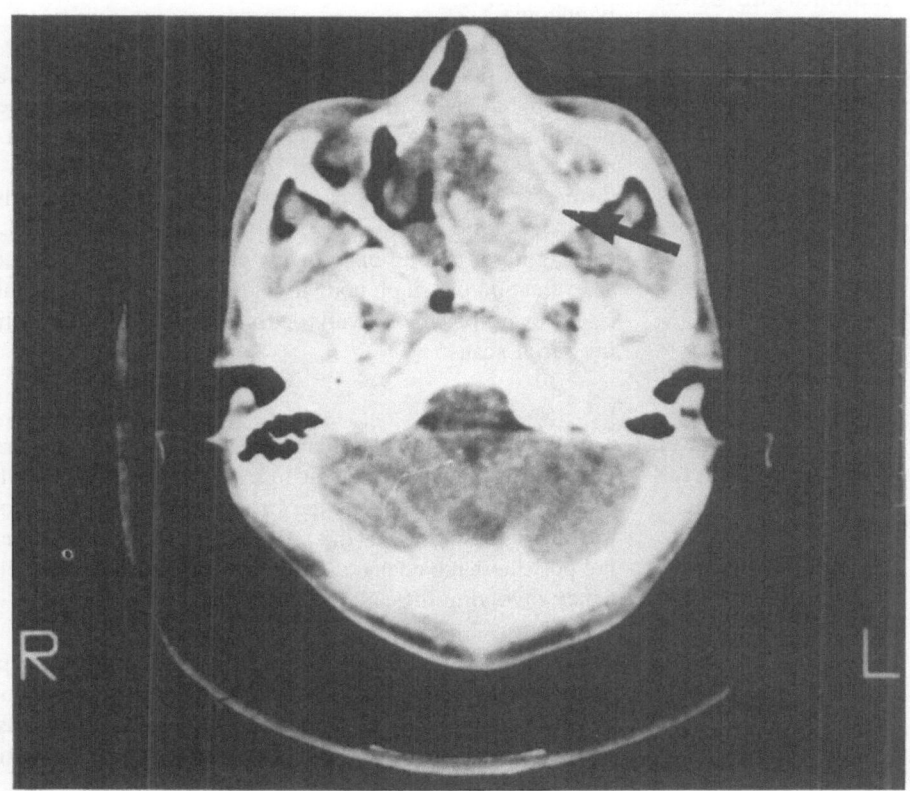

Figure 10-6. Extensive polypoid rhinosinusitis with mucocele (arrow) in left maxillary antrum eroding into ethmoids.

Neoplasia

CT is the preferred means of preoperatively staging the local extent of neoplasms originating in or involving the paranasal sinuses (Figs. 10-7 and 10-8).[6] Unresectability, such as that caused by invasion into the middle cranial fossa via the pterygoid plates, can be easily determined, and this will assist in the determination of appropriate therapeutic modalities. Local lymph node involvement can be determined. Serial scans performed following therapy are useful to follow progression or regression of the primary tumor and lymph nodal involvement.

SALIVARY GLAND– PAROTID ENLARGEMENT

Radionuclide Study

The salivary gland scan utilizing pertechnetate is an infrequently performed study that may be useful as a screening procedure in the detection of functioning (Warthin's) tumor versus nonfunctioning tumors such as carcinoma or lymphoma.[8]

Computerized Tomography

CT with or without utilization of sialographic contrast medium has been useful in distinguishing between focal parotid masses (Fig. 10-9) and diffuse enlargement such as may be seen in inflammatory disease. It can also aid in differentiating between parapharyngeal lesions extending into the parotid and masses originating in the parotid.[7] Local staging of parotid malignancy can be performed as well as evaluation of lymph node involvement. Patients can then be followed postoperatively or following irradiation utilizing serial scans.

LARYNX AND PHARYNX

Prior to the development of CT, the larynx and pharynx were somewhat difficult to evaluate radiographically. Plain-film tomography of the neck supplemented by contrast laryngography was the procedure of choice in evaluating posttraumatic changes, inflammatory disease, or malignancy involving these structures.

Trauma

Computerized Tomography

Although plain-film radiography is a fairly simple method of evaluating the possibility of cartilaginous injury and prevertebral soft tissue swelling, the excellent cross-sectional anatomic display offered by CT can more easily demonstrate the presence of injuries to the neighboring soft tissue structures of the neck such as the esophagus or great

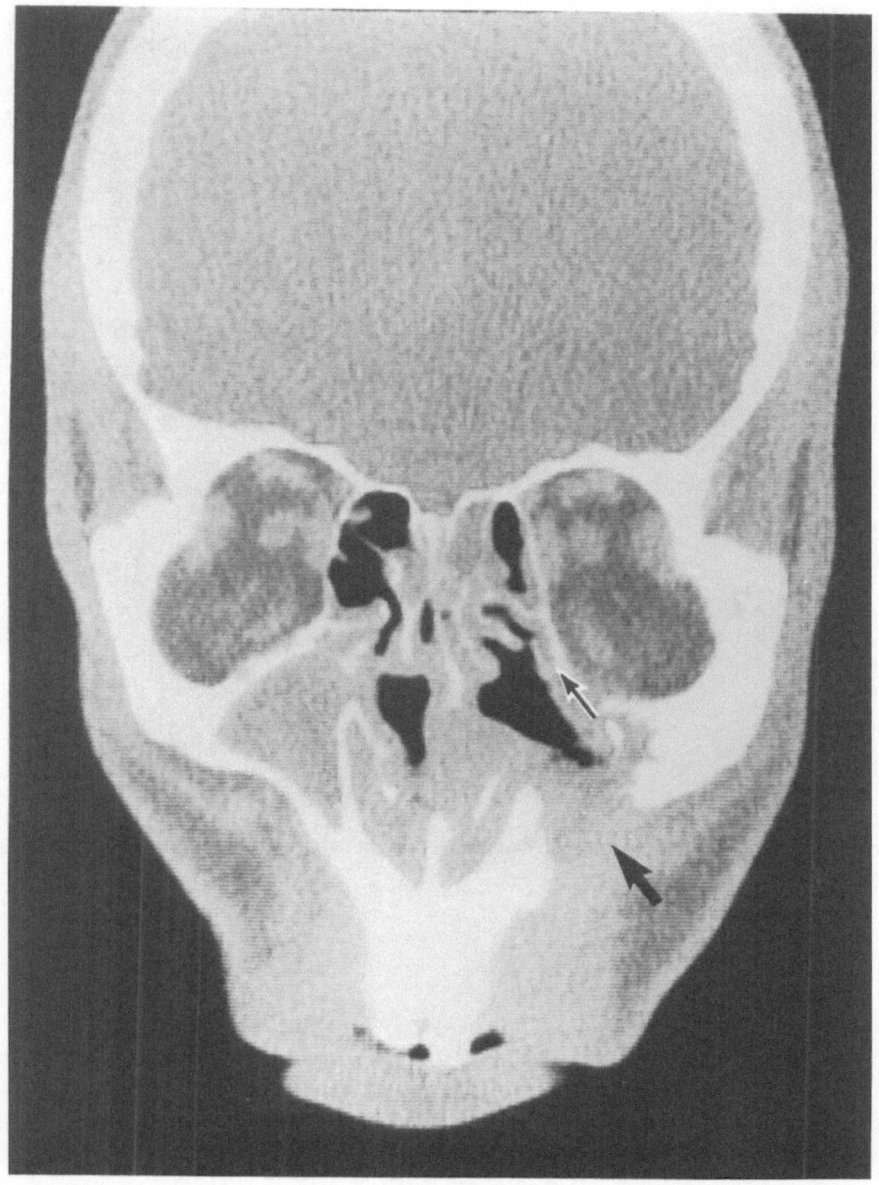

Figure 10-7. Coronal computerized tomography demonstrating lymphoma involving the maxill-ary and ethmoid sinuses. Destruction of alveolar ridge (arrow) by tumor.

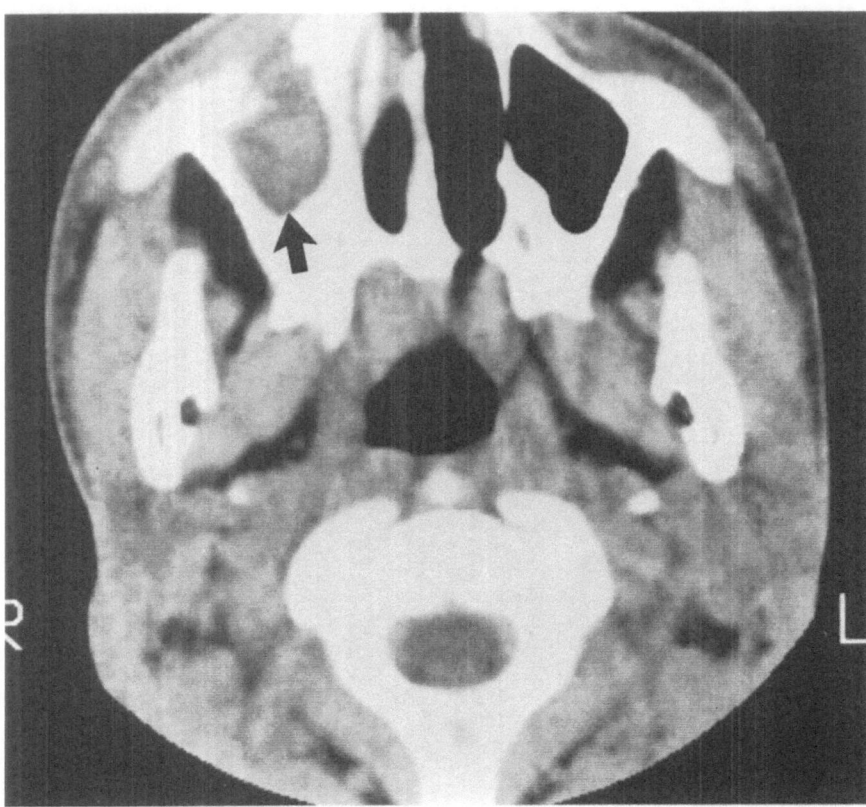

Figure 10-8. Axial scan of patient with carcinoma of right maxillary sinus destroying anterior wall of sinus (arrow).

vessels. More subtle degrees of cartilaginous injury or compromise of the airway can be detected utilizing this technique supplemented by reconstructed images in other projections.

Malignancy   Determination of malignancy in the larynx or pharynx is essentially a clinical diagnosis and usually requires a biopsy. However, CT, although nonspecific, has greatly aided in the local staging of known laryngeal or pharyngeal

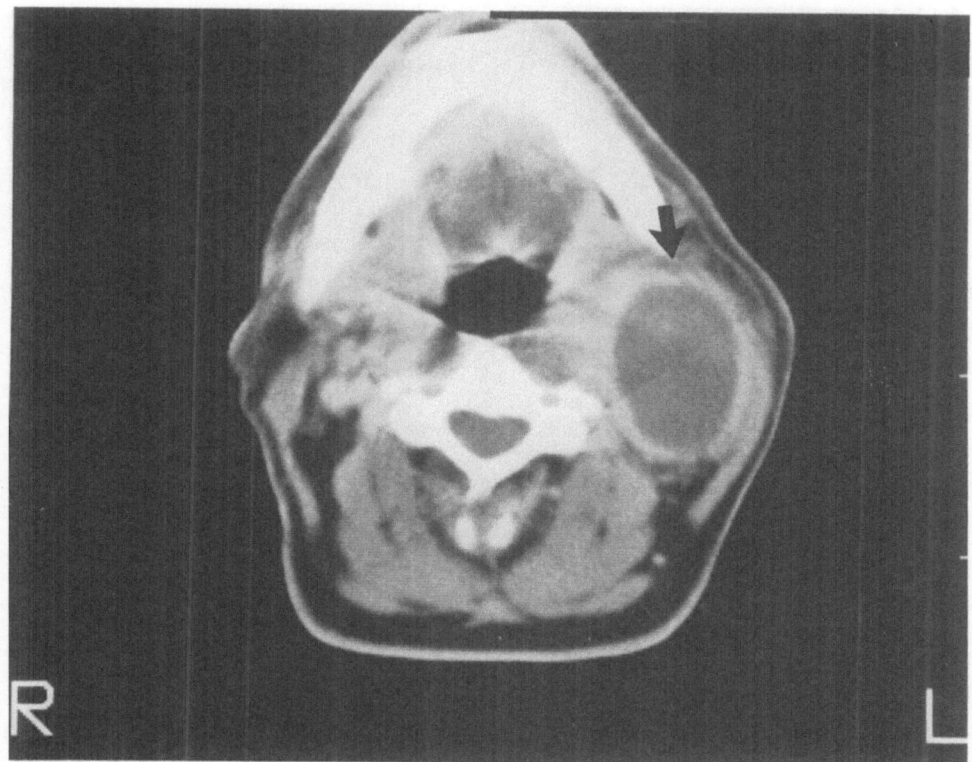

Figure 10-9. Large benign cyst of left parotid gland (arrow).

neoplasm (Figs. 10-10 to 10-12). The possibility of resection can be determined.[5] Both palpable and nonpalpable cervical lymphadenopathy can be detected. Patients can be followed with serial scans postoperatively or following irradiation to detect the progression or regression of the local disease and lymph nodal involvement.

Arthrography of the temporomandibular joint has been the standard radiologic procedure of choice for diagnosing internal derangements of the temporomandibular joints. Utilizing this procedure, information such as integrity of the meniscus and position of the meniscus can be obtained. The

TEMPORO-MANDIBULAR JOINT DYSFUNCTION

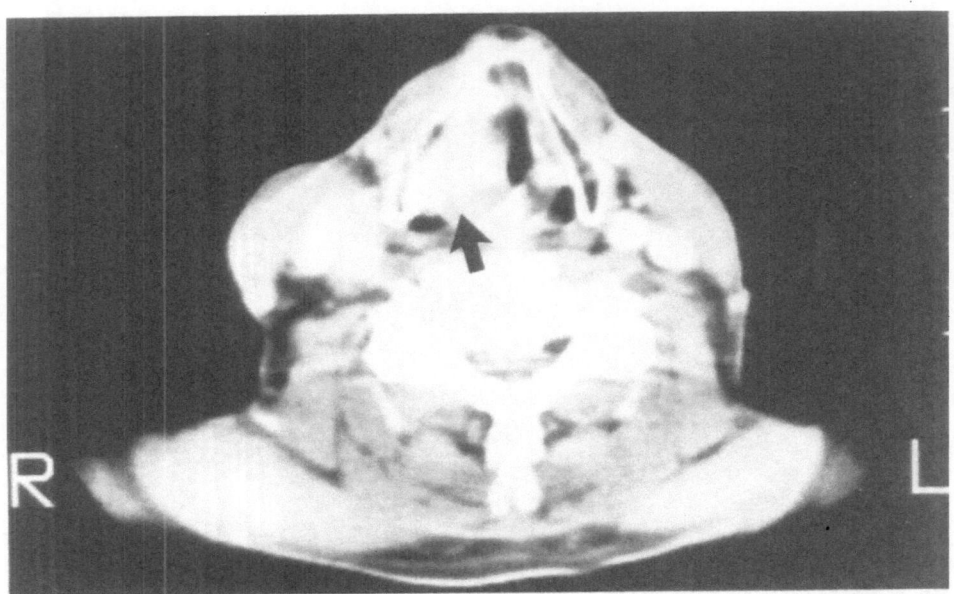

Figure 10-10. Extensive tumor involving right vocal cord and aryepiglottic fold (arrow).

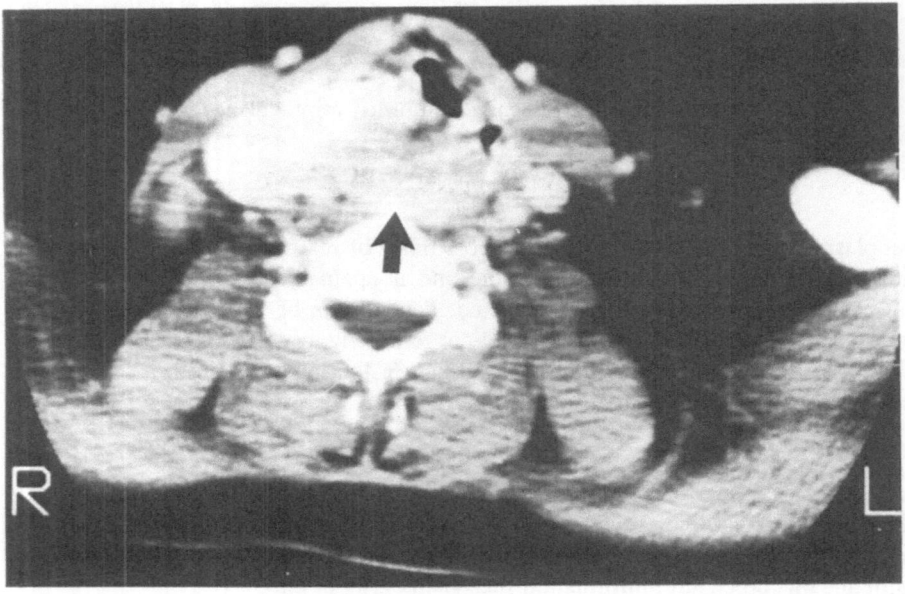

Figure 10-11. Large tumor involving piriform sinuses bilaterally (arrow) crossing midline posteriorly.

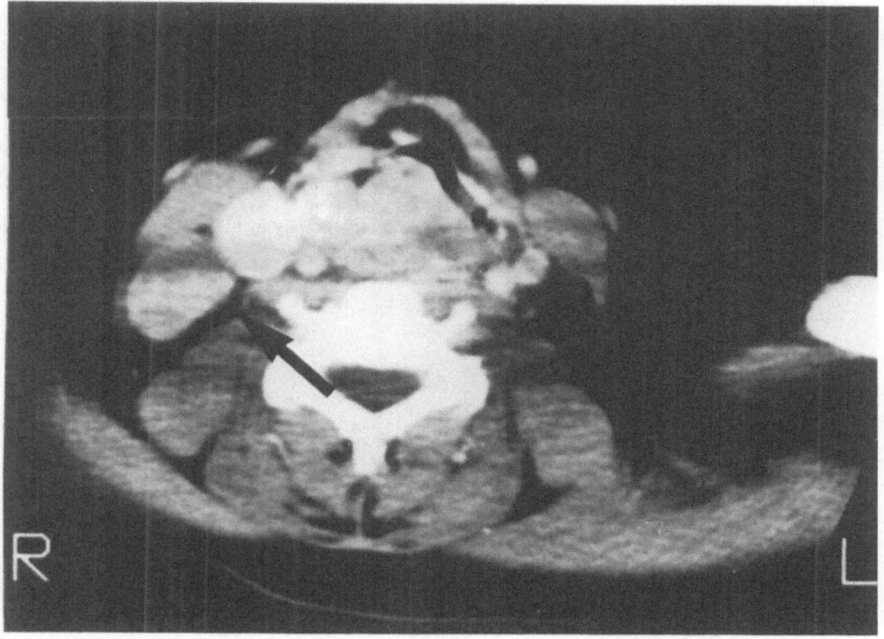

Figure 10-12. Same patient as in Fig. 11 with huge cervical lymphadenopathy (arrow).

procedure, however, is somewhat painful and is invasive. There is also a fairly high radiation dose delivered to the lens of the eye and thyroid gland depending on the quantity of fluoroscopy used and whether tomograms are necessary. CT utilizing sagittal reconstruction and the blink-mode software package have proved useful in diagnosing displaced temporomandibular joint menisci.[2]

REFERENCES

1. Citrin CM, Alper MG: Computed tomography of the visual pathways. *Comput Tomogr* 1979;3:305–331.
2. Helms CA, Vogler JB III, Morrish RB Jr: Temporomandibular joint internal derangements: CT diagnosis. *Radiology* 1984;152:459–462.
3. Hesselink JR, Davis KR, Dallow RL, et al: Computed tomography of masses in the lacrimal gland region. *Radiology* 1979;131:143–147.
4. Mancuso A, Hanafee W: *Computed Tomography of the Head and Neck*. Baltimore, Williams & Wilkins, 1982, p 211.
5. Mancuso AA, Hanafee WN: A comparative evaluation of computed tomography and laryngography. *Radiology* 1979;133:131–138.
6. Parson C, Hodson N: Computed tomography of paranasal sinus tumors. *Radiology* 1979;132:641–645.

7. Rice DH, Mancuso AA, Hanafee WN: Computerized tomography with simultaneous sialography in evaluating parotid tumors. *Arch Otolaryngol* 1980;106:472–473.
8. Schall GL, DiChiro G: Clinical usefulness of salivary gland scanning. *Semin Nucl Med* 1972;2:270.
9. Trokel SL, Hilal SK: Recognition and differential diagnosis of enlarged extraocular muscles in computed tomography. *Am J Ophthalmol* 1979;87:503–512.
10. Zilkha A: Computed tomography of blow-out fractures of the medial orbital wall. *AJNR* 1981;2:427–429.

11   Musculoskeletal System

Osteomyelitis is a difficult clinical diagnosis to make since there is always accompanying overlying cellulitis. Bone radiographs are useful in complementing the physical examination; however, the radiographic findings of osteomyelitis are similar to changes produced by many primary and secondary bone neoplasms, making the radiographic diagnosis difficult at times. The newer imaging modalities such as bone scan, gallium scan, and computerized tomography (CT) have been very useful in augmenting the plain-film findings.

INFLAMMATORY DISEASE

The radionuclide bone scan is a more sensitive means of detecting osteomyelitis than plain radiographs with the scan becoming positive 1–2 weeks earlier than the radiographic findings in many instances. Occasionally, early osteomyelitis in its purely destructive phase may result in a cold defect (Fig. 11-1); however, once bone repair begins, a hot lesion will signal the presence of infection (Figs. 11-2 and 11-3).[4] The bone scan, although sensitive, is non-specific, and plain radiographs of the bones in question are necessary to exclude other diagnostic possibilities such as trauma or neoplasm. In addition, three-phase bone imaging

Nuclear Bone Scan

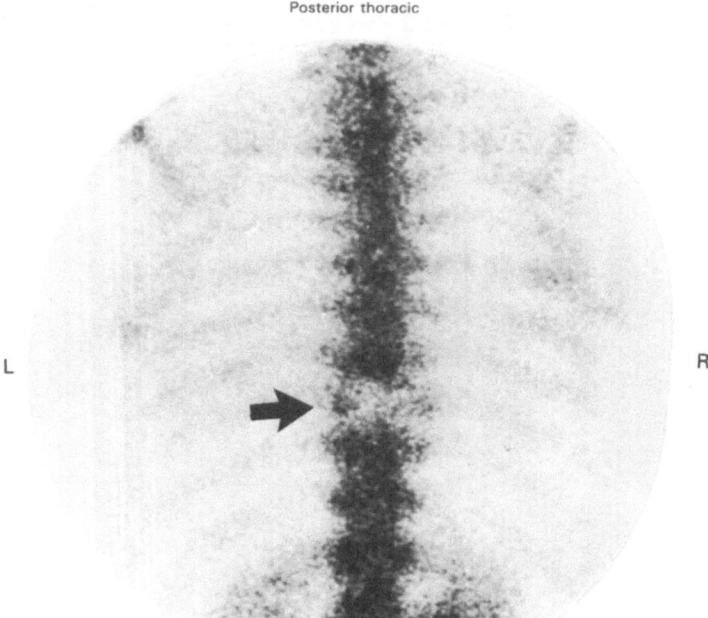

Posterior thoracic

L   R

Figure 11-1. Early destructive osteomyelitis in lower thoracic spine (arrow) depicted by cold spot on bone scan.

utilizing a vascular phase, immediate static images, and delayed static images is also useful in narrowing the differential diagnosis in many cases. Gallium scan is very useful for confirmatory evidence of osteomyelitis. This is especially true in younger children, who routinely have increased activity at the normal metaphyseal growth centers on their bone scans.

Computerized Tomography

CT has not proven generally necessary for documentation, localization, or diagnosis of infection because radiography and bone scan are usually adequate. However, CT can detect the earliest changes in medullary cavities of the bone and is very useful in evaluation of the anatomic extent of both bony and soft tissue spread of infection (Fig. 11-4).[6] In equivocal cases, CT-directed biopsy and aspiration is also quite useful.

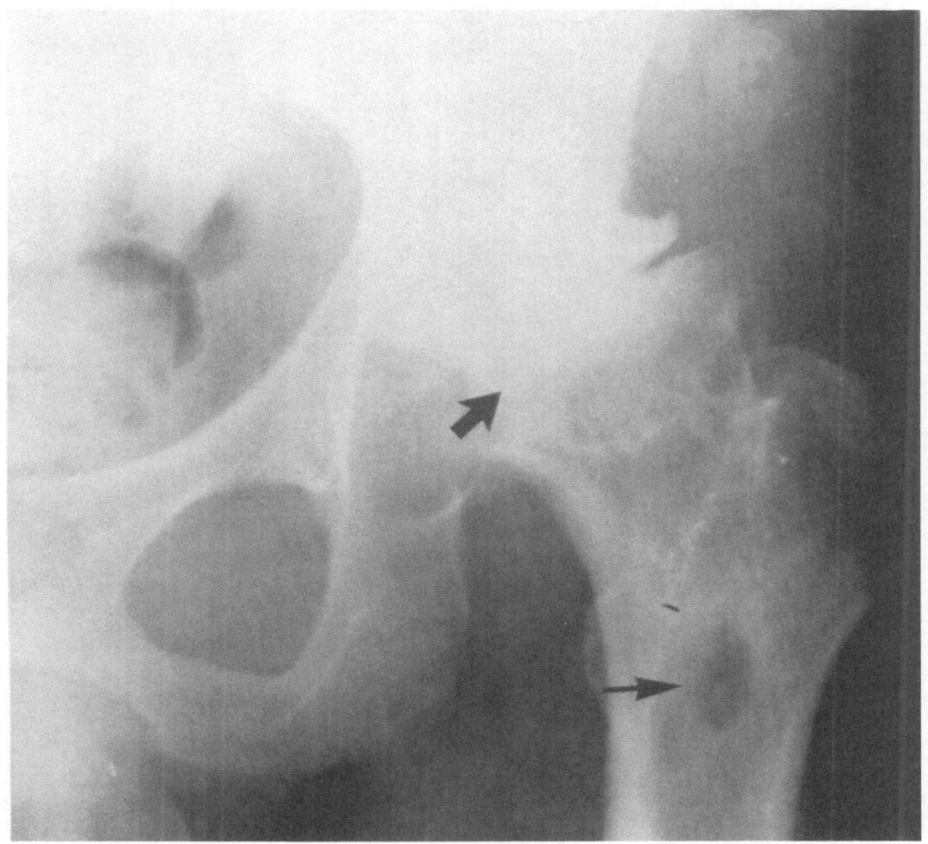

Figure 11-2. Lytic lesion (arrow) in subtrochanteric femoral shaft representing focus of osteomyelitis in patient with sickle cell anemia who also has aseptic necrosis of femoral head (arrow).

TRAUMA

In the acutely traumatized patient, the plain radiograph of the bone in question is usually sufficient to allow for diagnosis and description of the acute fracture. However, in many instances, such as stress fractures or in anatomically complex parts of the body such as the pelvis or hips, a fracture line is not well visualized, and further imaging modalities are necessary to confirm the presence of fracture.

Nuclear Medicine

In patients with suspected stress fractures, the initial radiograph may appear normal for several weeks until actual callous formation. The bone scan will show the fracture

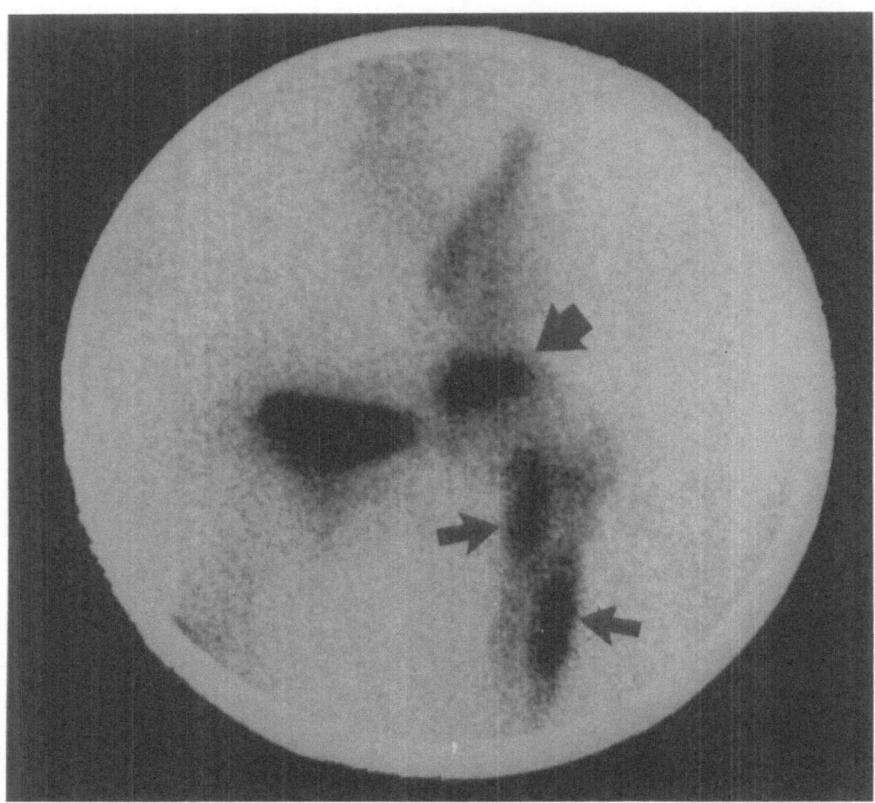

Figure 11-3. Bone scan showing increased activity (arrow) in femoral head representing avascular necrosis and lower area representing osteomyelitis (arrow).

almost immediately.[7] The bone scan is also useful in detecting recent fractures in areas that are difficult to study on plain radiography, such as low cervical spine, sternum, and acetabulum. A major complication of trauma is aseptic necrosis, which most commonly afflicts the hip or navicular bone of the wrist. The bone scan and flow study will detect the earliest signs of avascular necrosis, which will be manifested by decreased flow and areas of decreased activity within the afflicted bone prior to radiographic changes.

Computerized Tomography   CT has gained popularity in assessing trauma. The excellent cross-sectional display of anatomy and ability to reconstruct the images in multiple planes have made CT useful in the evaluation of facial trauma, especially in the

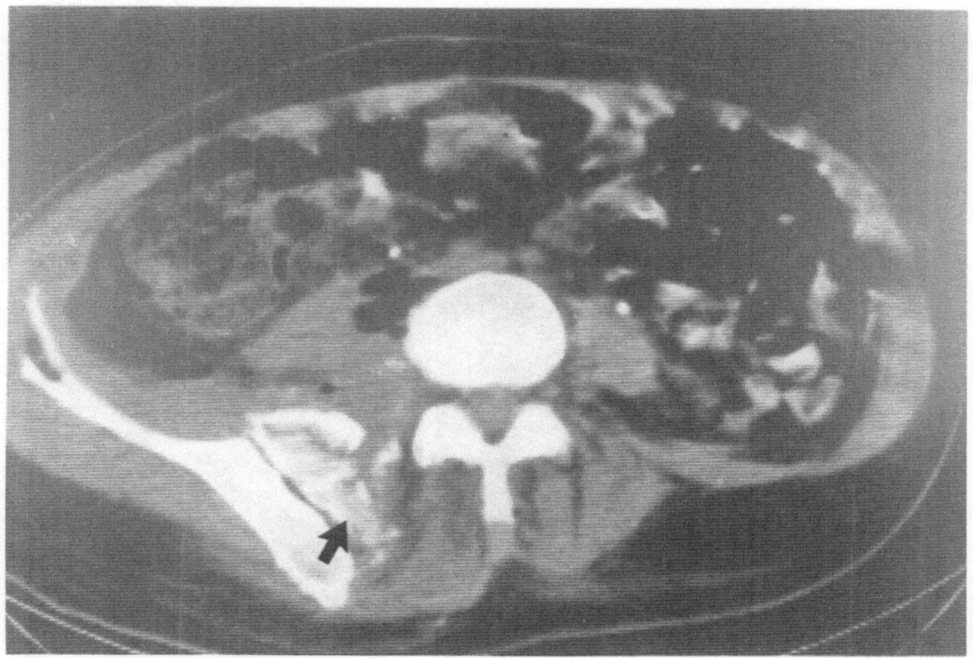

Figure 11-4. Extensive destruction of sacrum due to osteomyelitis (arrow) with retroperitoneal abscess.

evaluation of orbital injury to diagnose the presence of a blowout fracture or to assess patency of the optic canal in patients with decreasing vision following facial trauma.

CT is helpful in diagnosing cervical spine injuries and assessing the extent of the injury as well as stability of the fractures. The involvement of posterior neural arch structures and patency of the spinal canal are easily assessed (Fig. 11-5). CT is especially helpful to orthopedists trying to assess acetabular fractures, which are not easily seen on plain radiographs (Fig. 11-6). The presence and extent of accompanying soft tissue hematomas adjacent to vital structures, both intraabdominal and intrapelvic, can be assessed and evaluated utilizing this procedure.

PAINFUL PROSTHESES

With the increasing average age of the adult population, joint prostheses are more frequently utilized. The patient with a painful prosthesis presents a complex problem

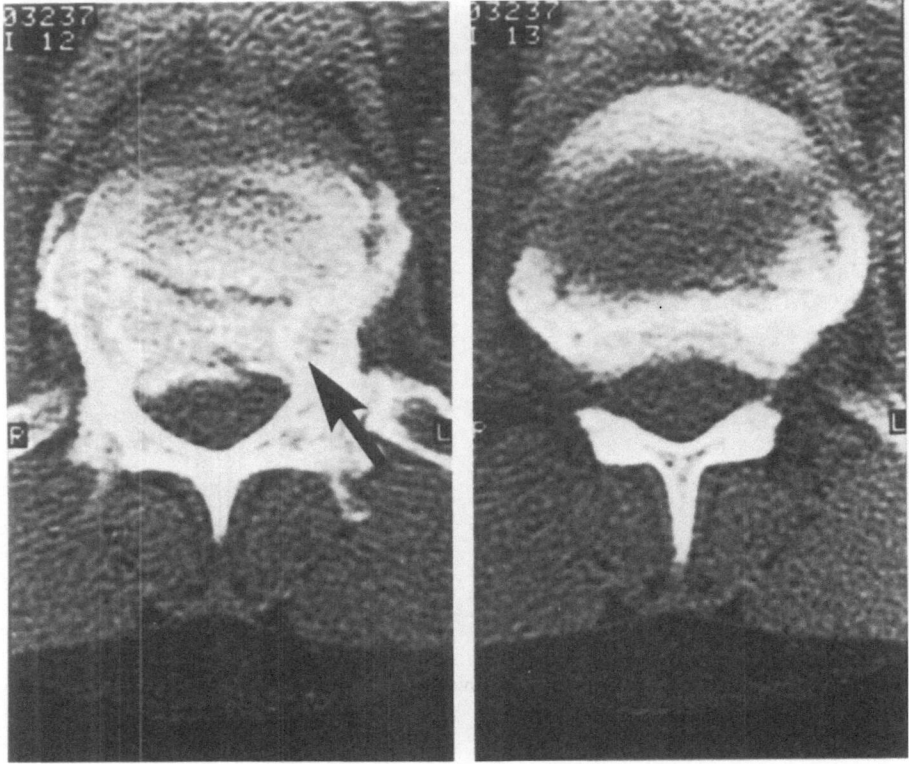

Figure 11-5. Compression fracture of vertebral body with displaced bone (arrow) fragment in spinal canal.

to the orthopedist. Many cases of loosening or infection can be easily diagnosed using plain radiographs or single-contrast arthography. However, in negative or equivocal cases bone scanning is a sensitive and sometimes more specific means of evaluating the source and cause of pain.[3]

NEOPLASMS

Primary Bone Lesions

The most specific means of diagnosing and classifying a primary bone tumor is the plain radiograph, which in most cases will result in a tissue-specific diagnosis. Radionuclide scans and CTs are complementary procedures and should not replace the plain radiograph as the primary diagnostic study.

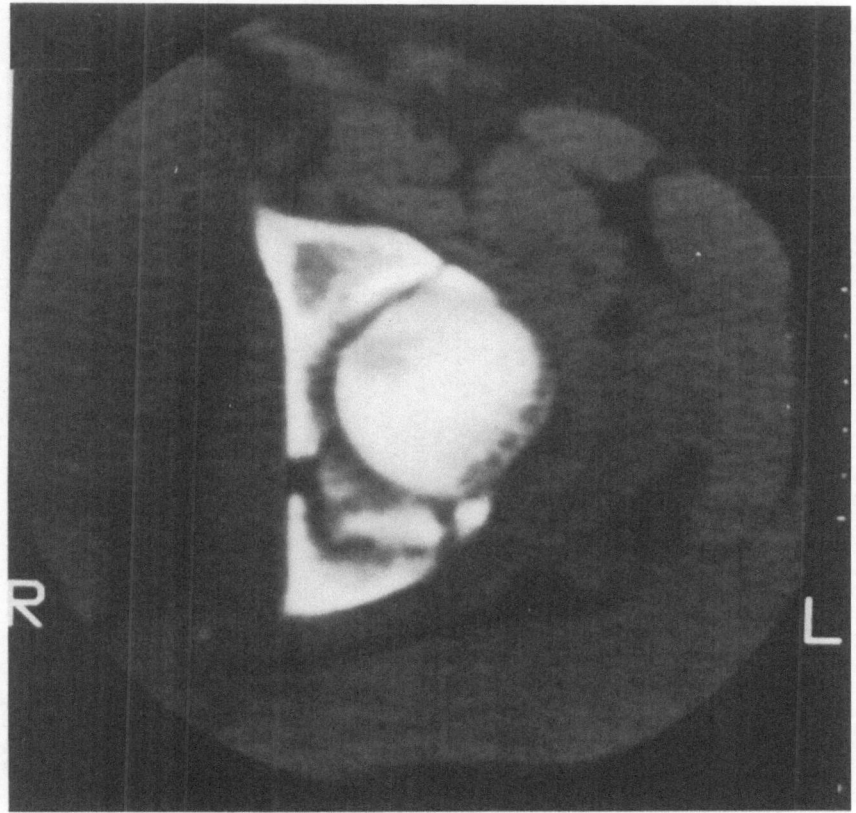

Figure 11-6. Extensive fracture of acetabulum (arrow) demonstrated on computerized tomography.

The primary role of bone scanning in a patient with a primary bone tumor is to evaluate the possibility of other occult bony lesions (Fig. 11-7). Occasionally, in patients with osteosarcoma, the bone scan tracer may localize in organs with bony metastases such as the liver or lungs.

Nuclear Medicine

The primary role of CT is to localize the anatomic spread of the bone tumor and soft tissue extent, if any (Fig. 11-8). The vascularity or hypovascularity of the lesion can be determined utilizing intravenous contrast. In addition, optimal sites for percutaneous biopsy can be determined.

Computerized Tomography

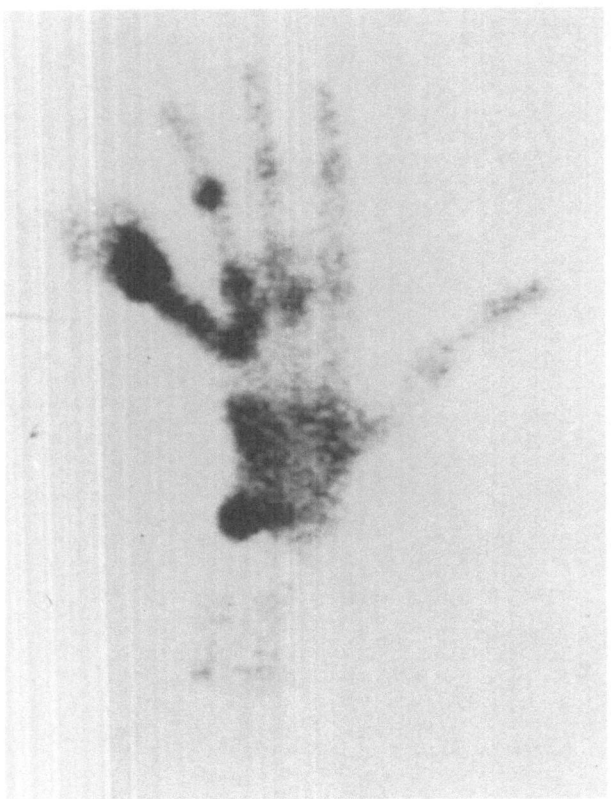

Figure 11-7. Multifocal giant cell tumors in hand and wrist of patient with previously detected tumor of distal femur.

Metastases

The metastatic plain-film bone survey was utilized in the past in patients with tumors that had a high propensity for spreading to the bone such as breast, lung, thyroid, and renal tumors. However, the bone scan has replaced the bone survey in detecting metastases owing to improved sensitivity.

Nuclear Medicine

The bone scan is a much more sensitive means of detecting bone metastases in staging tumors prior to therapy as well as following therapy (Fig. 11-9).[1] However, owing to the nonspecificity of positive bone scans, all positive areas must be evaluated with recent plain films. In addition, clinically suspected areas of metastasis should be radiographed in the event of a false-negative bone scan.

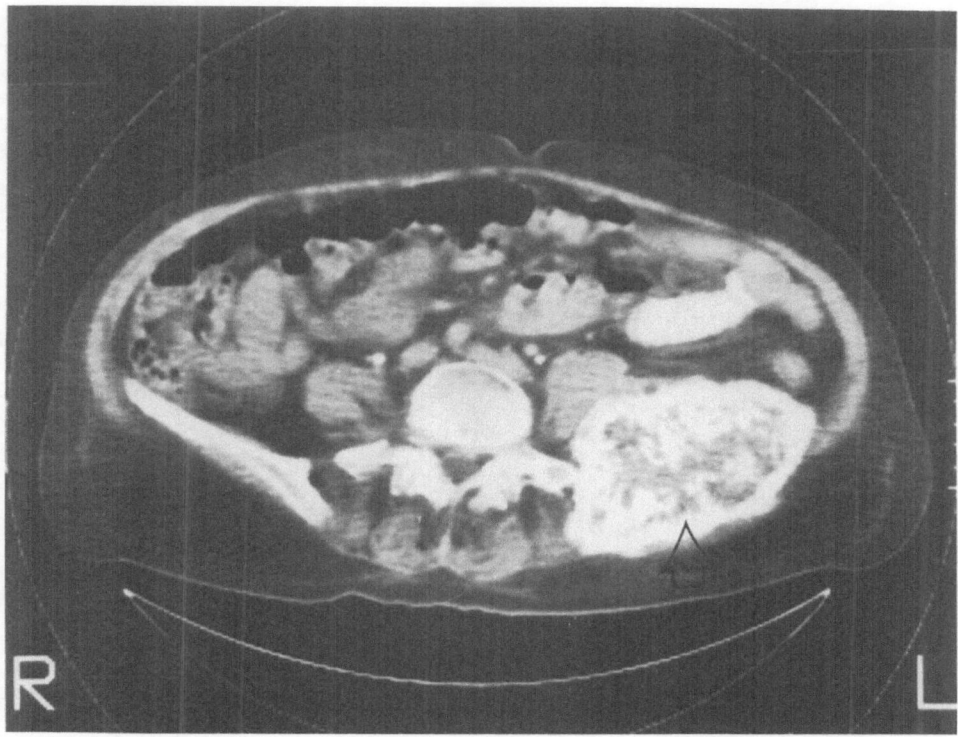

Figure 11-8. Computerized tomography demonstration of large chondrosarcoma (arrow) involving left iliac wing without soft tissue involvement.

Computerized Tomography

CT has a very limited use in the evaluation of bone metastasis. The major use would be in patients with equivocal lesions in whom percutaneous-directed biopsy is necessary. The other situation in which CT may be useful is in evaluation of the soft tissue extent of a known metastasis and to assess the effects exerted on neighboring structures such as spinal cord impingement by metastasis arising within a vertebral body.

SOFT TISSUE MASSES

Soft tissue masses have in the past been evaluated utilizing plain films and angiography. The newer imaging modalities have all but eliminated the need for more invasive diagnostic studies at this time.

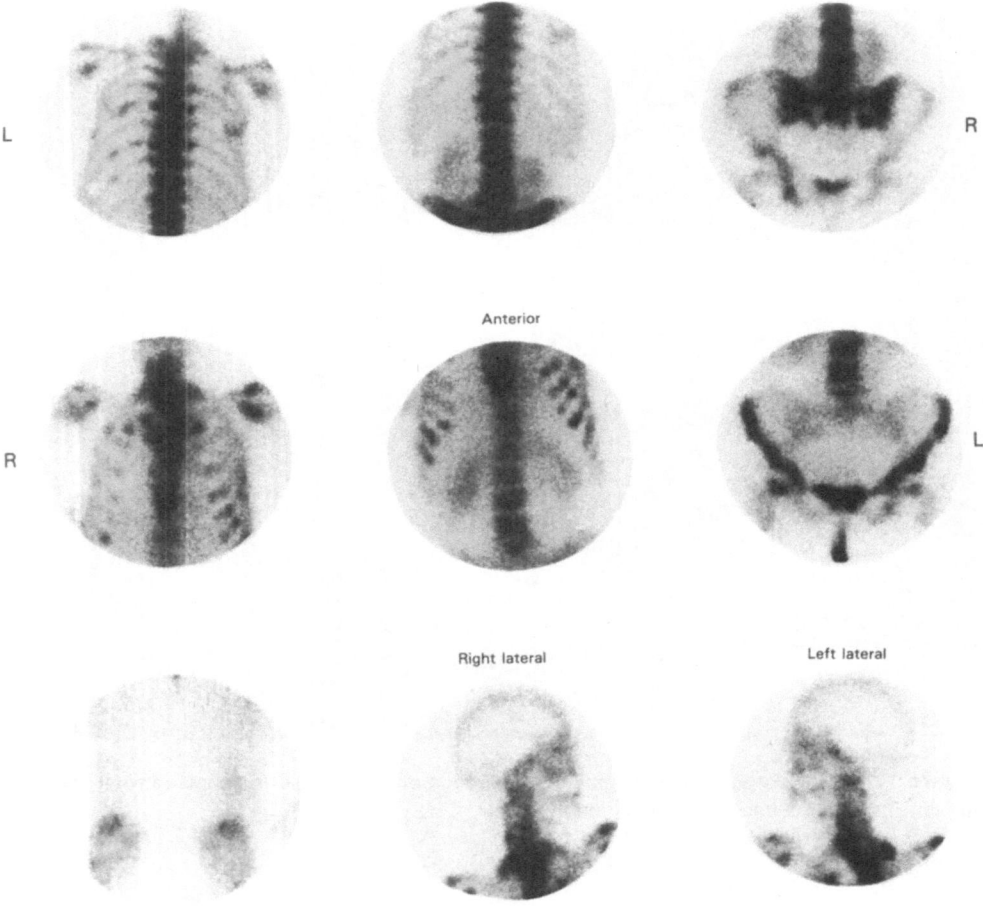

Anterior

Right lateral   Left lateral

Figure 11-9. Bone scan revealing multiple metastases in patient with breast carcinoma.

Bone Scan   Bone scanning in patients with soft tissue masses is a sensitive means of evaluating the possibility of local bone invasion or distant skeletal metastases. Increased activity in a bone adjacent to a soft tissue tumor implies direct invasion.

Ultrasound   Ultrasound is useful in detecting and differentiating between fluid-filled and solid soft tissue masses. It has been especially useful to orthopedists in patients with palpable soft tissue masses in the popliteal fossa and will confidently noninvasively detect Baker's cyst (Fig. 11-10). Ultrasound is also useful for localization of percutaneous biopsy of soft tissue masses.

CT gives the most detailed anatomic information and provides precise definition of radial spread of soft tissue lesions. One can obtain information about tumor tissue density and can show vascularity or avascularity of lesions as well as the relationship to bony structures (Fig. 11-11).[2] Percutaneous biopsy procedures may be done utilizing CT guidance.

Computerized Tomography

The usual radiographic means of evaluating joint pain is the plain film. However, in many instances there may be pain accompanied by joint effusion but no detectable bony abnormalities. Newer imaging modalities have markedly

JOINT PAIN

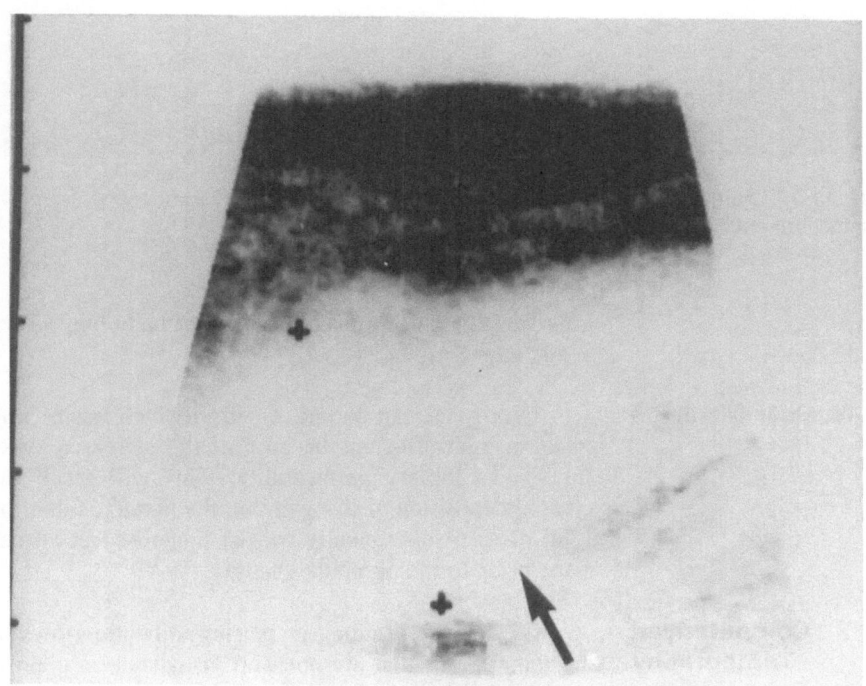

Figure 11-10. Sonographic demonstration of large Baker's cyst (arrow) in popliteal fossa.

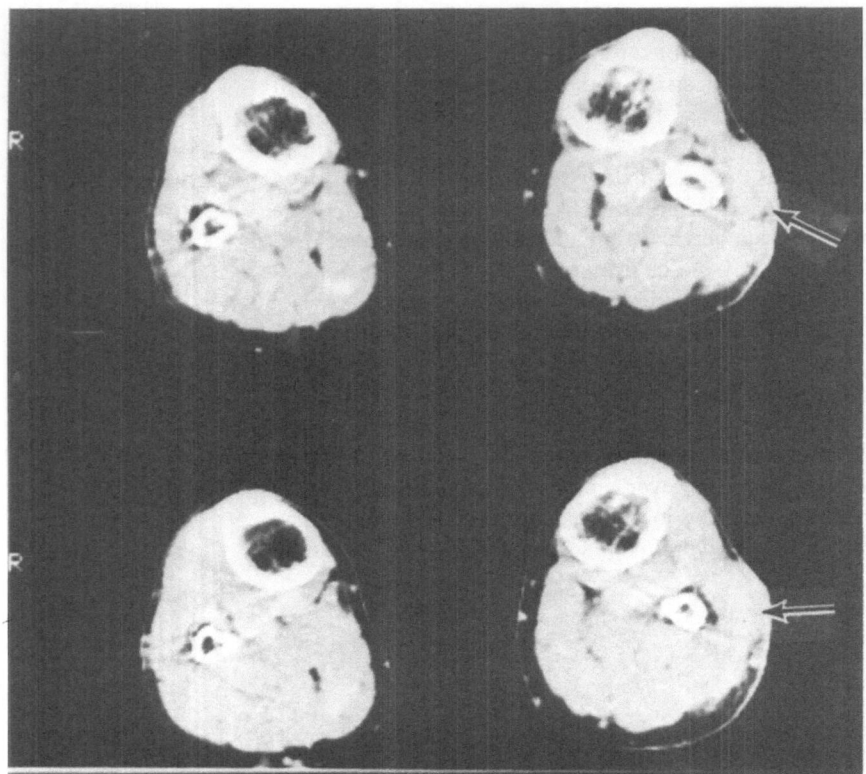

Figure 11-11. Soft tissue mass with increased vascularity (arrow) representing fibrous histrocytoma. No bone invasion seen.

improved the earlier detection of joint pathology in recent years.

Nuclear Medicine

Joint scans can be performed in which tracer concentrates in joint effusions because of the increased synovial flow and capillary permeability. This will result in increased deposition of the agent on the juxtaarticular bone.[5] Joint disease subsequently can be diagnosed at an earlier stage prior to radiographic changes.

Computerized Tomography

CT has been finding increasing utilization in evaluating joint spaces that are not well visualized on plain radiographs such as the temporomandibular joints, sacroiliac joints, the knees, hips, and sternoclavicular joints.

The bone scan is a more sensitive means of detecting bones involved with metabolic disorders such as renal osteodystrophy, hyperparathyroidism, or Paget's disease (Fig. 11-12), which, in many instances, will eliminate the need for a radiographic bone survey. As the findings are nonspecific, positive findings on the bone scan will need radiographic correlation. This will also result in a reduced radiation dose to the patient. In certain institutions the Norland-Cameron

GENERALIZED METABOLIC BONE DISEASE

Nuclear Medicine

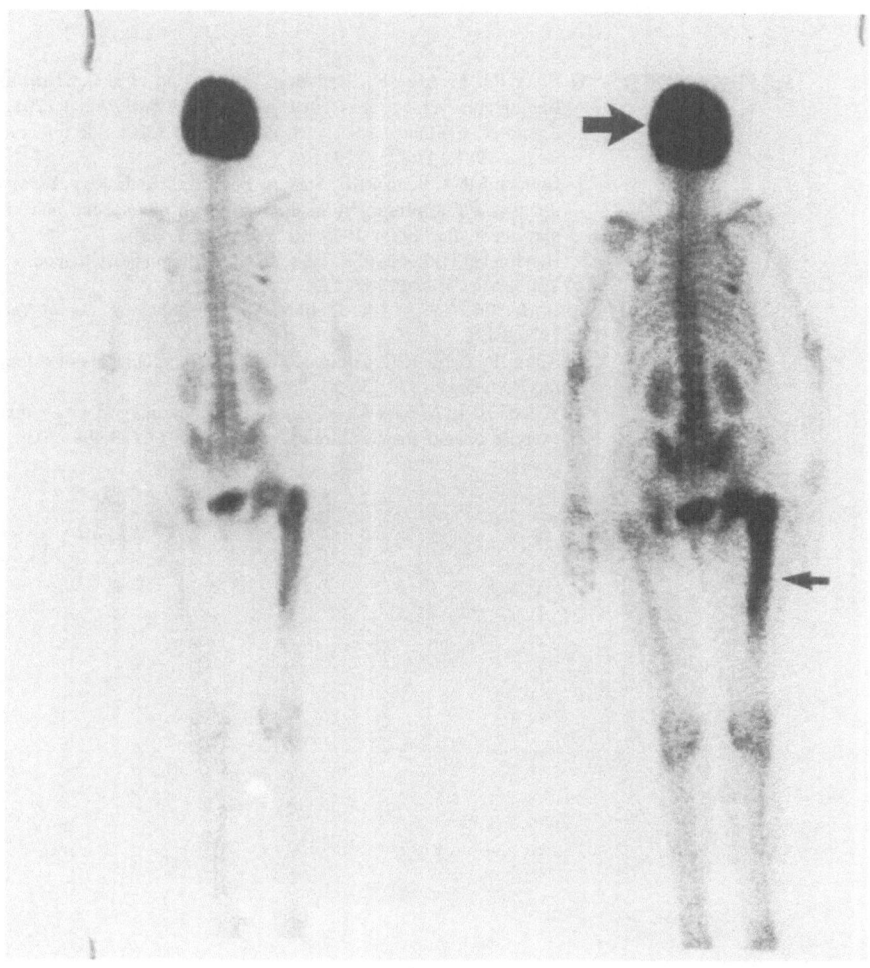

Figure 11-12. Bone scan revealing focal sites of Paget's disease involving right femoral shaft and skull (arrows).

bone mineral analyzers are useful in evaluation and quantitation of osteoporosis resulting in earlier detection of the disease, and subsequently improved treatment or prophylactic measures can be taken.

Computerized Tomography

There is very little utilization for CT in the evaluation of most generalized metabolic disorders affecting the bone. However, quantitative spinal bone mineral estimation can be performed with CT utilizing a special software package. This is limited to a few, select medical centers at this time.

REFERENCES

1. Blaur RJ, McAfee JG: Radiological detection of skeletal metastases: Radiographs versus scans. *Int J Radiat Oncol Biol Phys* 1:1201, 1976.
2. Egund N, Ekelund L, Sako M, et al: CT of soft tissue tumors. *Am J Radiol* 1981;137:725–729.
3. Gelman MI, Coleman RE, Stevens PM, et al: Radiology, radionuclide imaging and arthrography in the evaluation of total hip and knee replacement. *Radiology* 1978;128:677–682.
4. Handmaker H, Leonard R: Bone scan in inflammatory osseous disease. *Semin Nucl Med* 1976;6:95.
5. Hoffer PB, Genant HK: Radionuclide joint imaging. *Semin Nucl Med* 1976;6:121.
6. Kuhn JP, Berger PE: Computed tomographic diagnosis of osteomyelitis. *Radiology* 1979;130:503–506.
7. Wilcox JR Jr, Maniot AL, Green JP: Bone scanning in the evaluation of exercise-related stress injuries. *Radiology* 1977;123:699–703.

Breast

The primary screening procedure and most accurate technique for evaluating the breast has been plain-film mammography. In recent years, ultrasound has been a useful procedure in conjunction with mammograms, especially in younger patients or those in whom cystic and solid lesions must be differentiated. Occasional masses have been detected on computerized tomography (CT). It is now hoped that magnetic resonance imaging may be able to supplement or perhaps even replace mammography in more definitive evaluation of breast lesions.

ULTRASOUND

Ultrasound has proven to be a useful complementary study to mammography in the study of breast disease. Each examination provides a different type of information, and combination of the two studies yields a more complete evaluation of breast parenchyma.[5] Even on the mammogram with a dense glandular pattern, distinct lesions may be clearly seen sonographically that are not visualized radiographically. Sonographically, a malignant lesion may be distinguished by irregular margins[4] as opposed to the well-circumscribed borders of the benign lesions (Figs. 12-1 and

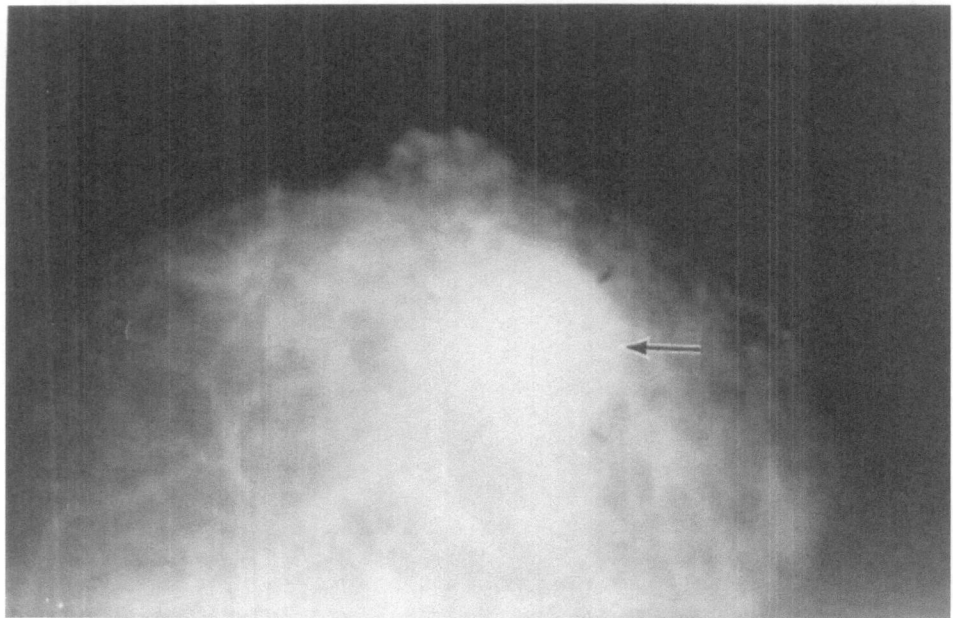

Figure 12-1. Large palpable mass in left breast with fairly well-circumscribed borders (arrow) in patient with fibrocystic disease.

12-2). In patients with mammographically detected microcalcifications and no detectable mass, sonography can demonstrate a mass effect although the calcification may not be visualized. Sonography is also useful in evaluating patients with palpable masses not seen radiographically.[2] Because of the lack of ionizing radiation, most patients under the age of 30 and all pregnant patients should undergo ultrasound as the primary screening procedure. Sonography is also very useful in patients who have had prosthetic implants.[3] The major limitation of ultrasound is in imaging totally fatty replaced breasts owing to the lack of resolution and detail present in images from more dense glandular patterns. However, these breasts are the ones in which lesions are most easily detected on mammography. The other limitation is that sonography is much less sensitive than mammography in the detection of microcalcifications in dense breasts (Figs. 12-3 and 12-4).

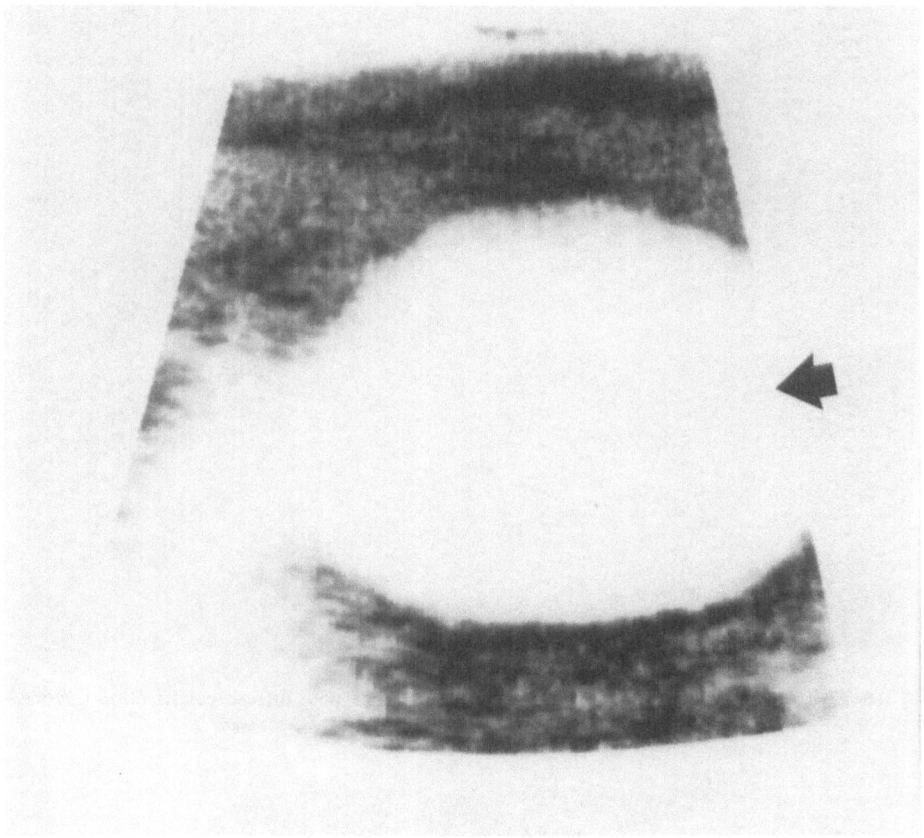

Figure 12-2. Typical sonographic appearance of benign cyst (arrow) in same patient as in Fig. 1.

COMPUTERIZED TOMOGRAPHY

CT may be helpful in evaluating patients with known or suspected breast cancer especially if the breasts are dense and mammography is equivocal. Carcinoma usually enhances markedly, enabling distinction from fibrocystic disease.[1] The retromammary space, axilla, and chest wall structures are well evaluated and the lesions can be locally staged. Possible destruction of ribs and other adjacent chest wall structures or infiltration into the pleural space can be detected (Fig. 12-5). This will aid in establishing radiation portals. Occasionally, an unsuspected incidental mass may be detected on CT performed for another purpose. CT,

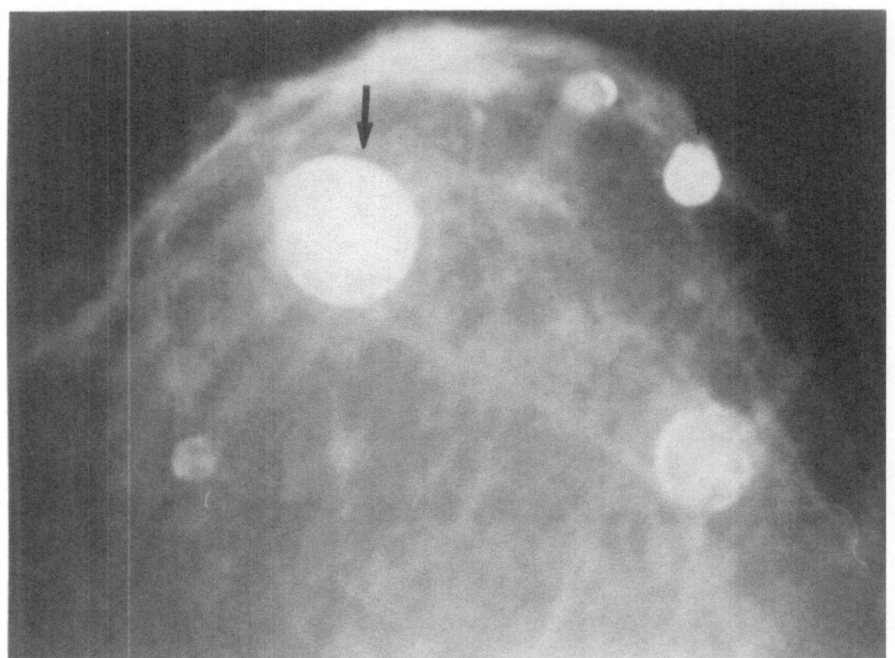

Figure 12-3. Mammogram demonstrating multiple lesions with diffuse calcification (arrows).

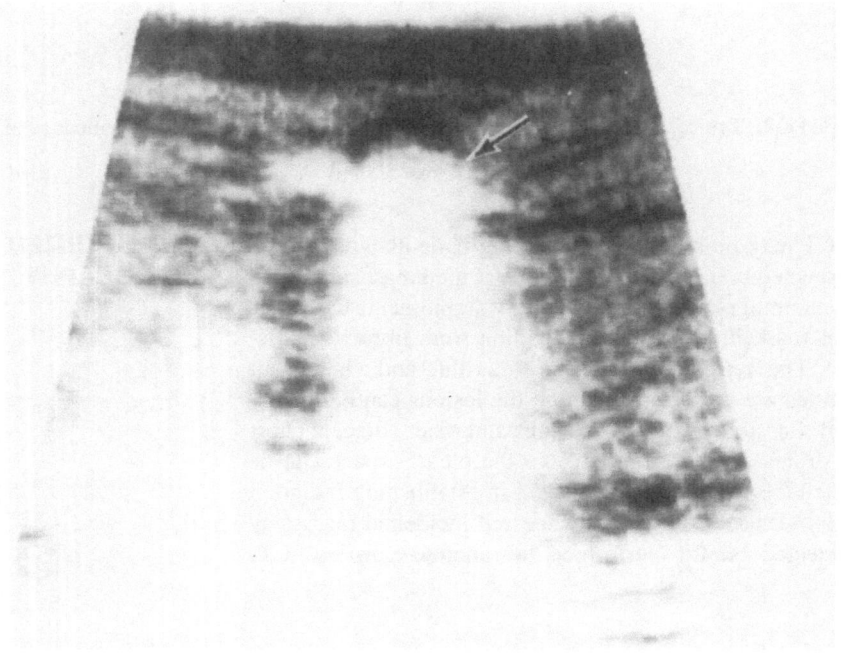

Figure 12-4. Nonvisualization of mass due to shadowing produced by calcification in lesion (arrow).

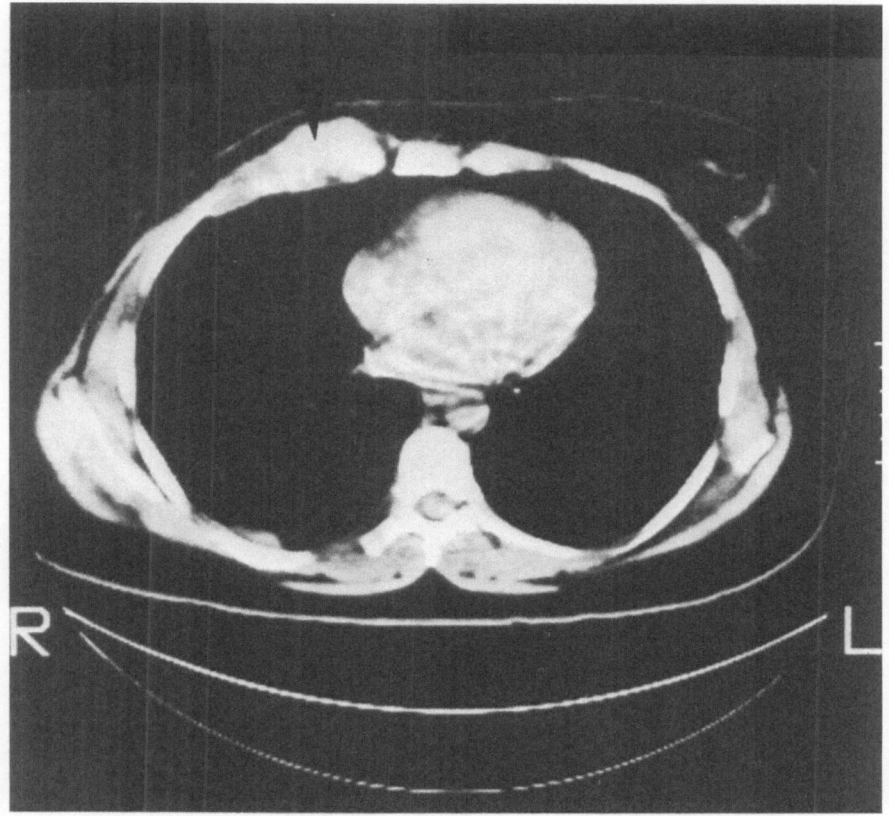

Figure 12-5. Recurrence of breast tumor (arrow) with invasion into thoracic cavity.

however, is more expensive and involves more ionizing radiation than plain-film mammography and should not be the routine screening procedure.

REFERENCES

1. Chang CHJ, Nesbit DE, Fisher DR, et al: Computerized tomographic mammography using a conventional body scanner. *Am J Radiol* 1982;138:553–558.
2. Cole-Beuglet C, Beiave RA: Continuous ultrasound B-scanning of palpable breast masses. *Radiology* 1975;117:123.
3. Harper P, Kelly-Fry E: Ultrasound visualization of the breast in symptomatic patients. *Radiology* 1980;137:465.
4. Kobayashi T: Grey scale echography for breast cancer. *Radiology* 1977;122:207.
5. Teixidor HS, Kazam E: Combined mammographic–sonographic evaluation of breast masses. *Am J Roentgenol* 1977;128:409.

13   Endocrine System

THYROID GLAND

The initial means and mainstay of thyroid imaging has been, and will for the foreseeable future remain, the nuclear isotope study utilizing radioactive iodine. Owing to the relatively easy accessibility of the radionuclide and primary role of iodine in thyroid metabolism, the iodine uptake and static scans can be utilized in evaluating both the physiology and morphology of the gland.

Hyperthyroidism

The 24-hr iodine uptake study performed with ^{123}I is used in conjunction with serum hormone levels T_3 and T_4 and other *in vitro* testing primarily to evaluate patients with clinical symptoms of hyper- or hypothyroidism. The static scan is obtained to supplement clinical palpation of the gland regarding the size and presence of palpable or non-palpable nodules. Anatomic localization of ectopic functioning tissue can also be performed. In the hyperthyroid patient, iodine scanning and uptake can provide differentiation between Graves' disease (Fig. 13-1) and nodular goiter with multiple hyperfunctioning nodules, which will subsequently aid in the determination of appropriate therapy. In the hyperthyroid patient with a single hot nodule, the scan

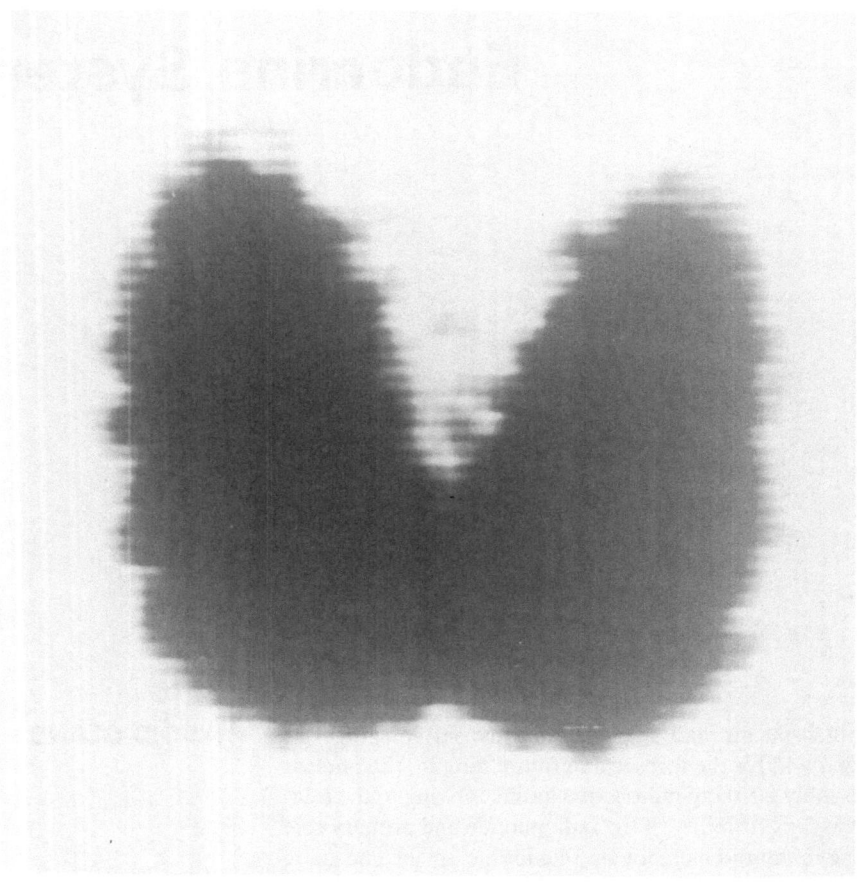

Figure 13-1. ^{123}I scan revealing diffusely enlarged thyroid gland with increased activity compatible with Graves' disease.

performed in conjunction with a T_3 suppression test (Fig. 13-2) can also help determine whether the nodule is autonomous with respect to thyroid-stimulating hormone (TSH), which will also be useful in determining whether surgical ablation or radiation therapy will be a better treatment modality. The uptake and scan is also used as a means to evaluate the effects of medical or surgical treatment on patients with known thyroid dysfunction.

Hypothyroidism   In patients who are clinically hypothyroid, the uptake and scan in conjunction with a prior intramuscular injection of TSH can help differentiate between primary hypothyroid-

Figure 13-2. Large hot autonomous hyperfunctioning nodule suppressing the remainder of the gland unresponsive to T_3 administration.

ism, such as that produced by Hashimoto's thyroiditis or congenital errors in thyroxine synthesis, and secondary or tertiary causes of hypothyroidism, such as that produced by pituitary or hypothalamic failure.[4] The uptake in conjunction with a perchlorate washout test has also been useful in the study of congenital goiters or Hashimoto's thyroiditis. This is based on the fact that perchlorate ions can replace iodide ions in the glands that trap iodine normally but do not organify the substance.

Enlarged Thyroid

Static images of the thyroid in conjunction with clinical palpation help differentiate between diffusely enlarged thyroid, such as that seen in thyroiditis or Graves' disease, and a multinodular gland. This scan is also useful in evaluation and screening of patients with prior external radiotherapy to the neck who are at increased risk for thyroid carcinoma, which will usually appear as a solitary cold nodule (Fig. 13-3). Patients with cold nodules are usually then evaluated with ultrasound to determine the cystic or solid nature of the lesion.[3] If the patient has a hot nodule, sonographic evaluation is not as critical in management owing to the very low incidence of functioning thyroid tumors.

Whole-Body Iodine Scan

The ^{131}I scan has a more limited use because of the higher radiation delivered to the patient per millicurie of substance. The scan, however, is useful in the detection of

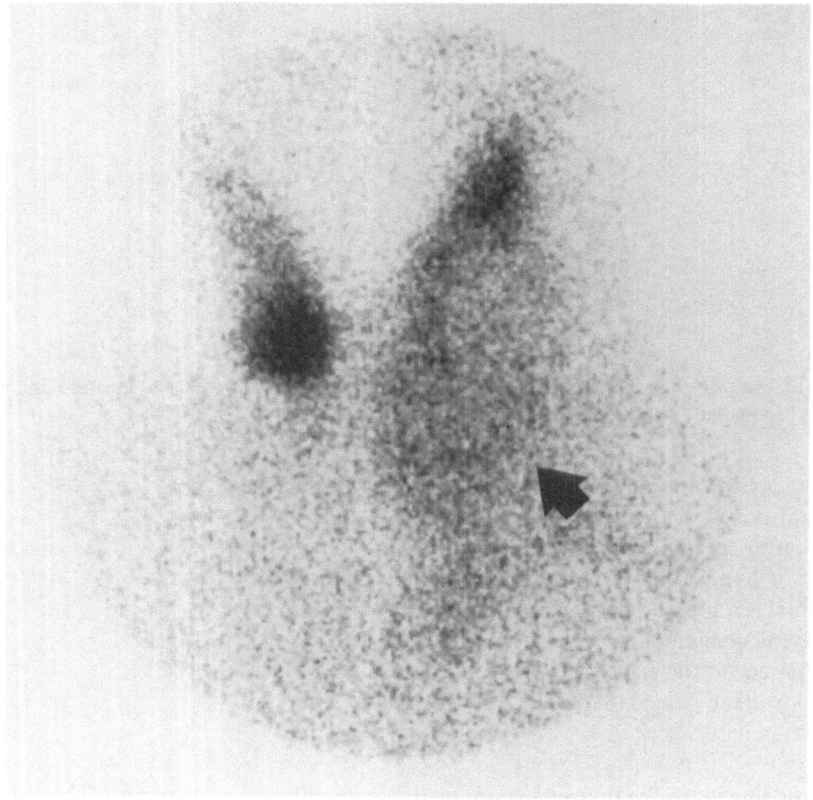

Figure 13-3. Large cold nodule in left lobe (arrow) in patient with papillary carcinoma of thyroid.

functioning thyroid cancer metastases or residual tumor following thyroidectomy. It is also utilized to help detect benign ectopic thyroid tissue such as that seen in patients with retrosternal goiter or ovarian thyroid tissue.

Radiotherapy

Being a very locally radioactive substance, ^{131}I is commonly used for internal radiotherapy for Graves' disease, Plummer's disease, the autonomous functioning nodule that suppresses the remainder of the gland, cardiac disease, and thyroid carcinoma with or without metastasis following initial surgery.[6]

Technetium Scan

The technetium scan is useful in pregnant patients because fetal thyroid tissue can trap radioiodide with resultant increased radiation dosage to the fetus. The technetium scan is also useful in patients who have previously had recent iodide ingestion or procedures utilizing iodinated contrast material, some of which may take months or years to clear. Differentiation between trapping and organification dysfunction, such as seen in hypothyroid patients due to congenital enzymatic defects in the latter condition, can be made.[5] Occasionally, tumors or adenomas may appear as hot on the pertechnetate scans but cold on the radioiodine scans.

Ultrasound

Ultrasound of the thyroid is used in most institutions as a complementary study in addition to rather than as a replacement for the radionuclide exam. Cold thyroid nodules on the isotope study can be characterized regarding possible solid component (Fig. 13-4) or cystic appearance (Fig. 13-5), and occasionally a solid tumor can be differentiated from a benign-appearing lesion. The sonogram is also useful in patients who have a clinically palpable nodule to detect the presence of other nonpalpable nodules. The possibility of a thyroid malignancy can also be diagnosed in patients who present with metastases to other organs such as the bone or lungs. In addition to actual thyroid masses, extrathyroidal lesions such as parathyroid adenomas or adjacent cervical lymphadenopathy can also be detected. The hot thyroid nodule is almost certainly an adenoma[1] and does not require ultrasound correlation unless the patient has had previous external radiotherapy and is at high risk for development of carcinoma.

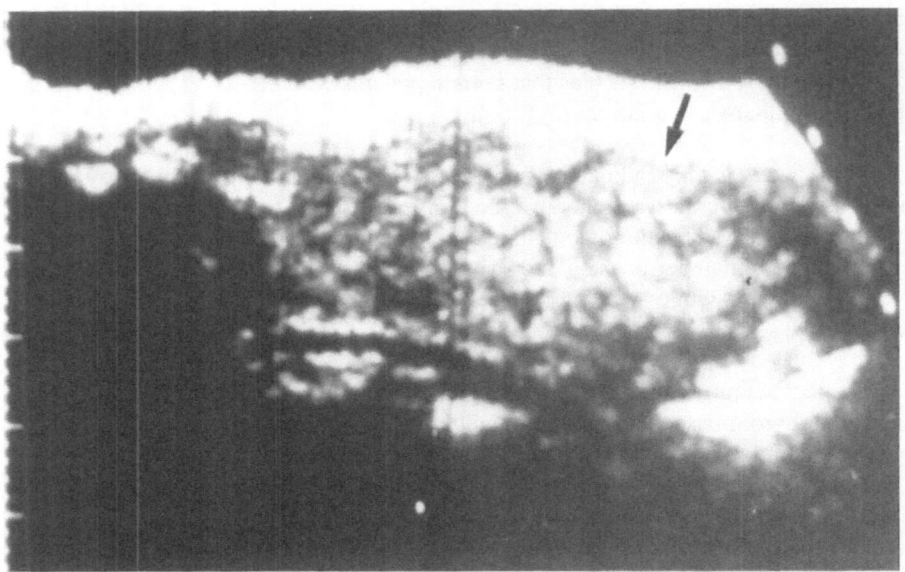

Figure 13-4. Large solid nodule (arrow) in left lobe of thyroid consistent with adenoma.

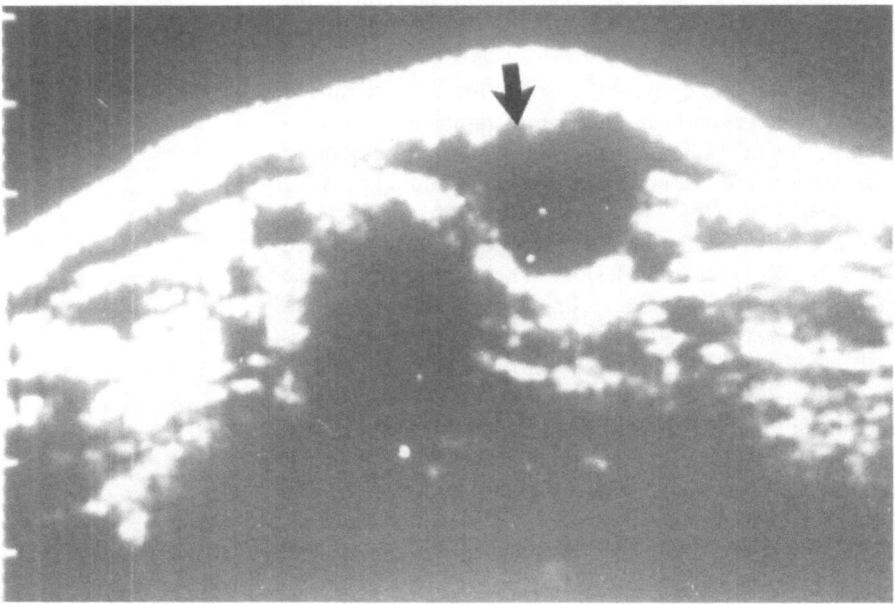

Figure 13-5. Benign cyst (arrow) in left lobe of thyroid.

There are several indications for computerized tomography (CT) of the thryoid at this time. These are largely limited to evaluation of known thyroid cancer in determining local invasion such as cartilage destruction and detection of local nonpalpable lymphadenopathy. The tumors can be studied both preoperatively and postoperatively for local recurrence, although the radionuclide scan is more sensitive and specific for this purpose. CT is also helpful in evaluating the extent of large goiters and determining possible intrathoracic substernal extension (Fig. 13-6).[2] It can also serve as a complementary exam to ultrasound when the solid or cystic nature of a lesion cannot be determined with certainty. Recent reports have advocated the use of CT in the evaluation of thyroid masses in preference to ultrasound; however, this is still a rather controversial issue.

Computerized Tomography

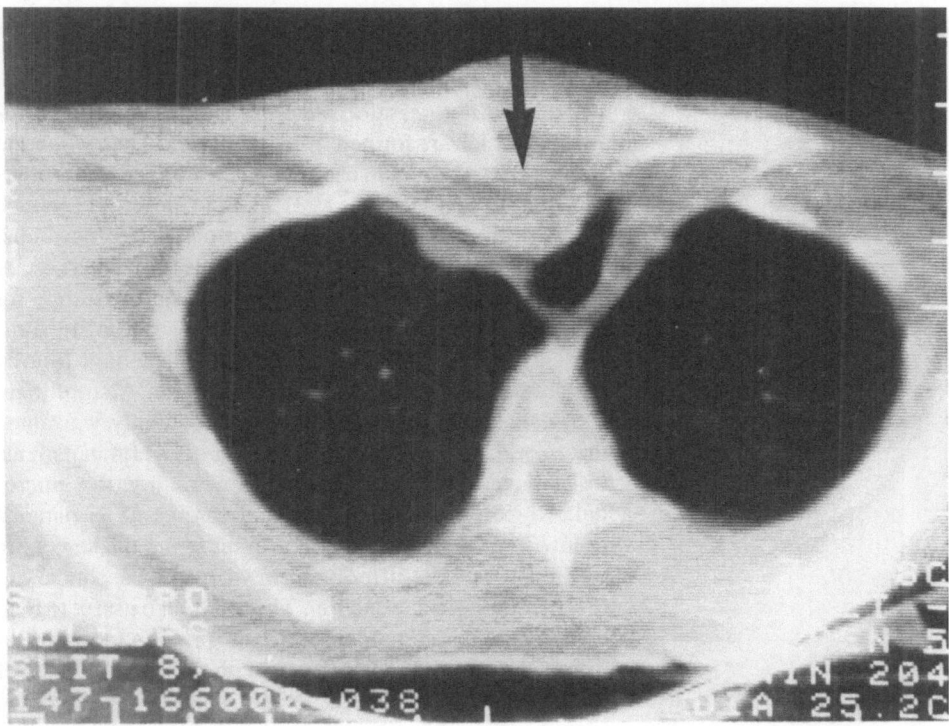

Figure 13-6. Large retrosternal goiter (arrow) deviating trachea.

REFERENCES

1. Atkins HL: *The Thyroid in Clinical Scintillation Imaging,* ed 2; Freeman LM, Johnson PM (eds). New York, Grune & Stratton Inc, 1975.
2. Josef RG, Sagel SS, Stanley RJ, et al: Computed tomography of the thorax. *Radiology* 1978;126:125–136.
3. Rosen IB, Walfish PG, Miskin M: Ultrasound of thyroid masses. *Radiol Clin North Am* 1979;59:19–33.
4. Tanton OD, McDaniel HC, Pittman JA: Standardization of TSH testing. *J Clin Endocrinol Metab* 1965;25:266.
5. Shambaugh GE, et al: Disparate thyroid imaging. Combined studies with sodium pertechnetate Tc-99m and radioactive iodine. *JAMA* 1974;228:866.
6. Young RL, et al: Effects of medical and surgical therapy on morbidity in papillary and/or mixed papillary-follicular thyroid carcinoma. *J Nucl Med* 1976;17:532.

ADRENALS
Nuclear Medicine

During the past 10 years, there have been revolutionary new developments in imaging of the adrenal glands. Previously, the adrenal glands could only be studied indirectly on excretory urograms and utilizing relatively invasive procedures such as retroperitoneal pneumography, angiography, or venography. Adrenal nuclear imaging is based on the function of the adrenal cortex, which composes approximately 90% of the gland and is responsible for production of glucocorticoids, mineralocorticoids, and sex hormones almost all of which are formed from a cholesterol base. For that reason, the first adrenal-scanning agent utilized was a cholesterol-based agent such as [^{131}I]19-iodocholesterol, which has now been replaced by 6-β-19-nor-cholesterol. Adrenal nuclear imaging has very limited use and is utilized in certain centers only because of the lack of approval of isotope for routine use by the Food and Drug Administration. In addition, delayed scanning times necessitating 4–6 days following administration of the agent are necessary. Also, utilization of dexamethasone suppression is frequently warranted in these patients.[1] The study has been quite useful in patients with adrenal hyperfunction in differentiating the micronodular hyperplasia, adenomas, and carcinoma in patients with low-renin hypertension, as well as being the screening procedure in women suffering from virilization secondary to excessive androgen production. The test is also useful to help lateralize adrenal pheochromocytomas prior to more invasive procedures although imaging with a new isotope ^{131}I MIBG, which localizes in the adrenal medulla, has also been used within the past year. Adrenal remnants can be detected status postadrenalectomy. This study is also useful in diagnosing hypofunction of one gland secondary to suppression by an adenoma. The procedure is also useful in patients allergic to iodine or in situations in which the adrenal gland cannot be studied owing to unsuccessful catherization.

Ultrasound

Ultrasound has found increasing use in the evaluation and characterization of patients with clinically suspected adrenal masses or in patients with adrenal masses incidentally discovered on the intravenous pyelogram (IVP) or abdominal radiograph. The lesions can be classified as to cystic or solid in nature,[7] and directed biopsies can be performed for cytologic diagnosis. In patients with adrenal tumors local extent or spread can be evaluated as well as the possibility of lymph node involvement or metastases. Progress of the lesions can be followed status posttherapy. Owing to the usually small size,[6] most normal adrenal glands are somewhat difficult to localize sonographically, especially the left adrenal gland, which is limited by artifact secondary to the overlying ribs or bowel gas. Since there is no ionizing radiation involved in the procedure, ultrasound should be the procedure of choice in the initial evaluation of children or pregnant women with suspected adrenal lesions. In the pediatric patient, ultrasound can visualize neonatal adrenal hemorrhage (Fig. 13-7) and can help to differentiate this lesion from neuroblastoma.[3] Local staging of neuroblastoma can also be performed preoperatively and followed postoperatively. In patients presenting with low-density masses on CT scan, ultrasound can help differentiate a low-density adenoma from a true cyst.

Computerized Tomography

CT is the procedure of choice in imaging adrenal lesions with both glands being identified in 99% of patients.[2] Owing to the accurate visualization of normal adrenals, CT is not only useful to detect and characterize masses but is also able to exclude lesions. In most cases of hyperadrenalism, CT findings are nonspecific but, with the appropriate biochemical tests, can help in making histologic diagnosis. Hyperplasia is usually represented by bilateral thickening, whereas the adenoma (Fig. 13-8) or other benign lesions are usually unilateral[2] (Fig. 13-9). Malignant lesions, either

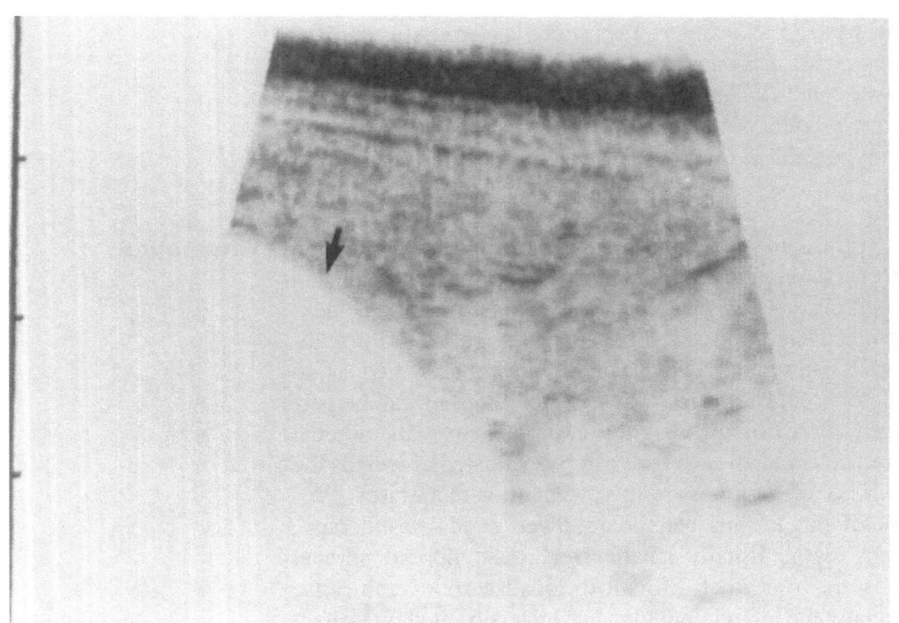

Figure 13-7. Large sonolucent suprarenal mass (arrow) representing neonatal adrenal hemorrhage.

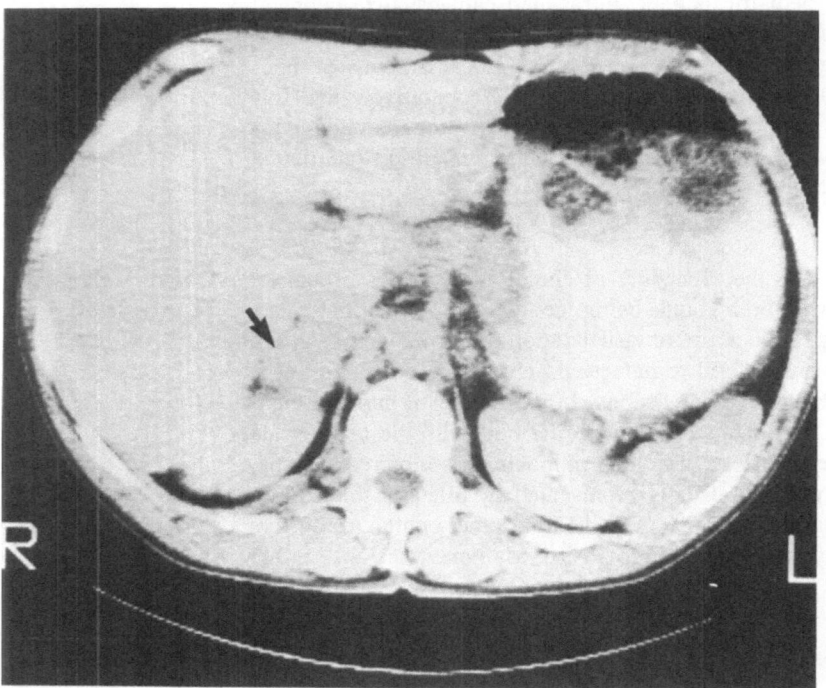

Figure 13-8. Large right adrenal mass (arrow) in patient with virilism representing adenoma.

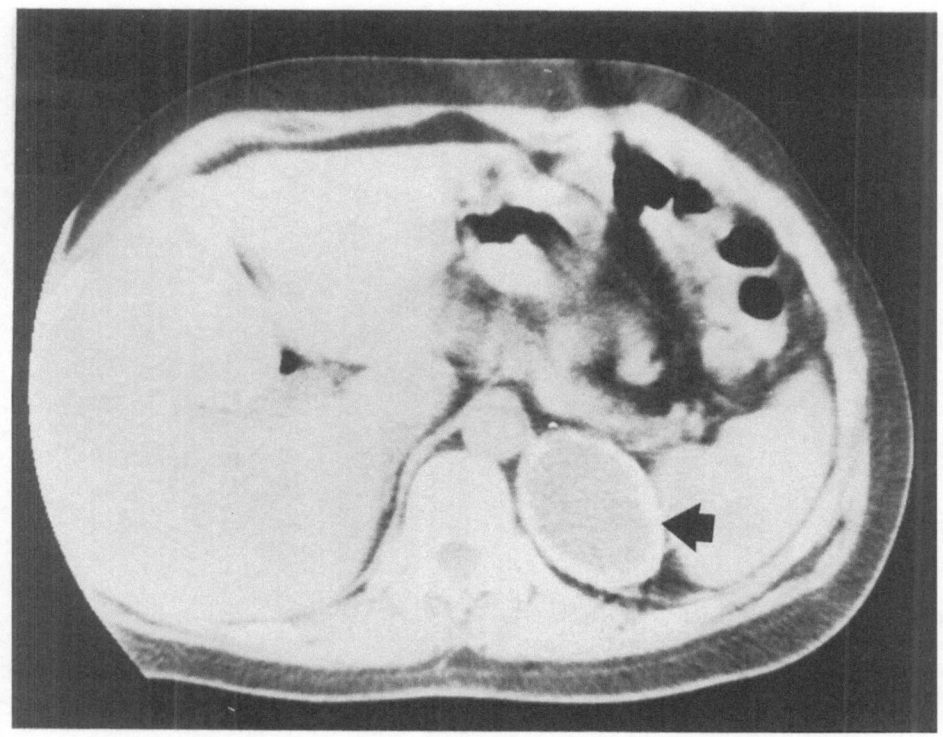

Figure 13-9. Calcified adrenal hematoma (arrow) found incidentally in patient evaluated for liver disease.

primary (Figs. 13-10 to 13-12) or metastases (Fig. 13-13), tend to be larger masses. Pheochromocytoma can also be large and may be bilateral in 10–20% of cases although the diagnosis is usually already known clinically prior to the examination.[5] CT is also very helpful in the detection of extraadrenal pheochromocytomas.[4] Unfortunately, 50% of patients with clinical signs of hyperplasia will demonstrate normal-appearing glands on the CT scan. CT, however, is also useful in evaluating suspected suprarenal masses and in differentiating true adrenal masses from pseudomasses seen on IVP.

The advantages of CT over nuclear medicine are the production of less radiation to the adrenals, not having to wait 4–6 days prior to scanning, and more routine availability of CT than the radioisotopes. CT is also easier to perform and interpret than ultrasound with more accurate re-

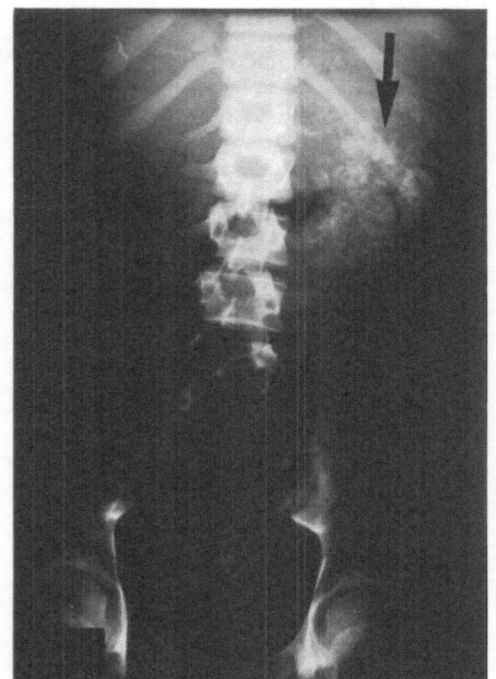

Figure 13-10. Large mass with calcifications (arrow) in left upper quadrant of 10-year-old child.

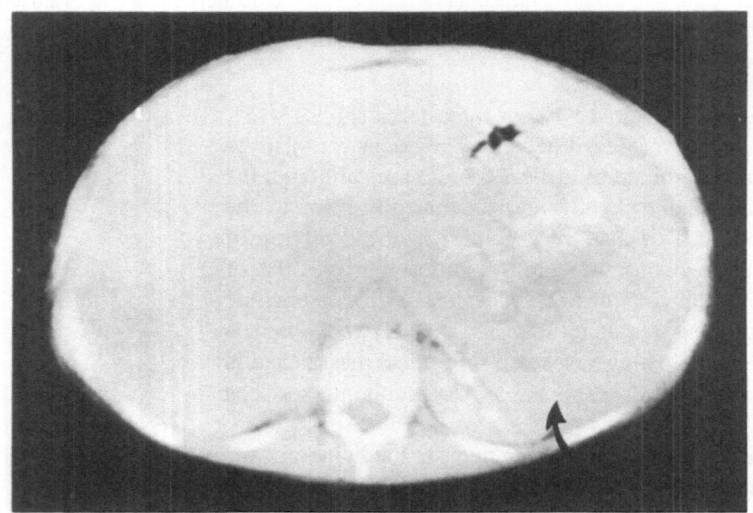

Figure 13-11. Computerized tomography revealing extensive neuroblastoma with calcifications (arrow).

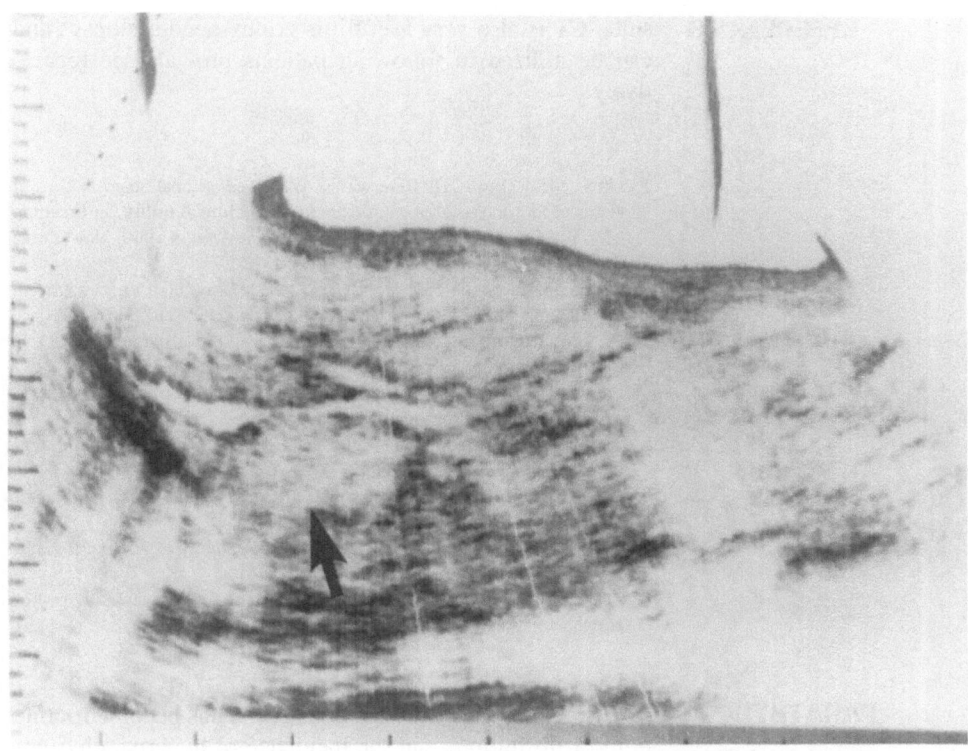

Figure 13-12. Large adrenal metastasis (arrow) compressing the inferior vena cava (IVC).

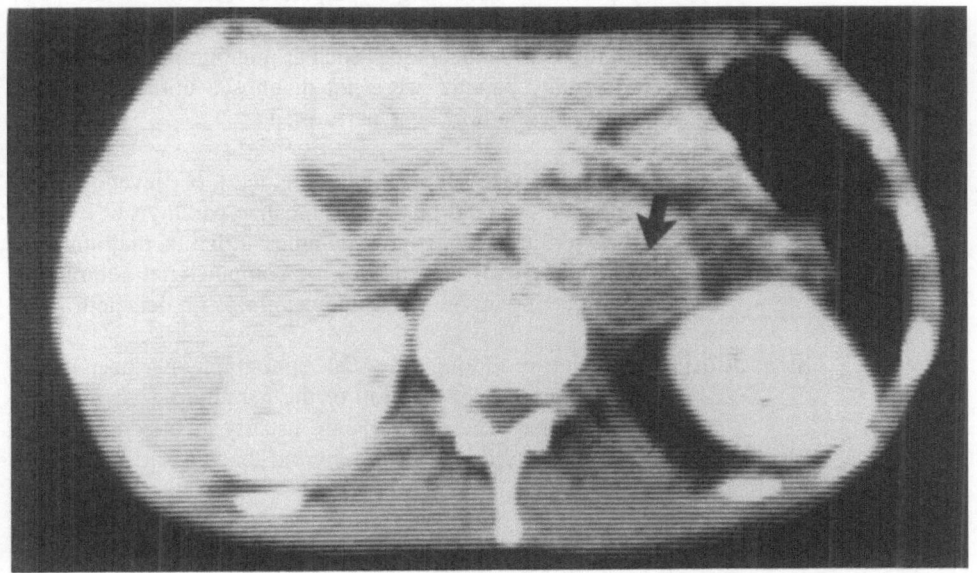

Figure 13-13. Primary adrenal carcinoma (arrow) with mild rimlike calcification.

REFERENCES

sults. CT is also very useful for skinny-needle biopsy[8] and can be utilized in following patients pre- and postoperatively.

1. Gross MD, Thrall JH, Bererwaltes WH: The adrenal scan: A current status report on radiotracers, dosimetry and clinical utility, in Freeman LM, Weissmann HS (eds): *Nuclear Medicine Annual 1980*. New York, Raven Press, 1980, pp 127–175.
2. Korobkin M, White EA, Kressel HY, e al: Computed tomography in the diagnosis of adrenal disease. *Am J Radiol* 1979;132:231–238.
3. Pery M, Kaftori JK, Bar-Maor JA: Sonography for diagnosis and followup of neonatal adrenal hemorrhage. *JCU* 1981;9:397.
4. Stewart BH, Bravo EL, Hacega J, et al: Localization of pheochromocytoma by computed tomography. *N Engl J Med* 1979;299:460–461.
5. Thomas JL, Bernardino ME, Samaar NA, et al: CT of pheochromocytoma. *Am J Radiol* 1980;135:477–482.
6. Yeh HC: Sonography of the adrenal glands: Normal glands and small masses. *Am J Radiol* 1980;135:1167–1177.
7. Yeh HC, Mitty HA, Rose J, et al: Ultrasonography of adrenal masses: Usual fgatures. *Radiology* 1978;127:467.
8. Zornoza J, Ordanez N, Bernardino ME, et al: Percutaneous biopsy of adrenal tumors. *Urology* 1981;18:412–416.

PARATHYROID

Hyperparathyroidism

Since screening for hypercalcemia has become routine in most institutions and the incidence of hyperparathyroidism may be as high as 1 in 2000 people, it has become increasingly important to be able to detect the presence of parathyroid hyperplasia or adenomas in patients clinically suspected of harboring hyperparathyroidism. In the past, the radiographic detection of parathyroid lesions was limited to invasive techniques such as angiography or venography. Many patients were not diagnosed until exploratory surgery of the neck was performed.

Nuclear Medicine

In the past, selenomethionine and [^{57}Co]cyanocobalomine studies could be used to localize parathyroid lesions. However, now with newer studies utilizing thallium and technetium with the addition of computerized subtraction techniques, parathyroid lesions can also be detected.

Ultrasound

High-resolution gray-scale sonography has been useful in preoperative localization of the parathyroid adenoma or hyperplasia.[2] These lesions are usually localized posterior to the inferior aspect of the thyroid lobes and have a fairly

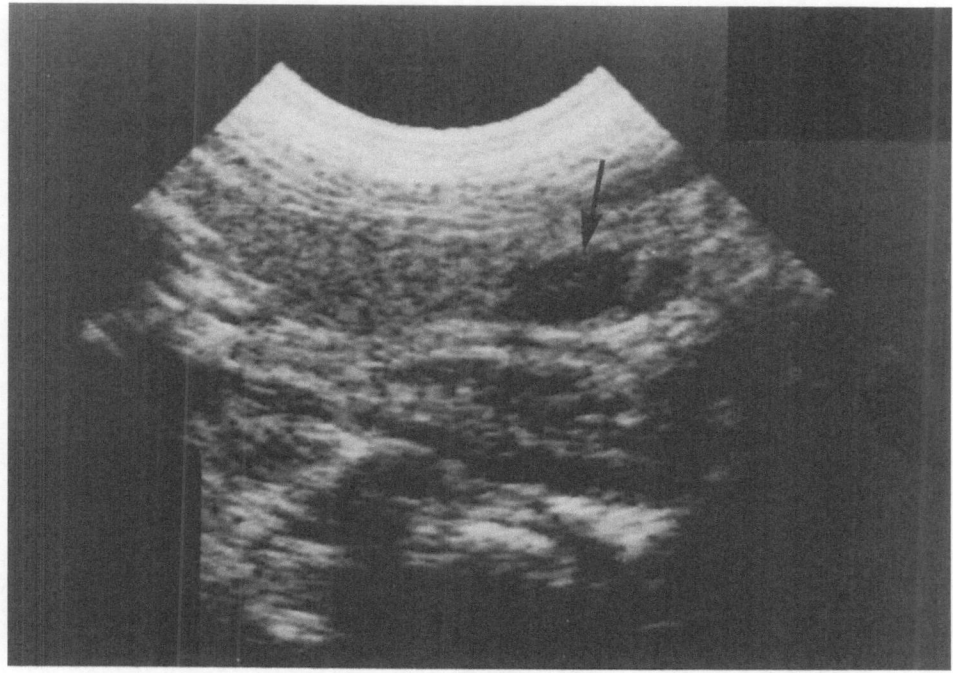

Figure 13-14. Relatively sonolucent parathyroid adenoma (arrow) along inferior lobe of thyroid.

characteristic appearance (Fig. 13-14).[1] The advantage of ultrasound is the lack of ionizing radiation. Disadvantages of the procedure are related to the confusion of parathyroid lesions with large thyroid lesions extending inferiorly, inability of the patient to extend the neck, and poor results in patients with excessively obese or scarred necks. The quality of scan that can be obtained is also based on operator experience.

In some patients with hyperparathyroidism, the parathyroid adenoma may be in an ectopic location usually within the superior mediastinum (Fig. 13-15). CT is a useful, adjunctive procedure in patients with negative sonograms or failed neck exploration in the search for a parathyroid adenoma. Infusion of contrast medium is helpful to opacify the lower neck and mediastinal vessels, thus aiding in the detection of such a lesion.[3]

Computerized Tomography

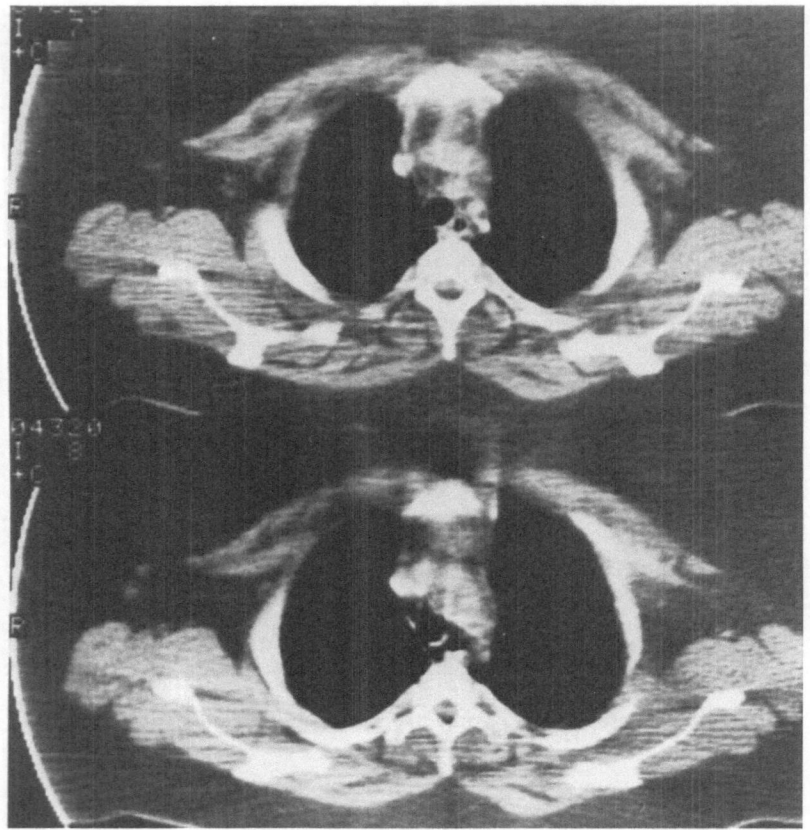

Figure 13-15. Small soft tissue nodule (arrow) in superior mediastinum representing ectopic parathyroid adenoma.

REFERENCES

1. Crocker EF, Bautovich SJ, Jellins J: Grey scale echographic visualization of a parathyroid adenoma. *Radiology* 1978;126:233.
2. Duffy P, Picker RM, Duffield S, et al: Parathyroid sonography: A useful aid to preoperative localization. *JCU* 1980;8:113.
3. Krody AG, Doppman JL, Brennan MF, et al: The detection of mediastinal parathyroid glands by computerized tomography, selective arteriography and venous sampling. *Radiology* 1981;140:739–744.

14 Magnetic Resonance Imaging of the Body

As described previously, magnetic resonance imaging (MRI) is a new imaging modality which does not rely on utilization of ionizing radiation but is based upon interaction of protons in the body with changing magnetic fields. MRI has proven to be more sensitive than computerized tomography (CT) in the detection of various intracranial abnormalities, specifically involving the brain stem, posterior fossa, and white matter disease. MRI is also effective in detecting spinal cord pathology and herniated discs at an earlier stage than computerized tomography.

There is currently much research utilizing MRI to help define further indications of this technique for detection of disease in other parts of the body. The spatial resolution of MRI is similar to CT and ultrasound, but the improved soft tissue contrast increases lesion detectability. Although tissue characterization of MRI on the basis of T_1 and T_2 relaxation parameters alone is in the early stages of development, the use of *in vivo* spectroscopy will improve MRI diagnostic capabilities.

Thoracic imaging with MRI is currently contraindicated in patients with pacemakers. In addition, imaging of the chest is limited due to cardiac pulsation and respiratory movement. These limitations, however, are overcome using cardiac gating and respiratory-gated techniques. Recent studies have demonstrated utility of MRI in detecting myocardial ischemia as well as evaluating congenital cardiac lesions without having to resort to contrast angiography. There is also excellent delineation of hilar and mediastinal pathology due to the easy differentiation of solid tissue from vascular structures with flowing blood.

Imaging of the abdomen and pelvis is somewhat limited at this point in time due to inadequate oral and organ targeted contrast agents available for widespread use. However, liver metastases and primary tumors may be detected using various pulse sequences. Lesions in the porta hepatis and intravascular invasion of tumor may be detected without contrast agents. The high resolution helps in the identification and characterization of renal mass lesions. Vascular involvement is easily detected. Retroperitoneal masses, lymphadenopathy, and other masses may also be detected without using intravascular contrast medium. Current studies have demonstrated good delineation of the normal pancreas and pancreatic lesions utilizing ferrous gluconate as an oral contrast agent.

Multiplanar imaging and varying pulse sequences enables MRI to be very sensitive in the early detection of skeletal tumors, osteomyelitis and avascular necrosis, although the lesions do not have a specific appearance.

The use of surface coils has improved the spatial resolution and lesion detectability in other organs such as the thyroid, parathyroid and breast.

It is the general consensus that the future of MRI is bright in some instances, complementing and even surpassing CT in the early detection of disease. Unfortunately the high cost of the equipment will limit availability of this technique to larger metropolitan areas and major medical centers for some time.

Appendix
Summary of Indications for Testing

Endocrine system

- Thyroid studies
  ^{123}I Uptake and scan
  Indications
  1. Assess goiter
  2. Palpable nodules in neck
  3. Clinical hypo- or hyperthyroid state
  4. Follow progress of thyroiditis
  5. History of prior neck irradiation
  6. Evaluate substernal mass
  7. Pre- and postoperative assessment
  8. Postoperative therapy for thyroid carcinoma
  9. Evaluate effects of thyroid medications

- TSH stimulation test
  Permits differentiation of primary and secondary hyper-thyroidism

- T_3 suppression test
  Evaluation of hot nodules

- Perchlorate washout test
  Useful in some forms of thyroiditis

INDICATIONS FOR NUCLEAR MEDICINE STUDIES

- Technetium scan

  Indications
  1. Useful in pregnant patients
  2. Useful in patients with previous iodine ingestion or injection
  3. May be helpful to differentiate between trapping and organification dysfunction

- ^{131}I whole-body scan

  Indications

  Detection of functioning thyroid carcinoma metastases or residual tumor following thyroidectomy

- ^{131}I therapy

  Indications
  1. Graves' disease
  2. Plummer's disease
  3. Thyroid carcinoma

- Adrenal scans

  Indications
  1. Screening procedure after initial history, physical, and preliminary hormonal studies indicate abnormality of adrenal gland or ovary prior to more invasive and costly procedures
  2. Differentiate between micronodular hyperplasia, macronodular hyperplasia, adenoma, and carcinoma in patients with low-renin hypertension
  3. Aid in diagnosis of diminished function of one adrenal gland
  4. Detect postoperative remnants following adrenalectomy
  5. Screening procedure to detect source of androgen in women who have masculine secondary sex characteristics
  6. Lateralization of pheochromocytoma now done by computerized tomography (CT)
  7. Patients in whom the adrenal vein is technically difficult to catheterize
  8. Allergy to iodinated contrast precluding vascular studies

CT is the procedure of choice for detecting adrenal masses, but these are nonspecific in nature. Nuclear adrenal scanning will aid in determination of the actual pathology owing to the physiologic nature of the study.

Bone and joint scans

Indications

1. Radiographically occult fractures following trauma (stress fractures, may be important medicolegally)
2. Primary bone neoplasm
3. Localization of osteomyelitis
4. To confirm bone or joint pathology to explain etiology of pain
5. Vascular insult—infarcts, aseptic necrosis, radiation necrosis
6. Staging neoplasms by detection of metastases prior to and following therapy (most useful in lung, breast, and prostate tumors in adults, neuroblastoma, leukemia in children)
7. Detect and evaluate the extent of metabolic bone disease (hyperparathyroidism), osteoarthropathies, Paget's disease, etc.
8. Evaluate extent and activity of arthritis as well as results of therapy
9. Detection of extraosseous calcifications (pulmonary, splenic, soft tissue, hepatic, cardiac, etc.)
10. Complications of prostheses—loosening or infection
11. Will occasionally demonstrate gross pathology of genitourinary tract coincidentally

Bone scans are more sensitive than radiographs in most cases, but are nonspecific necessitating the comparison of scans with radiographs of symptomatic areas or positive regions on the scan.

Gallium scans

Indications

1. Abscess detection and localization
2. Tumor localization and staging—specifically good for lymphoma (Hodgkin's), hepatoma, melanoma, lung and primary bone tumors
3. Response of tumor to therapy and recurrence
4. Benign processes
   a. Osteomyelitis
   b. Sarcoid
   c. Tuberculosis—active
   d. Gall bladder empyema
   e. Acute pyelonephritis

Genitourinary

Indications
1. Determine vascularity of known renal masses
2. Detection of renovascular hypertension

• Renal function (renogram)
Indications
1. Quantitative analysis and comparison of bilateral renal function secondary to various disease processes (obstruction, trauma, infection, metabolic disorders, etc.)
2. Diuretic function study—to distinguish between ureteral stasis and actual obstruction

• Renal architecture
Indications
1. Congenital malformations
2. Mass lesions detection (tumor, trauma, column of Bertin)
3. Renal infarct detection
4. Patients allergic to iodinated contrast

• Renal transplant scans
Indications
1. Renal flow
2. Assess transplant function
3. Complications (acute tubular necrosis, rejection states, masses, lymphocele, urinoma, hematoma)

• Cystogram (direct and indirect)
Indications
1. Computerized quantitation of bladder emptying
2. Vesicoureteral reflux detection (effective in pediatric age group owing to decreased radiation and simplicity)

• Scrotal flow and static scan
Indications
Distinguish between testicular torsion and acute epididymitis

Hematologic procedures

1. Red cell survival
2. Splenic sequestration
3. Red cell mass
4. Blood volume determination
5. Bone marrow scans

Indications

1. Selection of sites for bone marrow aspiration and biopsy
2. Assessment of myeloproliferative disorders
3. Acute versus chronic anemia
4. Detect focal disease in bone marrow (metastases)
5. Possible aid in staging lymphoma
6. Possible aid in monitoring response to therapy

Gastrointestinal studies: in vivo procedures

- Esophageal studies

  Indications
  1. Detect obstruction
  2. Detect small fistulae (more sensitive than barium study)
  3. Peristaltic disorders
  4. Detect and quantitate gastrointestinal reflux (more sensitive than barium swallow, less radiation)
  5. Detect ectopic gastric mucosa of Barrett's esophagus

- Gastric studies

  Indications

  Detect functioning gastric mucosa postoperative gastrectomy; gastric emptying—solids and/or liquid

- Gastrointestinal bleeding

  T_cS_c—rapid localization of gastrointestinal bleed—better for heavier bleeding (more sensitive than angiography)

  T_c—labeled red blood cells—localize sites of slower bleeding

- Meckel scan

  Detect presence of Meckel diverticulum with ectopic gastric mucosa

- Hepatobiliary

  Liver–spleen scan

  Hepatic indications
  1. Evaluate liver—size, shape, and position
  2. Evaluate diffuse hepatic disease
  3. Focal space-occupying lesions
  4. Evaluate metastases pre- and posttherapy
  5. Hepatic flow study to determine vascularity of known hepatic masses

High-resolution ultrasound and CT are more sensitive than liver scan for detection and follow-up of focal lesions

Splenic indications
1. Evaluate splenic size
2. Suspected trauma
3. Stage neoplasms and evaluate response to therapy
4. Asplenia
5. Detect accessory spleen (heat-treated red blood cells)
6. Detect situs inversus

- Biliary studies
Indications
1. Detection of acute cystic duct obstruction
2. Jaundiced patients to evaluate ductal obstruction
3. Postcholecystectomy patients to detect cystic duct remnant or biliary fistula
4. Evaluate biliary enteric bypass procedures
5. Detect traumatic biliary fistulae
6. Evaluate biliary reflux following Billroth II
7. Evaluate neonatal jaundice to distinguish between neonatal hepatitis and biliary atresia

Gastrointestinal studies: in vitro studies

- Gastrointestinal malabsorption
1. Schilling test, with or without intrinsic factor to determine etiology of B_{12} deficiency
2. Protein loss detection
3. Lipid loss detection

- Pancreas scan
1. Evaluate function and size of organ
2. Detection of masses intrinsic or extrinsic to pancreas

Largely replaced by ultrasound and CT

Central nervous system

- Brain scan with or without flow study
Indications
1. Neoplasm detection—benign, malignant, metastatic
2. Infectious processes—abscess, encephalitis, meningitis with empyema
3. Vascular disorders—arterial–venous malformation, aneurysm (huge), cerebrovascular accident (CVA), intracranial bleed
4. Trauma—subdural and intracerebral hematoma

5. Miscellaneous—demyelinating diseases, possibly useful to determine brain death

Most of the above-listed pathologic states may be more rapidly and easily diagnosed by CT. The most efficacious use of radionuclide brain scanning now is limited to situations in which one would like to assess both intracranial and extracranial flow (symmetry, detection of gross stenosis) prior to contrast examination. It can also be used to differentiate CVA from tumor frequently.

- Cisternography

Indications

1. Suspicion of block in subarachnoid cerebrospinal fluid (CSF) pathway (subarachnoid adhesion secondary to surgery or inflammation)
2. Document and localize CSF leak—otorrhea, rhinorrhea
3. Communicating hydrocephalus—normal pressure hydrocephalus, subarachnoid block, failure of CSF reabsorption
4. Determination of shunt patency and complications of shunting
5. Porencephalic cyst determination
6. Estimate ventricular size

CT will demonstrate morphologic abnormalities of the ventricular system; however, cisternography is better to evaluate physiology of the subarachnoid spaces and ventricular system.

It will also assist in the determination of when a shunt will be an effective means of treating patients with communicating hydrocephalus in addition to evaluating shunt patency.

Pulmonary studies

- Perfusion

Indications

1. Detection of pulmonary emboli and evaluate status posttherapy
2. Assist in diagnosis of congenital pulmonary anomalies
3. Evaluate extent of lung tumor (resectability)

- Ventilation

Indications

1. Evaluation of chronic obstructive pulmonary disease

2. Evaluation of ventilatory function prior to thoracotomy

All perfusion scans should be evaluated in conjunction with recent radiographs. Owing to nonspecificity of perfusion abnormalities, most, if not all, positive perfusion studies should be evaluated with a ventilatory scan.

Cardiac studies

- Radionuclide angiocardiography
  Indications
    1. Diagnose congenital heart lesions—shunt lesions, valvular
    2. Evaluate acquired valvular lesions
    3. Pericardial effusion detection (ultrasound more effective)
    4. Detection of pseudoaneurysms
- Avid infarct scans (pyrophosphate)
  Indications
    1. Detecting acute infarcts in patients with questionable clinical findings, enzyme levels, and equivocal electrocardiogram (left bundle branch block)
    2. Localization and estimation of infarct size
- Thallium—rest and/or stress
    1. Detection and estimation of size of ischemic or infarcted region
    2. Determine effects of stress on ischemic regions
    3. Evaluate myocardial perfusion prior to and postcoronary bypass
- Gated studies—rest and/or stress
  Indications
    1. Evaluate left ventricular function with and without stress (by calculation of ejection fraction and demonstrating abnormal cardiac wall motion)
    2. Evaluation of right ventricular function
    3. Monitor cardiac status of patients on cardiotoxic drugs (Adriamycin)
    4. Assist in distinguishing between diffuse cardiomyopathy and ischemic heart disease
    5. Detection of areas of dyskinesis (localized aneurysms)
- Miscellaneous procedures: Dacryocystography
  Indications
    1. Evaluate patients with epiphora in whom routine

clinical tests cannot determine etiology and site of obstruction
2. Determine presence of nasolacrimal abnormalities
3. Evaluation of postoperative patients with persistent tearing
4. Performance of physiologic and pharmacologic investigations
5. Determine relationship of ductal system to orbital mass

Liver–lung scan
Indications
1. Specifically demonstrates juxtadiaphragmatic pathology—e.g., subphrenic abscess
2. Most useful in patients who are difficult to scan with ultrasound. CT has largely replaced this study, although it may be useful in children and pregnant women where one wants to reduce irradiation.

- Radionuclide venogram
Indications
1. Simple way to detect deep venous thrombosis
2. Detect superior vena caval obstruction
3. Useful in patients allergic to iodine
4. Can be performed at time of pulmonary perfusion scan

- Salivary gland scan
Indications—limited
1. May aid in detection of certain tumors as preliminary screening procedure (functioning versus nonfunctioning)
2. Assess function of salivary glands—in patient with xerostomia—e.g., Sjögren syndrome

Liver
1. Hepatocellular disease versus metastases
2. Focal lesions—cystic versus solid
3. Guided biopsies
4. Metastases detection—pre- and posttherapy
5. Staging lymphoma
6. Inflammatory disease—intrahepatic versus subphrenic versus subhepatic
7. Postoperative trauma

INDICATIONS FOR ULTRASOUND

Gall Bladder and Biliary System
1. Rule out cholelithiasis versus polyps
2. To *aid* in detection of acute cholecystitis
3. Rule out ductal dilatation
4. Medical versus surgical jaundice

Pancreas
1. Inflammatory disease versus tumor
2. Complications of pancreatitis—pseudocyst versus phlegmon versus abscess

Abdominal Aorta
1. Atherosclerotic disease
2. Aneurysm detection
3. Complications of aneurysm—dissection
4. Status of grafts and complications

Spleen
1. Evaluate size
2. Focal lesions—cystic versus solid
3. Neoplasm
4. Inflammation
5. Trauma

Renal
1. Congenital anomalies
2. Hydronephrosis
3. Infectious disease
4. Renal masses on intravenous pyelogram—cystic versus solid
5. Diffuse renal disease
6. Complication of transplant—hydronephrosis, hematoma, abscess, lymphocele, urinoma
7. Renal failure—medical versus obstructive

Adrenal
1. Mass lesions—cystic versus solid

Retroperitoneal
1. Detection of lymphadenopathy
2. Fluid collections
3. Retroperitoneal fibrosis
4. Retroperitoneal neoplasms

Testicle

1. Epididymitis versus torsion
2. Masses
3. Fluid collections

General Abdominal

1. Ascites detection
2. Abscess or hematoma localization
3. Peritoneal (mesenteric) disease
4. Bowel lesions

Neck

1. Thyroid masses—cold nodules on isotope scan
2. Parathyroid masses—adenoma
3. Evaluate goiter
4. Extrathyroidal masses—cysts versus solid
5. Adenopathy
6. Vascular—carotid disease screening

Lower Extremity

1. Popliteal cyst
2. Aneurysm
3. Abscess and hematoma
4. Soft tissue tumors

Pelvis (Female)

1. Locate intrauterine device
2. Rule out intrauterine pregnancy
3. Uterine neoplasm
4. Ovarian masses—cystic versus solid
5. Localize hematoma or abscess
6. Pelvic inflammatory disease
7. Lymphadenopathy

Nongynecologic lesion
1. Bladder and prostate lesions
2. Congenital anomalies—pelvic, kidney, uterine—bicornuate
3. Anomalies

Obstetrical

1. Rule out IUP
2. Gestational age
3. Abnormal gestation sac—blighted ovum, missed abortion, molar pregnancy

4. Placenta localization—placenta previa
5. Placental abnormalities (tumors)
6. Ectopic pregnancy versus ovarian lesions
7. Incompetent cervix
8. Fetal death
9. Fetal anomalies
10. Amniocentesis

INDICATIONS FOR COMPUTERIZED TOMOGRAPHY

Head

1. Trauma—sites of bleeding, fracture location
2. Neoplasm—primary or metastatic
3. Congenital anomalies
4. Inflammatory disease—abscess localization
5. Vascular lesions—AVM, aneurysm
6. White-matter disease
7. CVA—hemorrhagic versus ischemic
8. Orbital pathology
9. Detect hydrocephalus
10. Postoperative follow-up
11. Internal auditory canals
12. Sellar pathology

Neck

1. Paranasal sinus pathology
2. Facial trauma
3. Parotid gland pathology
4. Cervical-spine trauma—rule out spinal cord involvement, determine the extent of fracture
5. Staging of tumors of larynx, pharynx
6. Laryngeal trauma
7. Neck mass localization

Chest

1. Search for pulmonary metastases
2. Evaluate pulmonary nodule
3. Evaluate widened mediastinum
4. Stage esophageal and lung tumors
5. Evaluate aortic aneurysms
6. Detection of lymphadenopathy (hilar or mediastinal)

Abdomen

- General
  1. Abscess localization
  2. Bowel or mesenteric involvement by tumor

3. Staging lymphoma
4. Guided biopsy—skinny needle
- Retroperitoneum
  1. Nodal evaluation
  2. Aortic aneurysm and complications
  3. Aortic graft and complications

Pancreas

1. Evaluate and stage pancreatic carcinoma
2. Complications of pancreatitis
3. Jaundice of unknown etiology

Liver–spleen

1. Localized masses
2. Evaluate metastases pre- and posttherapy
3. Suspected trauma of liver or spleen

Adrenal–renal

1. Evaluate renal masses—cystic versus solid
2. Stage renal tumors
3. Screening for adrenal masses
4. Evaluate renal trauma

Pelvis

1. Stage bladder tumors
2. Define gross extent of pelvic tumors
3. Search for undescended testes
4. Lymph node evaluation
5. Pelvic trauma—specifically acetabular fracture definition and pelvic hematoma detection.

Index

Raynaud's phenomenon, 120
Rectal tumor, 90–91
Renal agenesis, 82
Renal cell carcinoma, 122–123
Renal failure, 58
Renal mass, 61–66, 69, 208
Renal scan, nuclear, 61
Renal transplant, 68, 70
Renal vascular hypertension, 53–55
Respiratory system
  inflammatory disease of, 93–95
  lung neoplasm, 97–99
  mediastinal widening and mass, 95, 99–103
  pulmonary embolus, 94–101
  pulmonary metastases, 99–100, 102
Reticuloendothelial system: see Spleen and reticuloendothelial system
Retinal detachment, 158
Retinoblastoma, 160
Retroperitoneal nodes, 9, 12
RH incompatibility, 84

Sacroiliitis, 154
Salivary gland–parotid enlargement, 164, 167
Sciatica, 154
Scrotum, 72
  inflammatory disease vs. torsion of testicle, 73–75
  painless enlargement of, 75–76
  undescended testes, 76
Sellar lesions, 144–146
Seminal vesicles, 71–72
Sinusitis, 162–163
Skull fractures, 128
Soft tissue masses, 179–182
Sonography: see Ultrasound
Spinal bone mineral estimation, 184
Spinal dysraphism, 151–152
Spine
  inflammatory disease of, 152–154
  low-back pain, 152, 154–155
  magnetic resonance imaging of, 155–156

Spine (cont.)
  neoplasm of, 150–153
  trauma to, 149–151, 175–176
Spleen and reticuloendothelial system
  accessory spleen, 50
  asplenia, 48, 50
  polysplenia, 50
  splenic enlargement, 46–48
  trauma to, 44–46
  vein occlusion, 122, 124
Spondylolysis, 154
Stomach, 4–5
Sulfur colloid examination, 1, 26, 50
  in gastrointestinal bleeding, 5–7
Syringomyelia, 150

Tagged red blood cell study, 120
  in gastrointestinal bleeding, 5–7
  spleen scans with, 50
Technetium-IDA agents, 26–27
Technetium scan, 195, 204
Temporal lobe, 147–148
Temperomandibular joint, 167, 169, 182
Testes
  inflammatory disease vs. torsion of, 73–75
  undescended, 76
Thallium scans, 108–110, 204
Thoracic imaging, 2, 207
Thoracotomies, 100
Thrombophlebitis, pelvic, 124
Thymic tumor, 101
Thyroid gland, 169
  computerized tomography of, 197
  enlarged, 193–194
  hyperthyroidism, 191–193
  hypothyroidism, 192–193
  magnetic resonance imaging of, 208
  radiotherapy for, 195
  technetium scan of, 195
  ultrasound of, 194–197, 204–205
Thyroid-stimulating hormone (TSH), 192

Tomograms, 169
Transplants, renal, 68, 70
Turner's syndrome, 82

Ulcer disease, 4–5
Ultrasound
  of adrenals, 199–200
  of aortic aneurysm, 118–119
  of biliary malignancy, 34–35
  of biliary system trauma and postoperative complications, 32–33
  of bowels, 8–9
  of breast, 185–188
  in cardiomyopathy, 114
  in cerebrovascular disease, 137, 140
  in congenital heart disease, 109, 111–112
  of fetus, 81–84
  of gall bladder, 27, 29
  for intrauterine device localization, 89–90
  in ischemic heart disease, 111
  in jaundice, 29–30
  in liver enlargement, 20
  in liver neoplasm, 21–24
  in liver trauma, 17–18
  of orbits, 158
  in pancreatic inflammatory disease, 38–39
  of pancreatic neoplasm, 39–41
  of pancreatic trauma, 42
  of parathyroid, 204–205
  of pelvic masses, 85–89
  in pericardial disease, 115–117
  of peripheral vessels, 119
  of peritoneal cavity and abdominal wall, 10, 12
  of placenta, 81
  of presacral mass, 89
  of prostatic enlargement, 71–72
  in renal failure, 59–61
  in renal infection and reflux, 67
  of renal mass or enlarged kidney, 61–62, 64–65
  of renal transplant, 70
  of renal trauma, 56–57